FACING UP TO AIDS

Also by Alan Whiteside

INDUSTRIALIZATION AND INVESTMENT INCENTIVES IN SOUTHERN AFRICA (*editor*)
*TOWARDS A POST-APARTHEID FUTURE (*editor with Gavin Maasdorp*)

*From the same publishers

Facing up to AIDS

The Socio-Economic Impact in Southern Africa

Edited by

Sholto Cross
Senior Lecturer
School of Development Studies
University of East Anglia

and

Alan Whiteside
Senior Research Fellow
Economic Research Unit
University of Natal

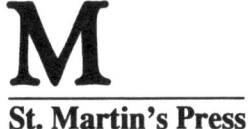

St. Martin's Press

Selection and editorial matter © Sholto Cross and Alan Whiteside 1993
Chapters 1–14 © The Macmillan Press Ltd 1993

All rights reserved. No reproduction, copy or transmission of this publication may be made without written permission.

No paragraph of this publication may be reproduced, copied or transmitted save with written permission or in accordance with the provisions of the Copyright, Designs and Patents Act 1988, or under the terms of any licence permitting limited copying issued by the Copyright Licensing Agency, 90 Tottenham Court Road, London W1P 9HE.

Any person who does any unauthorised act in relation to this publication may be liable to criminal prosecution and civil claims for damages.

First published in Great Britain 1993 by
THE MACMILLAN PRESS LTD
Houndmills, Basingstoke, Hampshire RG21 2XS
and London
Companies and representatives
throughout the world

A catalogue record for this book is available from the British Library.

ISBN 0–333–57817–1 hardcover
ISBN 0–333–57818–X paperback

Printed in Great Britain by
Mackays of Chatham PLC
Chatham, Kent

First published in the United States of America 1993 by
Scholarly and Reference Division,
ST. MARTIN'S PRESS, INC.,
175 Fifth Avenue,
New York, N.Y. 10010

ISBN 0–312–09106–0

Library of Congress Cataloging-in-Publication Data
Facing up to AIDS : the socio-economic impact in Southern Africa / edited by Sholto Cross and Alan Whiteside.
p. cm.
Includes index.
ISBN 0–312–09106–0
1. AIDS (Disease)—Africa, Southern—Social aspects. 2. AIDS (Disease)—Africa, Southern—Economic aspects. I. Cross, Sholto. II. Whiteside, Alan.
RA644.A25F33 1993
362.1'9698'9200968—dc20   92–2489
                                                      CIP

Contents

Preface vii

Acknowledgements ix

Notes on the Contributors x

Part I Setting the Scene

1 Introduction
   Alan Whiteside 3

2 The Global Pandemic of AIDS
   David FitzSimons 13

3 Current Research on the Economic Impact of HIV/AIDS: A Review of the International and South African Literature
   Jonathan Broomberg 34

Part II Modelling the AIDS Impact in South Africa

4 South African Trends and Projections of HIV Infection
   Hilary Southall 61

5 The Demographic Impact of AIDS on the South African Population
   Peter Doyle 87

6 Modelling the Demographic Impact of AIDS: Potential Effects on the Black Population in South Africa
   Gwenda Brophy 113

Part III Economic Assessments for South Africa

7 A Socio-Economic Analysis of the Long-Run Effects of AIDS in South Africa
   Sholto Cross 137

8 The Economic Impact of the AIDS epidemic in South Africa
   Jonathan Broomberg, Malcolm Steinberg, Patrick Masobe and Graeme Behr 158

9 Some Reflections on a Human Capital Approach to the Analysis of the Impact of AIDS on the South African Economy
   George Trotter   191

Part IV   The African Experience

10 The Impact of AIDS on Industry in Zimbabwe
    Alan Whiteside   217

11 The Medical Costs of AIDS in Zimbabwe
    Richard Hore   241

12 Simple Methods for Monitoring the Socio-Economic Impact of AIDS: Lessons from Sub-Saharan Africa
    Tony Barnett and Piers Blaikie   261

Part V   Facing up to AIDS in South Africa

13 Lessons from Tropical Africa for Addressing the HIV/AIDS Epidemic in South Africa
    Alan Fleming   295

14 Facing up to AIDS
    Sholto Cross   318

Index   321

Preface

South Africa, as befits the most powerful economy on the African continent, has a large investigatory literature on its history and society. Much of this, as with the current concerns directed at that land, has its focus on politics. Yet while the political events which are unfolding as a new era is born will continue to dominate the debate, this is a widely diverse country – a crucible for social change – where many worlds meet. Insights into these changes which are captured through analysis may continue to have a general impact on the way in which her policies are shaped, and attitudes formed. Specifically, for issues of demography and health policy, they also have great potential significance for other lands with similar profiles. South Africa's role and influence within the sub-continent is a growing one, and initiatives taken here have the potential to spread widely within the region.

The AIDS pandemic now spreading throughout southern Africa is without parallel in modern times in terms of probable long-run impact. The purpose of this collection of studies on the socio-economic aspects of its impact is to contribute to the process of policy formulation. The study of HIV and AIDS has been dominated by medical epidemiology, and only to a limited extent have studies been published concerning either economic analysis, or an understanding of the social context. This may partly reflect the fact that in those countries with an effective research infrastructure the disease has been largely confined to specific sub-cultures. South Africa has both a research base and an expected national problem of major proportions.

This volume is concerned with the social, economic and ultimately behavioural analysis of the disease where it is no longer confined to small segments of a national population. The methodology for such studies is still in its infancy: but southern Africa offers a possible terrain for the investigation of AIDS which goes beyond the pathological dimension. We believe that the modification of behaviour, whether at the level of atomistic individuals, peer groups or wider social entities, is a major form of defence against its spread. This requires detailed understanding of a spectrum of aspects of AIDS ranging from the modelling of population dynamics through to research on individual sexual behaviour, and both micro- and macro-economic and sociological investigations of its impact.

A number of the contributors to this volume specify areas for further research; programmes of both national and local level activity are already being planned in South Africa at the time of writing this preface. If the discussion and analysis presented here can lead to a further vigorous development in public (and private) health policies, to preparatory research and planning for preventative strategies, and to successful intervention to minimise the spread of AIDS and to sustain those afflicted by the disease and its consequences, then the book will have served its intended purpose.

Monetary values in the text refer to mid-1991, when the following exchange rates prevailed: 5 Rand to 1 pound sterling; 2.9 Rand to 1 American dollar; 1.25 (3.7) Zimbabwe dollars to 1 Rand (1 American dollar).

SHOLTO CROSS
ALAN WHITESIDE

Acknowledgements

The conference on the socio-economic impact of AIDS in southern Africa, from which this book originated, was held in Durban in July 1991, under the auspices of the Economic Reseach Unit (ERU) of the University of Natal. The editors wish to express their appreciation to the members and staff of the ERU whose support made this publication possible, namely Professor Gavin Maasdorp, Director of the ERU; Bruce Page, administrative coordinator; and Amanda Cooper, Kay Pedley and Nick Wilkins.

We also wish to thank the sponsors of the conference, whose assistance enabled us to bring together a wide range of researchers, businessmen and health policy analysts. We hope that the first fruits of their investment, as represented by the contributions published in this book, will encourage them to continue their support for policy studies and reseach in this area. Naturally, the views expressed by the editors and contributors are theirs alone.

We wish to thank Barlow Rand Limited, the British Embassy in South Africa, the Canadian Embassy in South Africa, the Chamber of Mines of South Africa, the Development Bank of Southern Africa, Eskom, Fedlife Assurance Limited, Fluor South Africa (Pty) Limited, Liberty Life Association of South Africa Limited, Metropolitan Life Limited, Nedbank, Old Mutual, Pref-Stores (Pty) Limited, SA Permanent Building Society, Smith & Nephew Limited, Standard Bank Foundation, Swiss–South Africa Reinsurance Company Limited, Tongaat Hulett Group Limited, Toyota South Africa Limited, and Unilever South Africa (Pty) Limited.

The editors would also like to express their personal thanks to Ailsa Marcham, Jane Maasdorp and Clare Wace for their support in making the production of this book possible.

Three chapters have appeared elsewhere. We gratefully acknowledge permission from the Southern Africa Foundation for Economic Research (SAFER) to include Chapter 10, and the Department of Community Health, University of the Witwatersrand, for permission to use Chapters 5 and 8.

Notes on the Contributors

Tony Barnett and **Piers Blaikie** are respectively Reader and Professor at the School of Development Studies, UEA, Norwich, and members of the Overseas Development Group. They have recently published *AIDS in Africa* (1992).

Graeme Behr was employed as a researcher at the Centre for Health Policy at the University of Witwatersrand Medical School.

Jonathan Broomberg is a Lecturer at the Centre for Health Policy in the Department of Community Health of the Medical School of Witwatersrand University, Johannesburg. He is currently studying at the London School of Hygiene and Tropical Medicine.

Gwenda Brophy is a demographic consultant who has written extensively on the southern African region.

Sholto Cross is a Senior Lecturer in Development Studies at the University of East Anglia, Norwich (UEA), and a member of the Overseas Development Group. He is currently working with the Independent Development Trust, Cape Town, on its rural development programme. He has worked extensively on politics and development in central and southern Africa.

Peter Doyle is Chief Actuary for Metropolitan Life Association, Cape Town.

David FitzSimons is Director of the London Bureau for Hygiene and Tropical Diseases. He has published widely on endemic diseases, and maintains the major collection of AIDS data in the UK. He is the editor of *AIDS Newsletter*.

Alan Fleming is Professor of Haematology, practising at Baragwanath Hospital, Soweto, a member of the South African Institute for Medical Research, and also of the Medical School of Witwatersrand University, Johannesburg.

Notes on the Contributors

Richard Hore is Chief Executive of CIMAS Medical Aid Society, Harare, Zimbabwe.

Patrick Masobe is employed as a junior research officer at the Centre for Health Policy at the University of Witwatersrand.

Hilary Southall is at the Institute of Social and Economic Research at Rhodes University, Grahamstown.

Malcolm Steinberg is the Director of the AIDS Programme of the South African Medical Research Council in Cape Town.

George Trotter is Professor of Economics at the University of Natal, Durban. He has published extensively in the field of manpower economics.

Alan Whiteside is a Senior Research Fellow of the Economic Research Unit at the University of Natal, Durban. He is currently a visiting fellow at UEA, Norwich. He is a leading researcher on socio-economic aspects of AIDS in southern Africa, and editor of *AIDS Analysis*.

Part I

Setting the Scene

1 Introduction
Alan Whiteside

The disease known as acquired immune deficiency syndrome, or AIDS, has been recognised for 10 years. During this time it has been more intensively researched and studied than any other disease in the history of humankind. It seems likely that while medical and scientific research will continue to make progress during the 1990s, it is social, behavioural and economic research into the disease which will become increasingly important. Scientists have now unlocked many of the secrets of the virus and know how it is spread, where it comes from, and what it does; the challenge for them is to develop a cure and a vaccine. For social scientists, the task is to develop ways to cope with the continually spreading impact of the disease.

While the medical parameters are increasingly understood, the social, demographic and economic implications of the disease are uncertain, and this is the area in which much work will have to be done in the next decade. The disease is set to be the single most important issue for the 1990s in much of the developing world. Until a cure is found, the greatest challenge will be to encourage changes in behaviour to prevent its spreading further.

This book is a first attempt to look at the economic and social implications of the disease in southern Africa. It is a collection of chapters bringing together the work of economists, political scientists, demographers and medical specialists. The authors, although they represent a wide range of disciplines, share a common concern about the potential of the human immuno-deficiency virus (HIV) epidemic adversely to affect the southern African region. The chapters were first presented as papers at a workshop in Durban in July 1991. The contributors were given the opportunity to revise and rework their papers in the light of the discussions and the editors' comments.

The picture presented in the book is not one of unrelieved gloom. There is certainly more of a chance to address and prevent the epidemic in southern Africa than elsewhere on the continent. The first step is understanding AIDS and what it can do.

THE NATURE OF AIDS

AIDS is caused by HIV, a member of a family of viruses known as retroviruses. Species of retroviruses have long been known to infect man and animals, and are characterised by the insidious onset of the diseases they cause. Retroviruses are fatal in virtually all cases.

HIV, in common with all viruses, is a parasite. Upon entry into the bloodstream it invades specific blood cells (T-lymphocytes) which constitute the single key factor in the production of antibodies aimed at resisting disease. Once HIV has established itself within a T-lymphocyte, the virus is capable of altering the normal functioning of the cell, and induces the T-lymphocyte to produce more HIVs at the expense of antibody production. The newly replicated HIVs are released from the host cell and invade other healthy T-lymphocytes. The process ends in the complete destruction of T-lymphocytes within the body and a total inability of the body to produce antibodies.[1]

Infected persons will pass through a number of stages. Immediately after infection, there is a period during which the person is infected and infective, but does not have sufficient antibodies for the virus to be detectable through laboratory testing. This period is known as the seroconversion phase. This is followed by a phase during which the virus is detectable, the person is healthy and infective, but the virus is replicating and beginning its attack on the immune system. This is known as the latent phase. It is followed by the onset of the disease, possibly initially through 'AIDS Related Complexes' (ARC) and then full-blown AIDS ending in death.

Both seroconversion time and the latent phase vary from one infected individual to the next. On current medical evidence, seroconversion time can range from six weeks to 15 months. The mean seroconversion time is put at three months. The latent period – the time from HIV positivity to full-blown AIDS – can range from one week to 15 years, and possibly longer.

To date, two strains of HIV have been identified. These are HIV I (the most common form in the West and most of Africa) and HIV II (found mainly in West Africa). The HIV II virus is more difficult to detect and may take longer to affect the carrier. Worryingly, there are a growing number of HIV II cases reported in Mozambique, and it has also been seen in South Africa and Zimbabwe. An additional source of concern is that both HIV I and HIV II mutate, and there are considerable variations even within one strain of the virus.

PATTERN OF SPREAD

The progress of the disease is being meticulously recorded in the developed world. Unfortunately, the methodology used and lessons learnt cannot readily be applied in southern Africa, the reason being that the pattern of the epidemic is very different in the West. A number of distinct patterns of spread have been identified. Pattern I is the variety prevalent in the West, Pattern II in sub-Saharan Africa and Pattern III in eastern Europe, North Africa, the middle East and Asia (although it appears Asia will be the main growth area for HIV spread in the 1990s). Latin America has a combination of Patterns I and II.

The key features of Pattern I are:

(a) it began to spread mainly from the late 1970s to the early 1980s;
(b) most cases are in homosexual/bisexual men and intravenous drug users, with few instances of heterosexual transmission;
(c) the male: female ratio is 10:1 (thus paediatric AIDS is uncommon);
(d) other transmission routes are uncommon;
(e) the level of HIV infection in national population is low.

Pattern II AIDS is the epidemiological pattern found in Africa. Here the key features are:

(a) it began to spread in the late 1970s and early 1980s;
(b) most cases are among heterosexual men and women;
(c) the male: female ratio is about 1:1 (thus paediatric AIDS is common);
(d) transmission via contaminated blood and blood products remains significant in many of these countries;
(e) national prevalence of HIV infection can exceed 1 per cent, and in some urban areas up to 25 per cent of those aged 15–49 years are infected.[2]

Until to 1987 South Africa experienced Pattern I AIDS, and white homosexual males comprised the majority of victims. Since then Pattern II AIDS has been the main mode of spread in South Africa. By contrast, the rest of southern Africa has only experienced Pattern II AIDS, but it began to spread during the 1980s, rather later than in Central Africa.

MODES OF TRANSMISSION

This topic is discussed in Chapter 2. It should be noted that in excess of 70 per cent of HIV infections are sexually transmitted worldwide, both hetero- and homosexually, but heterosexual transmission is the single greatest factor in the spread of the disease.[3]

The fact that it is mainly sexually transmitted makes the disease particularly significant for any society. It means that the people who will be infected and eventually die will be those in the economically active age group. These are the very people that one would least expect to be a burden on society in terms of needing medical care and social services. Furthermore, this group comprises the employed, the educated and experienced: in other words, the sector we can ill afford to lose.

Intravenous drug abuse involving contaminated needles and syringes account for some 30–40 per cent of HIV transmission in the United States and Europe. In southern Africa at present, intravenous drug abuse is virtually unknown.

The situation regarding transmission in southern Africa, and Africa as a whole, is markedly different from that in the West. Transmission in the Third World is largely one of disease transfer via heterosexual and mother-to-child dissemination. Again, this makes AIDS therefore markedly different from other endemic diseases in that it attacks specific age and sex cohorts and has an adverse effect on the next generation. Other transmission factors include transfusion of contaminated blood, and non-sterile medical instruments (especially needles and syringes).

Aggravating transmission via contaminated blood is the unavoidable 'window period' during which a blood donor will be HIV negative on pre-donation screening (that is, within the seroconversion time period) yet harbouring a sufficiently high HIV viral population to infect the recipient. The window period pertains to all blood transfusion systems, even those operating in the sophisticated countries. In the global pandemic setting, therefore, all blood transfusions carry a risk. This risk is directly related to the overall incidence of HIV within a given population in which the transfusion service operates. In Malawi, for instance, it is reported that there is a 1 in 100 probability of being transfused with contaminated blood despite donor screening, as compared to South Africa where this probability is reduced to 1 in 1.5 million blood transfusions, the Western average. This situation will change as the level of incidence among blood donors rises.

Aside from blood, certain body fluids carry low viral populations. For instance, tears and saliva are known to harbour extremely small numbers of the virus in HIV-positive individuals and are thus not considered to be routes of transmission. Semen, by contrast, harbours viral populations as high as those encountered in the bloodstream.

Due to the sometimes prolonged latent period, HIV infection worldwide has taken on gigantic pyramidal proportions. For every case of full-blown AIDS there are estimated to be 50–100 HIV-positive asymptomatic individuals, and between the extremes 3–10 individuals with AIDS-related complex (ARC).

A further factor in the African HIV pandemic is the rapidly increasing incidence of endemic diseases previously reasonably well controlled. These include malaria, tuberculosis (TB) and, in HIV-positive infants, measles. Inoculation campaigns against these diseases are hampered by HIV infection in that the vaccine, instead of conferring immunity, can cause the disease. In fact, it is feared that inoculation programmes could spark off epidemics of the diseases they are designed to eradicate.

Finally, the HIV pandemic in less-developed countries has resulted in extremely high infant infections. In some African states this is calculated at 20–40 per cent of babies. HIV-positive infants have a 50 per cent life expectancy of three years with 100 per cent mortality in five years, although this may be shorter in Africa.

AIDS AND HIV INFECTION IN SOUTHERN AFRICA

The Southern African region has had a varied experience of the HIV epidemic to date. In Malawi and Zambia, levels of HIV infection in the general population are approaching those of Uganda and other Central African countries. Generally, however, the incidence is very much lower, and in South Africa and Lesotho it is among the lowest on the continent. Reported AIDS cases and estimated HIV positivity is shown in Table 1.1. Chapter 2 puts the southern African epidemic in the global context.

The epidemic in the rest of Africa is being extensively studied by medical personnel and behaviouralists. What has been lacking from

Table 1.1 World Health Organisation figures for AIDS cases in southern Africa (June 1991) and estimated levels of HIV positivity

Country	1980–7	1988	Cases per year 1989	1990	1991	Last Report	Cumulative Case Total	HIV+ in the sexually active population mid-1991
Angola	41	63	NR	NR	NR	31.12.88	104	5–8
Botswana	36	22	29	NR	NR	17.01.90	87	3–5
Lesotho	2	3	6	NR	NR	27.04.90	11	0.5
Malawi	1 002	3 034	3 124	NR	NR	30.06.90	7 160	20
Mozambique	4	23	37	98	47	31.12.90	209	8–10
Namibia	19	43	127	122	NR	31.05.90	311	3–5
South Africa	86	92	175	312	304	21.11.91	969	1.5
Swaziland	1	2	7	20	41	31.09.91	71	2–4
Tanzania	1 608	2 500	2 093	1 912	NR	19.02.91	8 113	12
Zambia	709	985	1 115	1 227	NR	31.12.90	4 036	20+
Zimbabwe	119	202	1 311	3 167	1 107	30.03.91	5 906	16–18
Totals	3 627	6 969	8 024	6 858				

NR = not recorded.

Source World Health Organisation, except for Swaziland figures provided by National AIDS Control Programme, and South African figures from Department of National Health and Population Development; also included are editors' estimates for HIV positivity.

the research is the input of the social scientists, economists and demographers, particularly those based in Africa. Furthermore, much of the research has been designed by and for donors and governments. The business sector has not been fully involved, and neither have most grass-roots organisations.

Southern Africa with its indigenous research capacity and its infrastructure, both physical and informational, is well placed to carry out uniquely valuable work on AIDS and its consequences. Furthermore, the business community is well aware of the dangers posed by the epidemic and is willing to support the research. The result is that the chapters in this book are both practical and useful.

The first problem faced by researchers is the availability and quality of data. The value of HIV and AIDS data and reporting problems are discussed by Southall, Brophy and Whiteside elsewhere in this volume. It should be noted that the region is fortunate in that many countries have a reasonably well developed infrastructure which means that the quality of data is fairly good. These countries include Botswana, Lesotho, Swaziland, Namibia, South Africa and Zimbabwe. Mozambique and Angola, with their long-running civil wars, have sparse data.

PREDICTING THE EPIDEMIC

The first step in facing up to AIDS is to understand its dimensions. For this it is necessary to model the likely trends. This is covered in Part II. Doyle, in Chapter 5, has developed and adapted an actuarial model which has gained international recognition and which is being increasingly used by social scientists and the business community. Brophy uses a large-scale simulation model to project the potential demographic impact of AIDS on the black population of South Africa. Southall's chapter sets the scene and provides much of the background data relevant to South Africa.

THE SOCIO-ECONOMIC IMPACT

Although parts of southern Africa are in the early stages of the epidemic, others appear to be nearing the peak, at least in terms of HIV positivity. There is thus an urgent need to assess the likely socio-economic consequences and Chapters 7–14 set out to do this. It may be helpful to set out in broad terms some of the reasons for this concern.

First, the disease will have an impact at all levels of society and on all aspects of the economy. One of the key issues addressed by the contributors is the fact that there are the obvious direct costs in caring for HIV-related illness. It must be recognised that health care is a peculiar business. In the West, it is big business with most rich countries spending nearly 10 per cent of their gross domestic product (GDP) on it. A survey of health care, by *The Economist*,[4] found that such expenditure is closely linked to the wealth of the country. The implication is that in much of the region the amount spent on health is, and will be, limited. In countries with an unequal distribution of wealth, particularly South Africa, Namibia and Zimbabwe, there are two medical systems: a private one serving a relatively small group of wealthy people and the state sector for the majority. Already, both systems are under tremendous pressure.

When HIV is entered into the equation, then a potential crisis will arise. Although treatment costs can (and will) be contained, the problem lies in the numbers of people who will be hit by the disease. Furthermore, it has to be remembered that HIV infection is not instead of, but is in addition to, other diseases. Thus if HIV infection is expected to precipitate a crisis in health care in the West, it can only be imagined how much worse this will be in the Third World with its greater numbers. South Africa is in the unenviable position of facing a Third World epidemic with a population that may expect First World resources to be devoted to the care of the sick.

This issue of direct costs is addressed by three contributors. Chapter 3 provides an overview of the international and South African literature on the topic. The potential direct economic impact on South Africa is explored by Broomberg and his colleagues in Chapter 8 while Hore's chapter 11 on the direct costs in Zimbabwe provides a very useful case study.

Another key issue involves the indirect costs (morbidity and mortality) which are extremely hard to calculate. It is possible that they may have even greater significance in Africa where skilled and trained manpower is in short supply and yet may be the first to be hit by the epidemic. This topic is touched on in Chapter 8 and discussed at greater length by Trotter in Chapter 9, on AIDS and human capital costs.

Third, HIV infection has major implications for government resource allocation. In many African countries the cost of an Elisa test will use up more than the per capitum allocation of funds for a patient. Expenditure on HIV-related illness is both costly and inefficient in the long term. There is a further danger that HIV-related illness will clog up the health care system, especially beds in the main referral hospitals. Decisions on how to allocate resources will have to be addressed in the context of the HIV epidemic. There will also have to be serious questions asked as to the cost-effectiveness of education campaigns.

Fourth, at a macro-level, economists question the effect on a country's economy. How will the epidemic distort spending and production? This will depend both on its magnitude and on the people worst hit. If skilled people are particularly susceptible then economic growth may be slowed. AIDS may also have an impact on the pattern of both subsistence and commercial agriculture, and this is explored by Barnett and Blaikie in Chapter 12, who draw on research from Central Africa.

Fifth, the economist should not lose sight of the fact that each AIDS patient has a family who will be affected by his/her death, both emotionally and financially. The impact of this disease at the household level needs to be explored further.

In addition, many firms and industries are increasingly concerned by the epidemic and its potential effect on their business. Areas for consideration are manpower; employee benefits including medical aid, insurance, pension funds and group life cover; and production and markets. Chapter 10 is a case study on AIDS and industry in Zimbabwe, and Whiteside draws out many of the concerns there.

Finally, the reader needs to at least consider the non-quantifiable costs. These could include the loss of elite cadres, the social consequences of a massive demographic unbalance, and a climate of blame, accusation and moral panic. This is assessed by Cross in Chapter 7. One of the more serious impacts is that AIDS spreads first in urban populations, where a disproportionate number of skilled and educated people will be infected. These are the very people a society can least afford to lose.

POLITICAL AND SOCIAL IMPLICATIONS

One scenario that has been postulated is that the disease and its spread will lead to blame being apportioned, with the ill seeking to avenge themselves on the healthy: the development of a siege mentality and a plague mentality. The psychological impact of AIDS in South Africa, with its divided and mutually suspicious sections of society, will cost a dark shadow over the era of post-apartheid reconstruction.

South Africans have seen examples in the press coverage which laid emphasis on the likely decimation of the black population, implying that whites may be somehow immune. Whites have portrayed AIDS as a solution to the problem of the black population explosion; blacks regard it as an imperialist conspiracy to reduce their numbers, and prevent them from enjoying sex. The only way to reduce tension will be for the government, all political groupings and all community organisations to work together. AIDS has to be lifted out of the political arena; it is a problem that transcends party politics and requires a concerted response by all leaders.

The need to begin planning now for the impact of HIV is well illustrated by Fleming in Chapter 13, who points (in a very practical way) to some of the lessons that the region can learn from Africa. The two overriding points to note are that, first, parts of the region – South Africa, Botswana, Lesotho, Swaziland and Namibia – are in the early stages of the spread of HIV, which means that there is a chance that further spread can be averted or at least slowed. To do this will require immediate and imaginative action. The second point is that the epidemic and its likely effects must be planned for.

It is hoped this book will provide a spur for the further research and policy-making which this programme of planned resistance will require. The work is presented here not as the last word on any topic but rather as a stimulant towards the opening up of a debate on one of the many critical areas which will affect the southern Africa of the 1990s.

References

1. C. Connor and S. Kingman, *The Search for the Virus* (Penguin: Harmondsworth, 1988).
2. P. A. Sato, J. Chin and J.M. Mann, 'Review of AIDS and HIV infection: clobar epidemiology and statistics', *AIDS*, 3, Suppl. 1 (1989), pp. S301–S307.
3. J. Chin and J.M. Mann, 'The global patterns and prevalence of AIDS and HIV infection', *AIDS*, 2 (1988), suppl. 1 pp. 247–52.
4. *The Economist*, London, 6–12 July 1991.

2 The Global Pandemic of AIDS
D.W. FitzSimons

The 1980s were years of the beginning or ending of eras. Towards the close of the decade socialism was rejected in a series of largely peaceful revolutions in Eastern Europe and their shock waves reached further afield. In Africa the ideal of democracy was rekindled in many countries, with the overthrow or rejection of dictatorial or one-party regimes. In South Africa apartheid was rejected and its structures began to be dismantled. In many countries citizens talked optimistically of building a new society, recognising that they had crossed watersheds although the territories they were entering were uncharted.

However, the decade had its darker side, too. The catalogue of civil wars, famines, natural disasters, all taking a heavy toll, continued at depressing length. Moreover the economies of many countries, already precariously balanced, were shackled by an international economic recession. To these traditionally recognised hazards was added a new and unimaginable threat in the first years: HIV infection and AIDS. Such is the subsequent scale and impact of this new disease that they are eliminating the gains in child mortality rates in many developing countries made through immunisation and other child survival programmes; adult mortality rates in some areas have trebled in just 5 years, the success of TB-control programmes is rapidly being undone, and the shape of some African societies is being distorted, with unnaturally large populations of young and old as the disease kills those in their middle years. No end is in sight. No cure is available. Prevention through changes in behaviour is the only weapon available to stop the continued sexual spread of the virus yet, despite all international efforts, there are few successes to be seen. The AIDS epidemic in Africa is being followed by one of TB, leading one group of researchers to ask the provocative question 'Is Africa lost?'[1] (the term 'lost' having been used at a World Health Organisation – WHO – meeting in 1990 to mean that there is no way of dealing with the combined effects of the two infections). Unfortunately the spread of the virus means that bad news is not the monopoly of Africa.

The direct costs of AIDS and HIV infection, already substantial, are likely to be dwarfed by the indirect costs, particularly those related to loss of income and decreased productivity. But it has been only latterly that these consequences have been generally recognised and heeded by many financial and political leaders: the warnings were spelt out at a special session on AIDS at a World Bank meeting late in 1991. A joint publication by that organization and the International Monetary Fund warned that the epidemic threatens to alter dramatically the economic and social fabric of many societies, raising serious questions about the development process itself. Many governments have been reluctant to recognise and admit the epidemic itself, so much so that at the end of 1991 the Director of the WHO's Global Programme on AIDS urged African political leaders who had not yet done so to make a strong commitment to tackling AIDS.[2]

THE EPIDEMIC

Ten years ago one would not have found AIDS in any medical dictionary. The first cases of what is now described as AIDS were described in a brief report in the US Centers for Disease Control's *Morbidity and Mortality Weekly Report* in June 1981.[3] A cluster of cases of pneumonia caused by *Pneumocystis carinii*, previously seen only in patients who were immuno-compromised for one reason or another – by disease or through operations – had been identified in five homosexual men in Los Angeles, all of whom were found to have abnormal immune function. The authors of the report cautiously suggested infection through sexual contact. More cases began to be recognised and reported until an identifiable epidemic was defined. Other rare features, such as a skin cancer called Kaposi's sarcoma, were found in association with the condition whose manifestations appeared in bewildering variety. Two years later, in 1983, a virus was identified by Professor Luc Montagnier at the Institut Pasteur in Paris, and further work by Dr Robert Gallo at the National Cancer Institute in the USA led to its recognition as the cause of AIDS and to the development of a blood test for antibodies to the HIV. In Africa cases of a wasting disease called 'slim' were increasingly being reported in Uganda and neighbouring countries, and an aggressive form of Kaposi's sarcoma was seen in cases of what turned out to be AIDS, but these early signs of the epidemic were ignored internationally as attention focused on the spread among homosexual men in North America and Europe. Since those first reports in the USA cases have been detected from the middle of the 1970s and possibly earlier. The origins of the epidemic remain obscure and the subject of much speculation, ranging from deliberate experiments in biological warfare and outer space to the use of monkey cells for polio vaccines and the introduction of monkey viruses related to HIV into humans during experiments on malaria several decades ago.[4] Some of the debates have been insulting and discriminatory (in the early years in the USA Haitians were singled out as a separate risk group) and much of the early research, based on what are now seen as primitive assays, yielded results that were unquestioningly accepted and generalised. The confusion and ignorance surrounding AIDS led to the pointing of fingers at Africa as the source of the epidemic, an accusation that still rankles and causes ill-will. (Indeed, in the aftermath of the riots in Zaire in September 1991 when many expatriates working on Projet SIDA, a major research programme funded by the Americans and the Belgians, left or were withdrawn, accusations were made about the precipitate nature of their leaving, and memories of the earlier researchers' behaviour – typically seen as flying in, collecting blood samples, leaving, writing a rapid paper and being seen no more – were rekindled.) The important question must be not where did the virus come from, but where is the epidemic going?

The spread of the virus has been rapid, and seems inexorable. At present nobody knows how many people are infected with the virus and the epidemic is measured by the number of reported cases of AIDS, the clinical manifestation of the culmination of HIV infection (normally seen about 10 years after infection with the virus). The WHO has established a monitoring system through its Global Programme on AIDS, to which 163 countries had reported at the end of 1991. The bald figures, more than 446 000 cases, are presented in Table 2.1;[5] but of greater epidemiological significance than cumulative totals (although one has to bear in mind that each case is an individual) is the incidence: Table 2.2 shows various national rates which illustrate the extent of the problem – nearly three reported cases of AIDS for every 200 people in Malawi and one for every 1000 people in Tanzania. In fact, the most accurate picture will come not from the reported AIDS cases but from estimates made from seroprevalence studies, projections and mathematical models.

Table 2.1 Cumulative totals of AIDS cases reported to the WHO as of 30 September 1991

Location	Number of cases
Africa	120 547
Tanzania	21 208
Uganda	21 719
Zaire	14 762
Americas	237 436
USA	191 601
Brazil	19 631
Asia	1196
Europe	56 178
France	15 534
Italy	9792
Spain	9112
Oceania	2839
Total	418 196

Source *Weekly Epidemiological Record*, 66, 40 (1991), pp. 289–90.

Standards of reporting vary across the world, and even in the developed countries of USA and Europe rates of underreporting are believed to be between 0 and about 20 per cent. Consequently the WHO has estimated that, since the beginning of the pandemic, some 1.5 million people (including 500 000 children) have been infected with HIV and developed AIDS. Some 6–7 times more people, up to 11 million people, are thought to be infected with HIV worldwide, with the number increasing by about 5000 a day. In sub-Saharan Africa alone the WHO believes that about 900 000 children have already been born infected with HIV, and in some countries in East and Central Africa about one-third of sexually active adults are infected. By the end of the century its conservative estimate is that there will be 30–40 million infections in men, women and children globally, and about 12–18 million cases of AIDS; as the director of the WHO's Global Programme on AIDS, Dr Michael Merson, put it: 'we are today really only at the beginning of the pandemic'.

The regular reporting of cases has enabled the course of the epidemic to be traced. Dr Roger Bernard, an epidemiologist in Geneva, has used the WHO's data to plot and chart the spread of HIV as reflected by reported AIDS cases. These analyses show the very rapid initial spread as HIV enters high-risk populations, followed in most cases by a gradual decline in the rate of growth of the

Table 2.2 Incidence rates of reported AIDS cases
(a) Africa

Country	AIDS cases	Rate	Date of last report
Algeria	45	0.2	20 May 90
Angola	104	1.2	31 Dec. 88
Benin	158	3.6	30 June 91
Botswana	216	18.0	31 July 91
Burkina Faso	978	11.1	11 June 90
Burundi	3 305	70.1	31 Aug. 90
Cameroon	429	3.9	30 Apr. 91
Cape Verde	32	30.7	30 June 90
Central African Republic	1 864	71.5	30 June 90
Chad	130	2.6	25 June 91
Comoros	2	0.5	30 Apr. 90
Congo	2 405	138.2	31 Dec. 90
Côte d'Ivoire	8 297	82.5	30 June 91
Djibouti	104	24.2	31 Dec. 91
Egypt	30	0.1	1 Dec. 91
Equatorial Guinea	7	6.9	27 June 89
Ethiopia	1 534	3.5	31 Oct. 91
Gabon	117	10.2	31 Dec. 90
Gambia	141	20.3	30 July 91
Ghana	2 474	18.2	30 June 91
Guinea	338	5.6	1 July 90
Guinea-Bissau	157	17.6	26 Mar. 91
Kenya	9 139	44.9	31 May 90
Lesotho	11	0.8	27 Apr. 90
Liberia	12	0.5	1 Sep. 91
Libya	1	0.0	14 Feb. 90
Madagascar	2	0.0	26 Nov. 90
Malawi	12 074	151.3	31 Oct. 90
Mali	338	4.1	30 June 90
Mauritania	26	1.4	31 July 91
Mauritius	5	0.5	5 Apr. 90
Morocco	90	0.3	1 Dec. 91
Mozambique	272	1.9	30 Sep. 91
Namibia	311	26.3	31 May 90
Niger	352	5.6	30 June 91
Nigeria	84	0.1	29 Jan. 91
Reunion	49	8.8	17 May 90
Rwanda	5 100	84.0	31 Mar. 91
São Tomé	2	1.9	30 Sep. 91
Senegal	552	8.4	18 July 91
Sierra Leone	40	1.1	30 Apr. 91

cont. on page 18

(a) Africa cont.

Country	AIDS cases	Rate	Date of last report
Somalia	13	0.2	23 Dec. 90
South Africa	1 019	3.1	21 Nov. 91
Sudan	476	2.2	1 Dec. 91
Swaziland	71	9.7	30 Sep. 91
Tanzania	27 396	126.1	31 Aug. 91
Togo	100	3.3	1 June 90
Tunisia	82	1.1	1 Dec. 91
Uganda	21 719	132.4	31 Dec. 90
Zaire	14 762	42.6	31 Dec. 90
Zambia	4 690	70.4	31 May 91
Zimbabwe	7 411	82.3	30 June 91
Total	129 066		

(b) Americas

Country	AIDS cases	Rate	Date of last report
Anguilla	4	57.1	30 Sep. 90
Antigua	6	7.5	31 Dec. 90
Argentina	1 019	3.3	31 Mar. 91
Bahamas	659	278.0	31 Mar. 91
Barbados	208	82.2	30 June 91
Belize	12	7.2	31 Mar. 91
Bermuda	178	317.9	30 June 91
Bolivia	28	0.4	31 Mar. 91
Brazil	21 023	15.5	31 Aug. 91
British Virgin Islands	3	23.1	31 Dec. 90
Canada	5 246	20.7	31 July 91
Cayman Islands	10	40.2	31 Mar. 91
Chile	280	2.3	30 June 91
Colombia	1 483	5.6	31 Mar. 91
Costa Rica	276	9.8	30 June 91
Cuba	84	0.8	30 June 91
Dominica	12	15.8	30 June 90
Dominican Republic	1 535	23.9	30 June 91
Ecuador	134	1.4	30 June 91
El Salvador	370	6.8	30 June 91
French Guiana	232	269.8	30 Sep. 90
Grenada	27	2.4	30 June 91
Guadeloupe	195	58.4	24 Apr. 90

(b) Americas cont.

Country	AIDS cases	Rate	Date of last report
Guatemala	176	2.2	30 June 91
Guyana	177	22.4	30 June 91
Haiti	3 086	46.9	31 Dec. 90
Honduras	1 306	29.9	30 June 91
Jamaica	216	9.2	31 Mar. 91
Martinique	181	54.7	30 June 91
Mexico	8 720	11.1	30 Oct. 91
Montserrat	1	8.4	30 Sep. 90
Netherlands Antilles & Aruba	77	30.7	15 May 91
Nicaragua	16	0.5	30 June 91
Panama	280	12.6	30 June 91
Paraguay	28	0.7	30 Sep. 91
Peru	457	2.3	30 June 91
St Kitts & Nevis	33	73.2	30 June 91
St Lucia	36	26.1	30 June 91
St Vincent & The Grenadines	31	29.8	30 June 91
Surinam	83	20.2	31 Dec. 90
Trinidad & Tobago	785	66.2	31 Mar. 91
Turks & Calcos Islands	20	142.9	31 Mar. 90
Uruguay	200	6.6	31 Aug. 91
USA	202 843	87.8	30 Nov. 91
Venezuela	1 201	6.9	31 Mar. 91
Total	252 977		

(c) Asia

Country	AIDS cases	Rate	Date of last report
Bangladesh	1	0.0	30 Nov. 90
Brunei	2	0.8	31 Jan. 91
China	6	0.0	20 Apr. 91
Cyprus	20	2.9	31 Dec. 90
Hong Kong	49	0.9	31 May 91
India	85	0.0	30 Sep. 91
Indonesia	16	0.0	30 June 91
Iran	33	0.1	1 Dec. 91
Iraq	7	0.0	1 Dec. 91
Israel	153	3.5	30 June 91
Japan	405	0.3	31 Aug. 91

cont. on page 20

(c) Asia cont.

Country	AIDS cases	Rate	Date of last report
Jordan	13	0.4	1 Dec. 91
Korea (South)	8	0.0	10 July 91
Kuwait	1	0.1	14 Feb. 90
Lebanon	29	1.1	1 Dec. 91
Macau	0	0.0	30 Aug. 91
Malaysia	28	0.2	13 June 91
Nepal	5	0.0	31 Aug. 91
Oman	24	1.6	1 Dec. 91
Pakistan	17	0.0	1 Dec. 91
Philippines	53	0.1	28 Aug. 91
Qatar	31	8.4	31 Dec. 90
Saudi Arabia	35	0.3	1 Dec. 91
Singapore	30	1.1	25 June 91
Sri Lanka	10	0.1	31 July 91
Syria	11	0.1	1 Dec. 91
Thailand	119	0.2	25 July 91
Turkey	55	0.1	30 Sep. 91
United Arab Emirates	8	0.5	21 Oct. 90
Total	1 254		

(d) Europe

Country	AIDS cases	Rate	Date of last report
Albania	0	0.0	31 Dec. 90
Austria	639	8.5	30 Sep. 91
Belgium	896	9.1	30 June 91
Bulgaria	12	0.1	30 June 90
Czechoslovakia	25	0.2	31 Mar. 91
Denmark	870	17.0	30 Sep. 91
Finland	94	1.9	30 Sep. 91
France	16 552	29.8	30 Sep. 91
Germany	6 968	9.0	30 Sep. 91
Greece	528	5.3	30 Sep. 91
Hungary	73	0.7	30 Sep. 91
Iceland	18	8.8	30 June 91
Ireland	215	6.1	30 Sep. 91
Italy	10 584	18.5	30 Sep. 91
Luxembourg	41	11.2	30 Sep. 91
Malta	20	5.8	30 June 91

(d) Europe cont.

Country	AIDS cases	Rate	Date of last report
Monaco	7	25.9	30 Sep. 91
Netherlands	1 857	12.7	30 Sep. 91
Norway	237	5.6	30 Sep. 91
Poland	78	0.2	30 Sep. 91
Portugal	746	7.3	30 Sep. 91
Romania	1 557	6.8	30 Sep. 91
San Marino	1	5.2	31 Dec. 90
Spain	10 101	26.0	30 Sep. 91
Sweden	617	7.4	30 Sep. 91
Switzerland	2 086	31.8	30 Sep. 91
UK	5 065	9.1	30 Sep. 91
USSR	66	0.0	30 Sep. 91
Yugoslavia	242	1.0	28 Nov. 91
Total	60 195		

(e) Oceania

Country	AIDS cases	Rate	Date of last report
Australia	2 813	16.9	30 Sep. 91
Fiji	3	0.4	31 Jan. 91
French Polynesia	27	15.7	19 Aug. 91
Guam	10	9.4	13 Sep. 91
Marshall Islands	2	4.4	22 Nov. 91
Micronesia	2	2.7	2 May 90
New Caledonia	18	11.8	16 July 91
New Zealand	274	8.3	18 June 91
Papua New Guinea	37	1.0	20 June 91
Samoa	1	0.6	11 July 91
Tonga	2	2.1	10 July 91
Total	3 189		

Notes Rates are given per 100 000 population. Rates of 0.0 mean less than 0.1.

Source WHO statistics, as at 1 January 1992, from *Weekly Epidemiological Record*, 67, 3, (1992), pp. 9–10: population data based on UN estimates.

incidence rate. Thus in the USA the time taken for the number of reported cases to double reached 12 months in 1985 and has lengthened since then. In Europe the doubling time is now much more than 12 months; the total number of cases reported at the end of June 1991 was just over a quarter greater (28 per cent) than at the corresponding juncture in 1990.[6] A glance at the shape of the curves for Africa shows that the pace of the epidemic shows no sign of diminishing, with doubling times of 12 months or less, and the picture is similar for the Western Pacific and Asian regions.

Although numerically the USA has the greatest number of cases and in cities such as New York the prevalence rate is similar to that in developing countries, the countries that are bearing the greatest burden at present are those in sub-Saharan Africa. The WHO projects that the rate of growth of AIDS cases will reach a plateau in North America and Europe at some point in the mid-1990s but it sees continued growth in Latin America, an accelerating growth of incidence in Asia and a continuing rise with some deceleration in Africa (see Figures 2.1 and 2.2). Indeed the recognition that HIV has established more than a toe-hold in Asia, that the spread of HIV infection is linked with poverty and the prevalence of sexually transmitted diseases (STDs) and that no society is immune has caused the WHO to dub Asia the sleeping giant of AIDS. Dr Merson of the WHO noted that more than half the world's population lives in South and South-East Asia, and that the population of sexually active adults in India is two-and-a-half times greater than the population of all of sub-Saharan Africa; the Indian government believes that already there may be a million people infected with HIV in the sub-continent. The annual incidence of HIV infections in Asia is expected to exceed annual incidence in Africa some time during the mid- to late 1990s.[7]

TRANSMISSION PATTERNS

The first cases of AIDS were seen in homosexual men in the USA and it soon became apparent that whatever was causing the condition was spreading like wildfire through these populations. The belief that it was a 'gay plague' became established and was fostered by much of the press, releasing a tide of discrimination and blame. Then cases began to be detected in haemophiliacs, whose lives had been transformed by the introduction of treatment with blood products. It now appeared that these very therapeutic agents were contaminated. Not

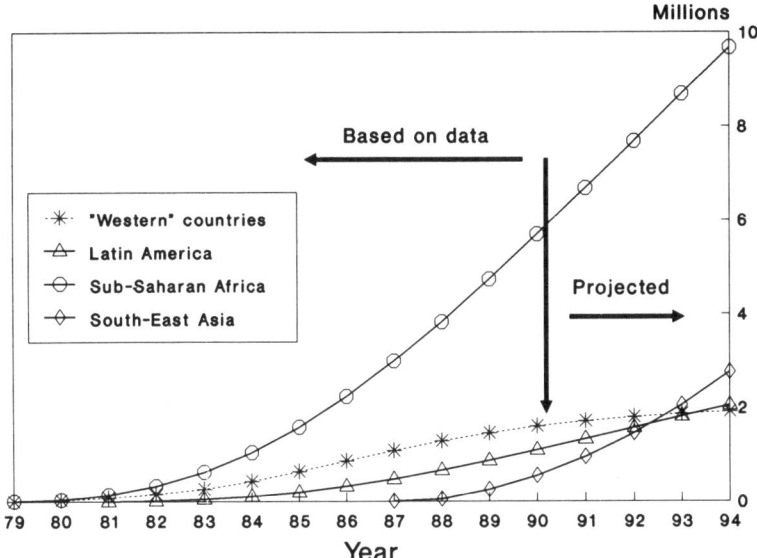

Figure 2.1 Estimates/projections of cumulative adult HIV infections
Source World Health Organisation, Global Programme on AIDS.

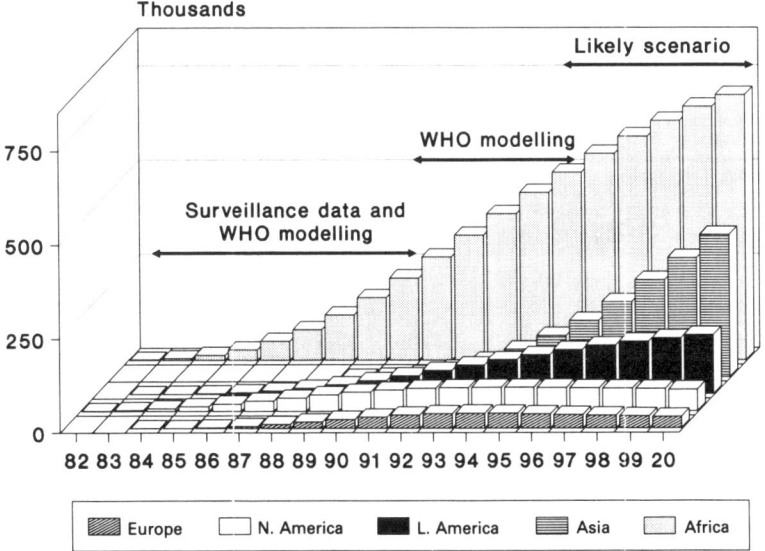

Figure 2.2 Distribution of estimated and projected annual adult AIDS cases
Source World Health Organisation, Global Programme on AIDS.

only haemophiliacs but recipients of blood transfusions began to be infected. In the USA donors were often paid for their blood but many homosexual men had been used to donating free blood. As a result the blood supply became contaminated until screening was introduced in 1985. Blood products made from this contaminated blood were exported widely across the world, leading to the appearance of cases of infection in many countries.

As in so many other areas, the events in the USA repeated themselves in Europe a couple of years later. Several countries reported increasing numbers of cases in homosexual men. Cases appeared in people who injected themselves intravenously with illicit drugs. This predominance of cases in homosexual men and intravenous drug users led to the belief, even in government circles in developed countries in 1985, that AIDS was restricted to these groups and of no concern to developing countries or even the rest of the population. Then it emerged that Belgium had a peculiarly large proportion of cases in people who were heterosexual. In the USA Haitians seemed to have been disproportionately affected but later links with sub-Saharan Africa emerged as important, a pattern seen also in Europe. With cases appearing in seemingly unrelated groups and types of people the fear in the latter part of the decade arose of a universal threat: a virus that caused a fatal illness, and against which there was no cure or protection, was sweeping across the world. Every report seemed to bring news of cases of AIDS or HIV infection in other countries and continents; cases occurred in doctors, health-care workers, priests, teachers, schoolchildren, babies; in fact, men and women generally.

The introduction of blood tests for HIV antibodies and further epidemiological studies led to the identification of the main routes of transmission and, by the time of the third International Conference on AIDS held in Washington, DC, in 1987, these had been determined; the conclusion of the conference was that, although the extent of the epidemic then was worse than imagined, at least the ways that the virus was transmitted were known and no unpleasant surprises had emerged in that regard.

The most common route of transmission is sexual intercourse, it being estimated that two-thirds of all infections are now being acquired through heterosexual intercourse (with rough proportions of 70 per cent for heterosexual and 10 per cent for homosexual intercourse). At the seventh International Conference on AIDS in Florence in 1991 Dr James Chin of the WHO's Global Programme on

Table 2.3 Routes and efficiency of transmission of HIV

Type of exposure	Efficiency per single exposure (%)	Percentage of global total
Blood transfusion	>90	< 3–5
Perinatal	30	5–10
Sexual intercourse	0.1–1.0	70–80
Vaginal		(60–70)
Anal		(5–10)
Injecting drug use – sharing needles etc.	0.5–1.0	5–10
Health care – needle – sticks etc.	< 0.5	< 0.01

Source World Health Organisation, Global Programme on AIDS.

AIDS surmised that 70–80 per cent of infections were acquired sexually, with vaginal intercourse predominating over anal intercourse (see Table 2.3), although the latter was probably a more effective means of transmission of the virus. The chances of infection lay in the range of between 1 in 100 and 1 in 1000, but the factors controlling transmission are largely unknown, as there have been documented cases of people becoming infected after a single episode of unprotected vaginal intercourse with an infected partner while other people have remained uninfected after hundreds of episodes of similar intercourse with an infected partner. The presence of other STDs, particularly those causing genital ulcers, is linked with an increased risk of infection; and the stage of infection in the infected partner is another factor. Research seems to indicate that men are more easily able to infect women through sexual intercourse than vice versa, but in many African countries the ratio of infected men to infected women is about equal. Of the two types of HIV, the most common, HIV I, is thought to be transmitted about three times more readily than the other form, HIV II, which also causes AIDS but which is largely restricted to West Africa.

Pregnant infected women can pass the virus to their unborn children, and about 5–10 per cent of cases of HIV infection globally are thought to be transmitted in this way. In developing countries about one-third of children born to infected mothers are actually infected themselves; in developed countries the proportion is lower, a figure of about 12 per cent being quoted from a European study but a higher one in the USA. The transmission rate appears to depend on social class, access to health care, health status of the mother, stage of infection in the mother and even, according to a recent report on twins, the order of birth.[8] Instances have been reported of transmission from infected mother to infant through breast milk, but this is considered to be a minor route and international agencies recommend that in countries where the incidence of HIV and the risk to children of diarrhoeal and respiratory diseases are high, infected mothers continue to breast-feed their infants.

Before screening of blood for HIV antibodies was introduced (from 1985 onwards), contaminated blood products and transfusions of contaminated blood caused many cases of transmission, and this route accounts for about 3–5 per cent of all present HIV infections in the world. Because of the quantity of blood, and therefore of the virus, given in transfusions the risk of infection is high, with the rate of infection estimated at more than 90 per cent. Screening alone for antibodies will not completely eliminate the risk of infection from donated blood as there is a period immediately after infection with HIV, the so-called 'window period' which lasts up to about three months, before antibodies are detectable.

In most countries donors are now advised about the risk behaviours associated with HIV infection and asked not to donate if they fall into that category. In one regional transfusional centre in France, for example, donors have been asked since 1989 to sign a declaration stating that they have read information given to them about HIV/AIDS and do not have any risk factors for HIV infection before being allowed to donate.[9] In the USA the American Red Cross, which supplies about half the national blood requirements, has begun a complete reorganisation of its collection and handling of blood in order to provide a major reassurance over the safety of the blood supply. For developing countries, where still not all blood is screened, guidelines have been drawn up to minimise the use of blood transfusions and it has been recommended that HIV screening programmes (with counselling as part of them) be included in primary health care (PHC) programmes.[10] In some countries where screening is not widely available it has been suggested that children and old people may usefully serve as likely uninfected donors, and in developed countries autologous donation – the giving of blood by a person who knows that he or she is scheduled for an operation for storage and use during that operation – has become more popular.

Although direct inoculation of HIV into blood is the most efficient method of infection (see Table 2.3), the risk from the sharing of injecting drug equipment or accidental injuries such as needlepricks to health-care workers is much lower because of the much smaller amounts of virus transmitted on each occasion. For intravenous drug users the risk is estimated to be about 1 in 100–200, and this group presents a major concern. At present intravenous drug users account for about 5–10 per cent of all infections in the world, but the rate is increasing and such people, frequently being young, sexually active and heterosexual, may act as a bridge into the general population. In the USA the growing use of crack, a form of cocaine which increases the sex drive and whose effects are short-lived, resulting in the need for addicts to inject with a much greater frequency than those who use heroin, is further spreading the virus, particularly among women who exchange sex for drugs.

Health-care workers known to be infected through occupational exposure make up a very small portion of the infected population, less than 1 in 10 000, yet they and their professional bodies have been very vocal in raising their concerns about the risks (which clearly will grow with the increasing numbers of infected patients receiving health care). These concerns are mainly expressed in developed countries whereas the greatest risks are being experienced in developing countries where facilities are inadequate. The converse, infection of patients from infected health-care workers, is so rare that only one documented case exists – that of a dentist in Florida who appears somehow to have infected at least three patients[11] – yet nevertheless this has caused considerable public alarm.

Even though early on in the epidemic it was established that HIV could not be transmitted through casual contact or through the bites of mosquitoes, there remain many people who still believe that these routes are possible, indicating the challenge that health educationalists face. Generally, however, the levels of knowledge about HIV and AIDS among the general populace are good, and the challenge for the 1990s is to translate knowledge about the dangers and risks into changes in behaviour and maintenance of those changes. Behavioural research is the Cinderella of AIDS, and few papers on social, prevention and control issues and the evaluation of preventive campaigns have been published compared with the now vast fields of virology and molecular biology (in 1990 some 8300 papers on HIV or AIDS were identified by the US National Library of Medicine).[12]

AIDS AND SOCIETY

In the space of 10 years we have moved from a condition being recognised by a few specialists and widely rumoured in the gay community to a known virus and defined disease syndrome known of from Murmansk to Maputo, from Mexico to Manchuria. Nearly every country has a national AIDS programme. There are international, regional and national conferences on all aspects of AIDS, from human rights to vaccines. One day in the year has been designated World AIDS Day (1 December), and the spread of events around it is such that the Minister of Health in the UK described it as the 'World AIDS Season'. Millions of pounds and dollars have been spent on education and research: $4000 million a year on research in the USA alone, President Bush announced defending his administration's record on research and prevention.[13]

Two drugs have been licensed, zidovudine and didanosine (the latter in the last half of 1991); these anti-viral agents do not cure AIDS but prolong the life of people with AIDS. More than 150 different experimental drugs have been or are being developed against HIV infection and its associated opportunistic infections. Nevertheless, it is a sad fact that most of these are beyond the reach of people infected with HIV or with AIDS in developing countries. At least 13 candidate vaccines are being investigated and the WHO, which recognised the difficulties in getting a vaccine into developing countries and the need to protect their populations from exploitation, has set up ethical committees and has been coordinating the activities of academe and industry. It has also nominated four countries that will serve as sites for the first field trials when a candidate vaccine or vaccines is chosen: Uganda, Rwanda, Brazil and Thailand. (Zaire would probably have been chosen had it not been for the riots in September 1991.)

AIDS has dramatically changed doctor–patient relations and has necessitated the redesign of clinical trials. Patients are now key members of the decision-making process about trials and treatments. Hospices, terminal care and community-care services are seen as crucial elements in the management of dying patients (even though they play, and have played, just such a role in cancer). Pressure groups and activists have had a major influence in putting these subjects on the agenda and the lessons of their success have been learnt and applied by other 'disease advocates': in the USA activists are now working on behalf of patients with breast cancer to speed the release of experimental drugs, just as they have been for AIDS, and to increase the amount of money and resources directed into research and, if possible, prevention; there are at least 15 national groups of cancer patients and their families whose intent is to provide support and to lobby for funding.[14] The reason for this may lie in the fact that the first patients were young, well-educated men who had learnt to articulate their demands and be assertive in the fight for gay rights.

Against all this there has been ignorance, prejudice and discrimination. Dr Jonathan Mann, founder and former director of the WHO's Global Programme on AIDS, identifies these attitudes as part of a third epidemic. He delineates the first as the largely hidden and rapidly accelerating spread of HIV. The second is the visible form of the infection, namely AIDS and related illness (that is, symptomatic infection). The third epidemic is social rather than medical; as HIV and AIDS spread, in their wake come denial, blame, stigmatisation, prejudice and discrimination. In a speech in 1987 Dr Mann told the United Nations: 'The third epidemic of social, cultural, economic and political reaction to AIDS . . . is as central to the global challenge as AIDS itself.'[15]

In developed countries the impact has been less economic than cultural and political, and has been a function of the main groups affected. In the USA the first wave of the epidemic struck the gay community, already well versed in the ways of protest, activism and organisation. Information about the disease spread rapidly through existing networks, and even before public health education started in earnest homosexual men had begun changing their sexual behaviour to what is now referred to as safer sex. While the public and politicians were concerned with the 'gay plague' and its implications, the epidemic spread into the disadvantaged, inner-city heterosexual populations, predominantly black and Hispanic, poor, with at best modest access to health care, and among whom the prevalence of sexually transmitted diseases and high-risk behaviour generally were higher than the national average, and whose women faced enormous pressures to bear children and great obstacles to enforcing safer sex. Whereas members of the gay community (or their insurers) were able to afford some of the costs of treatment, those in the inner cities are not and the economic burden of the epidemic is falling on the public sector. Such is the pressure and the increasing recognition of the existing inequities in the distribution of health services that demands for a form of national health-care provision are being seriously considered. Nevertheless, the initial doomsday scenarios of economic and social dislocation are appearing more and more unrealistic.

In Europe and other developed countries with solid economic bases the questions are similarly about re-allocation of funds for care, services, research and education with no major threats to the fabric of society now perceived. The epidemic is expected to peak in the mid-1990s, costs for care having risen to high but manageable levels.

In developing countries the picture is somewhat different. Existing health budgets are low, the average figure often quoted being about US$5 per person per year (which is roughly about the cost of two HIV antibody tests). Here AIDS promises to have a serious economic impact, not only through the direct costs of screening for infection, care, treatment and education, but also in the undoing of advances in primary health care and disease prevention. In addition there will be the costs of lost productivity, social dislocation, and the burden of care of children who have lost one or both parents to AIDS will devolve on to the extended family or the state. In a joint study on the impact of AIDS on agricultural production, the WHO and the Food and Agriculture Organisation (FAO) conclude that where rural infection rates are around 10 per cent the adult labour force could be reduced by a quarter by the year 2010; with seroprevalence rates often higher than this already in many areas the impact will be that much greater. The effects will be seen not just on the output of food but in nutritional status.

Already the demographic consequences are visible in sub-Saharan countries. In East and Central Africa child mortality rates have increased to their 1980 levels because of paediatric AIDS deaths, and mortality in adults has trebled in 5 years.[16] A recent review by leading epidemiologists of mathematical models of the spread of HIV in Africa shows that although it will vary considerably country by country, the general conclusion is that without major changes in behaviour or the advent of new drugs or an effective vaccine AIDS is likely to induce significant demographic changes in the worst affected countries.[17] Population growth rates are expected to be reversed from positive to negative in the worst-affected areas in a few decades, although this view is not shared by all researchers.[18] The WHO's demographic model prepared by the World Bank indicates that by the year 2010, instead of declining, crude death rates and both child and infant mortality rates will remain more or less constant or will increase slightly. Similarly, life expectancy will decrease slightly instead of increasing by a projected 20 per cent. The model projects only a lessening of total population growth, from 3 per cent to just under 2.5 per cent a year.

A similar picture may be seen in Asia in the first and second decades of the next century.[19] There the WHO estimates that already half a million people may be infected with HIV (and, in one report in November 1991, says that the Indian government has reported that there may be as many as one million infected people there already), some 200 000–400 000 in Thailand alone. The rate of new infections is expected to climb dramatically until early in the next century. Mechai Viravaidya, a minister in the Office of Thailand's Prime Minister who was prominent in the country's family planning programme (to such an extent that condoms are widely referred to as 'mechais'), has warned of the potential major impact of HIV on the economies of his and other developing countries, costing billions of dollars in lost earnings (Thailand presently earns $5000 million a year through tourism, $2000 million through direct foreign investment and $1000 million in remittances from Thai workers abroad) and medical care. He warned an Asia–Pacific conference that the impact of AIDS will be felt faster than anybody expects, as AIDS kills those in the most productive sectors of society. Those aged 25–40 will die after they have been trained and he noted that 'the only saving could be on the pension fund'.[20] Of course, Thailand and India are not alone. Indonesia, the Philippines and Pacific nations with high rates of STD will face problems if HIV establishes itself. Infections in intravenous drug users in southern China have been reported, and recent research in that country indicates that homosexual behaviour may not be as rare as its political leaders had led outsiders to believe.[21] Likewise Latin American countries face a major challenge with, for example, the same risk factors existing in Brazil as in Africa at present.

Dr Merson of the WHO warned the International Monetary Fund and the World Bank that AIDS had become a major factor in the world economy. He foresaw the deaths of as many as one-fifth of young and middle-aged adults over a short period of time leading to social turmoil, economic disruption and even political destabilisation in many countries. Whether these gloomy prognostications are borne out in practice remains to be seen. What is apparent is the wide variation between and within countries, making it extremely difficult to forecast effects; our lack of knowledge about the true extent of spread of HIV compounds these difficulties. How many forecasts are based on extrapolations from unrepresentative populations needs to be established before plans to cope with AIDS can be drawn up. The absence of hard data makes fertile ground for anecdote and rumour. For instance, what does one make of reports by reputable researchers that more than 40 per cent of a major rural population in a southern African country is infected, and that this is affecting agricultural output? A few years ago people who estimated the effects of a seroprevalence rate of 20–25 per cent were generally held to be extremely pessimistic, but now such rates are more widely accepted. What is needed in all these cases is careful definition of the populations studied.

Historically, societies have shown remarkable robustness in the face of adversity. Disasters, wars and epidemics have swept away many thousands and left devastation in their wake, yet extinctions of social groups or nations are rare. AIDS differs from other disasters and epidemics in its toll of the young, qualified and economically productive. Wars had similar consequences but did not leave the legacy of infected children. Nevertheless, human adaptability suggests that affected societies will survive, but they will not be the same. The global response to AIDS, the re-examination of attitudes towards issues such as human rights, sexuality, death, women and care that it has caused, and the vast scientific strides all show what can be done cooperatively between communities. The challenge is to maintain and strengthen this collaboration in the 1990s as the epidemic strikes hard at some of the societies least able to cope.

References

1. J.L. Stanford *et al.*, 'Is Africa lost?', *Lancet*, 338 (1991), pp. 557–8.
2. P. Brown, 'Poverty holds up Africa's fight against AIDS', *New Scientist*, 3 January 1992.
3. Centers for Disease Control, 'Pneumocystis pneumonia – Los Angeles', *Morbidity and Mortality Weekly Report*, 30 (1981), pp. 250–2.
4. C. Gilks, 'AIDS, monkeys and malaria', *Nature* (London), 354 (28 Nov. 1991), p. 262.
5. *Weekly Epidemiological Record*, 66 40, (1991), pp. 289–90.
6. European Centre for the Epidemiological Monitoring of AIDS, *AIDS Surveillance in Europe*, quarterly report no. 30 (1991).
7. 'Update on AIDS', *Weekly Epidemiological Record*, 66 48, (1991), pp. 353–7.
8. J.J. Goedardt *et al.*, High Risk of HIV-1 Infection for First-born Twin,' *Lancet*, 14 December 1991.
9. P. Moncharmont *et al.*, 'Intérêt de L'information et de la responsabilisa-

tion des donneurs de sang dans la prévention de la transmission du virus de L'immunodéficience Lumaine', *Pressé Médicale*, 20, 13 (1991), p. 1513.
10. I. N'tita *et al.*, 'Risk of transfusion-associated HIV transmission in Kinshasa, Zaire', *AIDS*, 5, 4 (1991), pp. 437–9.
11. 'Unreported findings shed new light on HIV dental case', *AIDS Alert*, 6, 7 (1991), pp. 121–44.
12. J. Elford *et al.*, 'Research into HIV and AIDS between 1981 and 1990: the epidemic curve', *AIDS*, 5, 12 (1991), pp. 1515–19.
13. *The Times*, 3 September 1991, p. 9.
14. *Journal of the National Cancer Institute*, 83, 8 (1991), pp. 528–9.
15. J. Mann, quoted in *The 3rd Epidemic: Repercussions of the Fear of AIDS* (London: The Panos Institute, 1990).
16. See n. 7.
17. R.M. Anderson *et al.*, 'The spread of HIV-1 in Africa: sexual contact patterns and the predicted demographic impact of AIDS', *Nature (London)*, 352, 15 August 1991, pp. 581–9.
18. N.J. Robinson, *AIDS Newsletter*, 6, 15 (1991), p. 24. See also n. 7.
19. See n. 4.
20. Several sources: see, for example, *AIDS Newsletter*, 6, 15 (1991), item 1043.
21. *Daily Telegraph*, 11 December 1991, p. 13.

3 Current Research on the Economic Impact of HIV/AIDS: A Review of the International and South African Literature
Jonathan Broomberg

RECENT RESEARCH TRENDS

The earliest reported studies of the social and economic impact of the HIV/AIDS epidemic date back to 1984, three years after the disease was definitively recognised. Since that time, extensive work on these issues has been undertaken in the USA and Europe. To date, however, only very limited work has been done on the social and economic impact of the disease in developing countries.

Most of the initial analyses of the economic and social impact of HIV/AIDS aimed to generate estimates of the total direct and (less frequently) indirect costs of the disease as a means of computing the total national economic burden of the disease. These results were then usually compared to total national health expenditures, as well as to expenditures on other important illnesses. While more recent work has continued to focus on the overall economic implications of HIV/AIDS, there has been much more focus on the more detailed micro-economic aspects of the disease. Examples here include cost-effectiveness, the impact of new treatment strategies, economic aspects of diagnosis, prevention and research, and the impact of the disease on specific economic sectors.

The concern with the overall economic burden of HIV/AIDS reflected the initial perception that the epidemic had the potential to overwhelm the health services, and to have a drastic impact on national economies. As it has become clear that, at least for the developed countries, this is not the case, economic research efforts have turned to more detailed questions of resource allocation within the health sector, and analysis of the impact of the epidemic at the micro-economic level.

Analysis of existing international research indicates three important limitations characterising most research conducted so far: these are the limited policy applicability of most studies, highly variable results, and the narrow scope of many studies.

Limited Policy Applicability

Only a small fraction of research conducted so far has had any practical policy implications. One obvious explanation for this is the focus on computing the total costs of the disease, rather than on more detailed cost-effectiveness, cost-benefit or sectoral impact studies.

Such 'burden of disease' data may provide valuable background information for policy-makers, and may be useful in stressing the urgency of the problem, but is ultimately not useful in determining the allocation of resources either to the health sector from outside, or within the sector itself.[1] This is so for several reasons: a high economic burden may reflect an already substantial consumption of resources. Even where this is not the case, there may be no effective interventions to lessen the high economic burden. Also, the simple addition of direct and indirect costs may involve distributional assumptions with which policy-makers may disagree. For example, the indirect costs of a disease that disproportionately affects lower socio-economic classes (with higher unemployment rates, and lower average earnings) will be lower than that of a disease that affects all classes equally. It is thus likely that the shift of recent work towards more detailed micro-economic analysis will be accompanied by greater policy applicability.

Variability of Results

Another reason for the limited applicability of research conducted so far is the high degree of variability in the results of most studies. Such variability occurs both within and between countries. In the USA, for example, the highest estimates of lifetime direct personal costs per AIDS patient are 7.3 times higher than the lowest estimates,[2] and differences between high and low estimates of direct costs per person per year, while varying less, are still substantial (3.8:1).[3] Interestingly, the variation between estimates for the USA is greater than that for different European countries.[4] Such variability results, in part, from problems in gathering reliable data, and from the highly dynamic nature of the HIV/AIDS epidemic.

One explanation for the problem of data reliability is the uncertainty of epidemiological predictions of the future course of the epidemic. This is especially true for developing countries where epidemiological data on HIV/AIDS is, for the most part, unreliable. This has led some health economists to suggest that in these countries only costs per infected person can be accurately calculated, and that the total burden of the disease can only be calculated on the basis of presumptive estimates of HIV prevalence.[5] Longer experience with the epidemic, and more reliable data collection, have made this less of a problem in the developed countries.

Another explanation is to be found in the different methodological approaches and the sampling problems described in the previous section. In addition, important differences in the samples selected for study may account for much of the variability. This problem of sample selection is illustrated by the fact that widest variability in results noted above was for estimates of lifetime costs. This is due to widely varying estimates of survival after being diagnosed as having AIDS between studies (from 7.1 to 24 months).[6] When this factor is eliminated by calculating direct personal costs per person per year, the variation is diminished.

The observed variability is also a result of the rapid changes in the disease profile, and in approaches to dealing with HIV/AIDS, which are often not taken into account when comparing different studies. Examples include the impact of new treatment strategies, such as AZT (an anti-viral drug that is being used with good effect in both the AIDS and pre-AIDs stages) on survival time, and changing practice patterns, such as increasing use of outpatient rather than inpatient care.

Limited Scope of Research

Most research on the economic impact of the HIV/AIDS epidemic has covered a narrow portion of the total costs incurred by individuals and by society. Most studies have looked only at direct medical care costs, although a few have included estimates of non-personal direct costs, and of indirect costs. Most other costs to individuals, external costs, and all intangible costs are omitted from all studies. These limitations are in part a result of inadequate data and in part a result of conceptual difficulties.

It is thus clear that, at present, neither developed nor developing countries have adequate data on which to base reliable estimates of current and future costs of the HIV/AIDS epidemic.[7] Until the limitations described here are adequately dealt with, all economic impact estimates should be treated with caution. The wide ranges of presently available estimates emphasises this point.

Results of Current Research: Developed Countries

Current research in developed countries suggests that HIV/AIDS will have a far smaller impact on the overall economy than was originally envisaged, and that health expenditures on the disease will represent a relatively small and manageable share of total national health care expenditures.

Table 3.1 shows some recent estimates, for the USA, of the share of total health expenditures accounted for by total personal medical care costs of AIDS, as well as of the share of gross national product (GNP) accounted for by the total national cost of AIDS. As noted in the table, personal medical care costs are estimated to account for a maximum of 1.5 per cent of total national health expenditures in 1991, while total costs are estimated to comprise a maximum of 0.2

Table 3.1 Costs of HIV/AIDS in relation to national health expenditures and GNP (USA)

Study	Year	Personal medical care (US$ bn)	%Total health expenditure	Total cost of HIV/AIDS US$ bn	% GNP
Bloom and Carliner	1986	1.7	0.4	8.5	
(1986 dollars)	1991	8.0	1.5	48.8	0.2
Scitovsky and Rice	1986	1.1	0.2	7.9	
(1986 dollars)	1991	8.5	1.4	45.6	0.19
Hellinger	1991	5.3	1.0		
(1988 dollars)					

Sources   D.E. Bloom and G. Carliner, 'The economic impact of AIDS in the US', *Science*, 239 (1988), pp. 604–9; F.J. Hellinger, 'Updated forecasts of the costs of medical care for persons with AIDS, 1989–93', *Public Health Reports*, 105, 1 (1990); A.A. Scitovsky and D.P. Rice, 'Estimates of the direct and indirect costs of acquired immunodeficiency syndrome in the United States, 1985, 1986, and 1991', *Public Health Reports*, 102, 1 (1987).

per cent of GNP in the same year. Note, however, that these estimates are significantly higher than the equivalent figures for 1986.

Contrary to original expectations, the cost of HIV/AIDS has turned out to be close to that of other serious, chronic illnesses in these countries. In the USA, for example, a 1985 estimate for the total costs of HIV/AIDS was given as $4.6 billion, while the equivalent costs for end-stage renal disease were $2.2 billion, motor vehicle accidents $5.6 billion, and lung cancer $2.7 billion. HIV/AIDS is thus estimated to cost more than each of these individually apart from motor vehicle accidents; and in terms of lifetime costs per patient, the evidence suggests that, aside from end-stage renal disease, the costs of the other diseases listed here ranged between 45 and 70 per cent of the costs of HIV/AIDS.[8] Nevertheless, the cost of HIV/AIDS remains small in comparison to total personal health expenditures and, while expenditures on HIV/AIDS will be large, they will remain sustainable.

Results of Current Research: Developing Countries

Far less data is available for developing countries. One study, conducted in Zaire and Tanzania, suggests that although the expenditures per patient with HIV/AIDS are unlikely to exceed those for other serious diseases, total expenditures on HIV/AIDS constitute a far greater proportion of per capitum health spending than is the case in the developed countries, and total costs constitute a greater proportion of GNP.[9] These observations suggest that the expenditures on HIV/AIDS, especially in the face of massive epidemics, are likely to be unsustainable for several of the developing countries. In terms of the health sector, there is likely to be a substantial shift of resources within the health sector away from PHC and towards the treatment of patients with HIV/AIDS, and ultimately significant numbers of patients are likely to be cared for in their communities rather than in the formal health sector.[10] The total economic burden of the disease is also likely to be far more significant in these countries. This is discussed in more detail in the section on indirect costs.

In comparing expenditures on HIV/AIDS in developed and developing countries, there is a predictable, approximately linear relationship between direct costs per case and GNP per capitum. This pattern is similar to that which connects general health care expenditure to GNP per capitum in all countries.[11]

DIRECT COSTS OF HIV/AIDS

The measurable direct costs of a disease usually consist of personal medical care costs, and non-personal costs, incurred by society (such as those of research, prevention and testing). Most studies have investigated personal medical care costs, although some of the more recent studies have included estimates of non-personal costs as well. Almost all studies have focused exclusively on the costs of AIDS, omitting the costs of the pre-AIDS phases of the disease.

Personal Medical Care Costs

Table 3.2 gives a range of estimates of direct medical care costs for both developed and developing countries. The table indicates the wide variations discussed above, and demonstrates that this variation is less when the effect of lifespan is corrected for in the estimates of cost per person per year. As the table also shows, the major causes of the divergent results are differences in assumptions as to the numbers of hospital admissions, average length of stay in hospital and hospital costs.

As the disease has been studied further, however, certain trends have emerged. There appears to be a convergence in the estimates for the number of hospital days per person per year (one review shows that seven out of ten recent studies in the USA found this to vary between 54 and 63 days per year[12]). One reason for greater uniformity may be the increased understanding of the disease and how to manage it that has come with more experience. This is also the explanation for the trend towards decreasing use of hospitalisation and increasing use of outpatient care in the management of AIDS patients. There is in fact substantial evidence from the USA that the general use of resources in treating AIDS declines as experience with the disease increases.[13]

Despite the wide variations in these results, there is now consensus among most health economists studying the problem that the personal costs of treating a patient with AIDS in the developed countries falls within the range of $30 000–$50 000 per year (1989 dollars). As noted above, this is comparable to the costs of treating most other serious illnesses in these countries.

Table 3.2 shows that the estimates derived from developing countries are substantially lower than those for developed countries,

Table 3.2 Review of international studies on the direct costs of HIV/AIDS

Source	Year of estimate	Mean cost per person per year ($US)	Lifespan†	Hospital days per person per year
USA				
Hardy	1986	135 690	13 months	155
Scitovsky*	1984	46 700	7.5 months	56
Seage	1984	46 505	–	62
Scitovsky and Rice	1986	31 902	–	63
Hellinger	1985	28 500	24 months	23
Kizer	1986	46 700	18 months	60
Pascal	1986	75 200	15 months	58
Lafferty	1985	32 100	7.2 months	47
Hay	1987	32 100	12 months	19
Kaiser Permanente	1987	24 200	15.1 month	N/A
Europe				
UK				
Johnson	1985	28 400	5.2 months	115
Cunningham	1986	46 800	12 months	30
Griffith				
Rees	1986	36 300	12 months	91
Germany				
Auguste-Viktoria	1987	29 900	18 months	80
Other Countries				
Australia				
Fanning	1986	26 400	7.2 months	58
Zaire				
Over	1986	1 600* / 100*	–	N/A
Tanzania				
Over	1986	600* / 100*	–	N/A
Jamaica				
Policy Reseach Institute	1987	2 700*	–	N/A
Brazil				
Ministry of Health	1987	18 000*	–	N/A

* Mean lifetime costs.
† Lifespan refers to the length of life after diagnosis of AIDS.

Sources Adapted from M.F. Drummond and L.M. Davies, *AIDS: The Challenge for Economic Analysis* (University of Birmingham, AIDS European Regional Programme, 1990); and A.A. Scitovsky and M. Over, 'AIDS:

cost of care in the developed and developing world 1988', *AIDS*, 2 (1988), Suppl. 1, s. 71–81. See also A.M. Hardy *et al.*, 'The economic impact of the first 10,000 cases of acquired immunodeficiency syndrome in the U.S.', *Journal of the American Medical Association*, 255 (1986), pp. 209–11; G.R. Seage, A.A. Scitovsky and D.P. Rice, 'Estimates of the direct and indirect costs of acquired immunodeficiency syndrome in the United States, 1985, 1986, and 1991', *Public Health Reports*, 102, 1 (1987); F.J. Hellinger, 'Updated forecasts of the costs of medical care for persons with AIDS, 1989–93', *Public Health Reports*, 105, 1 (1990); M. Over, S. Bertozzi, J. Chin, B. N'Galy and K. Nyamuryekung'e, 'The direct and indirect costs of HIV infection in developing countries: the case of Zaire and Tanzania', in A.F. Fleming, M. Carballo, D.W. FitzSimons, M.R. Bailey and J. Mann, *The Global Impact of AIDS* (New York: Alan R. Liss, 1988).

---

confirming the relationship between expenditure on AIDS and GNP per capitum in these countries. Another explanation for the low costs in developing countries may be the very low value of time spent by health personnel in these countries relative to developed countries.

The few studies that have been done in developing countries indicate a similar pattern of wide variation in cost estimates, both within and between countries. The reasons postulated by the authors of these studies are similar to those in developed countries. One additional factor, which is likely to be more important in developing than in developed countries, is the impact of differing socio-economic class on access to formal sector health services.[14]

Another issue requiring attention in developing countries is the cost of treatment forgone by patients who are 'crowded out' of the system as increasing numbers of people with AIDS are treated by the health services. There does not appear to have been any research conducted on this issue in developing countries thus far.

Personal Medical Care Costs in the pre-AIDS Phase

In developed countries, direct costs in the pre-AIDS phase will be largely those attributable to a range of outpatient care for those who are aware that they are HIV positive, and who are being treated and monitored by the health services. This issue has become increasingly important as evidence has accumulated of the efficacy of certain early drug interventions in prolonging life (see below). The difficulties in obtaining reliable data are even greater here than is the case in the

AIDS phase. One major problem is in projecting the number of HIV positives who will be aware of their disease, and who will need access to the health services. One estimate for the UK puts this figure at 10 per cent (Dr Padayachee, personal communication). It is also very difficult to determine the usage of services since these are likely to differ even more than is the case in the AIDS phase. One reason for this is that different stages of the disease require different intensities of monitoring.

These difficulties have meant that where attempts have been made to assess the direct costs of the pre-AIDS phase, these have been done through the construction of a hypothetical model of the use of services, and the application of the resulting costs to a series of assumptions about the percentage of HIV positives who will be exposed to the health services. One estimate for the USA suggests that the 1988 cost of early intervention was $9637 per person per year. On the assumption that 50 per cent of all HIV positives who do not have AIDS are treated in the pre-AIDS stage, the total national costs would have been $5.1 billion in 1988; this is almost twice the $2.6 billion given as one estimate of the total cost of treating people with AIDS in the same year.[15]

In the developing countries, the economic impact of the asymptomatic phase is equally important, although for different reasons. Most developing countries will not be able to afford the very expensive drugs now being used for early interventions, and neither will they be able to afford intensive laboratory monitoring of asymptomatic patients. However, the very high incidence of active TB among HIV positives (since the immune suppression resulting from HIV leads to the reactivation of latent TB) means that the pre-AIDS phase will have very serious direct and indirect costs in these countries.

The study in Zaire and Tanzania cited above suggests that, in 1985 prices, the total costs per asymptomatic HIV-positive person are approximately one-third of the direct medical costs per symptomatic HIV-positive case, namely between $47 and $560 (in Zaire), or between $37 and $223 (in Tanzania).

Non-Personal Medical Care Costs

The major difficulty in tracing the non-personal costs of combating a disease lies in tracing the numerous public and private sources of expenditure on testing, research, education and other interventions. Even where good public-sector data exist, the problems of obtaining private-sector data means that such estimates can, at best, be educated guesses. One US study estimated that, in 1986, 33 per cent of total direct costs were non-personal costs, and projected this forward to suggest that the figure for 1991 would be 21 per cent.[16] We have found no estimates for developing countries.

The difficulties in projecting such costs forward are compounded by uncertainty as to policy decisions that will affect such costs. This has led Rees to suggest that, since these expenditures are not demand-led, projections should be normative rather than positive; in other words, analysts should project what *ought* to be spent, rather than attempting to predict what will actually be spent.

INDIRECT COSTS

The standard approach to measuring indirect costs, adopted in all studies, is the human capital approach. This takes forgone earnings due to morbidity, disability and premature mortality as a proxy for lost production. The value of lost production is then usually discounted to the year under study using a social discount rate. Unfortunately, most studies count only the value of marketable production, thus omitting the value of household work, subsistence agriculture and other forms of non-marketed 'production'. Only two American studies that we have reviewed included this component in attaching a value to lost production.[17]

Another important problem is that, in the absence of reliable data to the contrary, all studies assume that individuals with HIV/AIDS resemble the general population in terms of average earnings, gender and age, and in terms of labour participation rates. In most countries this is obviously not the case. In the USA and Europe, for example, the disease is predominant among the relatively more employed, higher-earning male homosexuals, and among intravenous drug users, who are more likely to be unemployed and to earn less on average.

A consistent finding in most studies is that the indirect costs of HIV/AIDS account for 80 per cent or more of the total costs of the disease. This is in contrast to the pattern in other serious illnesses, in which indirect costs tend to account for 65–75 per cent of total costs.[18] This is explained by the fact that, on average, AIDS causes morbidity, disability and premature death among a younger, more productive population than is the case for most other serious illnesses which

Table 3.3 Data on indirect costs of HIV/AIDS

	Lifetime costs per person (US$)
USA	
Hardy et al.	623 000
Scitovsky and Rice	541 000
Tanzania	
Over et al.	5 093

Sources A.M. Hardy *et al.*, 'The economic impact of the first 10,000 cases of Acquired Immunodeficiency Syndrome in the U.S.', *Journal of America Medical Association*, 255 (1986), pp. 209–11; M. Over *et al.*, 'The direct and indirect costs of HIV infection in developing countries: the cases of Zaire and Tanzania', in A.F. Fleming, M. Carballo, D.W. FitzSimons, M.R. Bailey and J. Mann, *The Global Impact of Aids* (New York: Alan R. Liss, 1988), pp. 123–35; A.A. Scitovsky and D.P. Rice, 'Estimates of the direct and indirect costs of acquired immunodeficiency syndrome in the United States, 1985, 1986, and 1991', *Public Health Reports*, 102, 1 (1987).

have been studied. For the same reason, most studies have found that over 90 per cent of the indirect costs are accounted for by losses due to premature death, rather than due to disability or morbidity.[19]

The one reported study of the indirect costs of HIV/AIDS in developing countries yielded similar results. The figures for Zaire show that indirect costs account for between 79 and 95 per cent of total costs, while for Tanzania the range was 96–98.5 per cent.[20] Table 3.3 shows some results of the indirect costs per case, for the USA, and for the one African country mentioned here. The substantial discrepancies reflect the different unemployment rates, and vastly different average earnings in the different countries.

The approach adopted here takes labour participation rates into account in calculating forgone earnings due to HIV/AIDS. However, all the studies we have reviewed have omitted to include an adjustment for replacement of those disabled or dying prematurely by the unemployed. This may not be important in developed countries where employment rates are high, and where the costs of replacing most employees are significant. However, it is clearly of relevance in developing countries where high unemployment rates, particularly among the unskilled labour force (coupled with high rates of the HIV infection in this group), mean that a significant proportion of those ill and dying from AIDS could be replaced fairly quickly. This would mean that indirect costs to the economy may be much lower than would otherwise be predicted.

Another important omission from most studies, as noted in the case of direct costs, is the effect of morbidity and mortality in the asymptomatic phase of HIV infection. This is especially important in developing countries where TB is likely to contribute significantly to the overall burden of morbidity and mortality of HIV/AIDS.

SPECIFIC ISSUES IN THE ECONOMICS OF HIV/AIDS

In addition to research on the direct and indirect costs of HIV/AIDS, research attention has now shifted to more detailed aspects of the economics of this disease. Although a detailed review of this work is beyond the scope of this chapter, some of the major trends and important findings of this research will be briefly presented here.

The Economics of Treatment

Research on the economics of treatment has examined issues of cost-effectiveness of different treatment settings and different therapeutic interventions, as well as trends in the use of these settings and interventions.

Treatment settings
One debate has focused on whether people with AIDS should be treated by a 'cluster' approach (treating all people with AIDS in the same ward/hospital) or by a 'scatter' approach. The economic evidence accumulated so far shows neither to be conclusively more cost-effective.[21]

An important trend, noted earlier, has been the shift – particularly in the USA – towards increased use of outpatient rather than inpatient care for people with AIDS. This has resulted from a combination of increased understanding of the disease (and how best to manage it) as the epidemic has progressed, the availability of drugs such as AZT and pentamidine to prevent opportunistic infections, pressure from those who pay for health care, and the development of effective community care alternatives (such as hospices and community care groups).[22] This trend has not been as marked in Europe, where the epidemic is newer, and where there is less pressure to avoid hospitalisation, since hospitalisation costs are lower.

The increased use of outpatient and community services may be one important explanation for the observed decline in the direct costs of treating people with AIDS.[23] However, there is thus far only suggestive evidence as to the relative cost-effectiveness of these different treatment settings.[24] Even if it is clear that community-based alternatives are cost-effective, other non-economic considerations, such as the viability of community-based services in the face of a massive epidemic, will need to be taken into account. In addition, increasing reliance on such services increases the need for greater coordination and planning between multiple providers of care.[25]

There has been much less published work on these issues in developing countries. However, it is clear that, in many of these countries, outpatient and community care settings have already become the mainstay of care of people with AIDS since the formal hospital services are unable to cope with the load placed on them. For this reason, issues such as availability of community-based services, planning and coordination will be of great importance.

Therapeutic interventions

The range of available therapeutic interventions has widened significantly since the advent of the HIV/AIDS epidemic, and with this has come the need for assessment of the economic consequences of such interventions. Several drugs are now available for use in HIV/AIDS. AZT, which has been shown to prolong life in people with AIDS and in asymptomatic HIV positives, has been subject to extensive economic investigation. Of course, when a drug that is able to prolong life significantly is available, it becomes difficult to apply strictly economic criteria in evaluation. The additional years of life gained (adjusted for quality of life) and the side-effects are also relevant considerations. Research indicates that, in the USA, AZT costs approximately $8 000–10 000 (1988) per life year gained. Most research also concurs that the lifetime costs of treating a person with AIDS are approximately the same whether or not AZT is used. Reduced hospital costs are offset by the higher costs associated with a longer lifespan, and similar costs in the terminal phases of the disease.[26] Other drugs, such as pentamidine – which prevents *Pneumocystis carinii* pneumonia (PCP) – have been subjected to similar investigation.

No research on the cost-effectiveness of different interventions appears to have been done in developing countries. Although it is likely that AZT and other expensive medications will not be affordable for most counties, the potential costs and benefits should still be documented. In addition other interventions, such as the use of Izoniazid (INH) to prevent TB, and alternatives to pentamidine to prevent PCP, are available and are already in use. The cost-effectiveness of these interventions in developing countries requires urgent investigation.

The Economics of Prevention

Despite the range of interventions now available for HIV/AIDS, no cure has yet emerged, and it is clearly accepted that prevention of new infections should be a major priority. It is also clear that, in addition to securing safe blood transfusions, one important focus of such prevention should be on behaviour change. The potential benefits of expenditure on prevention can be crudely estimated on the basis of estimates of the number of lives saved and the total costs per life lost to the disease. However, the measurement of the relative cost-effectiveness of different prevention programmes is more complex. It is extremely difficult to measure the effects of prevention programmes on behaviours. Other questions include the relative gains for the individual and for society from prevention efforts, the very long time horizon over which benefits have to be assessed, and whether efforts should be applied to the whole society or to high-risk groups. Despite these complications, the importance of economic analysis of prevention efforts is obvious, and substantial research on this issue is now under-way.[27]

The Economics of Diagnosis

There has been a major debate on various aspects of HIV testing policy. One issue concerns the costs and benefits of screening the general population as opposed to only high-risk groups. Another is whether the partners of those infected should be traced and screened. There is general agreement that high-risk groups should be tested. However, current evidence suggests that general population screening is significantly less cost-effective (measured in terms of quality adjusted life years gained) than screening high-risk populations.[28] This suggests that, except on a limited scale, and for specific purposes (such as tracking the epidemic), population screening is unjustifiable from an economic point of view. As new, more effective interventions for asymptomatic HIV positives become available, however, arguments for wider screening may become more pressing.

Who Bears the Costs of HIV/AIDS?

Now that we have some idea about the magnitude of the direct and indirect economic burden of HIV/AIDS in developed and developing countries, attention has turned to the question of who will bear the burden of the various costs of the disease.

In most European countries which have well developed, equitable national health systems, this is less of an issue. However, in the USA, and certainly in most developing countries, two pressing concerns have emerged. The first is the issue of cost shifting between different responsible authorities. In the USA, for example, different payers attempt to limit their liability by shifting the burden of care elsewhere. This is very likely to occur in all countries, including developing countries, which have dual public and private health-care systems. The general pattern will be of the private sector attempting to shift the burden of care to the public sector. This will result in the public sector bearing a substantial share of the total costs of the disease.

The second issue concerns the economic consequences for infected individuals and their families. In the USA, the disease is now spreading primarily among those who are unlikely to have adequate private insurance coverage. This is likely to be true as well for those developing countries which do have private health sectors. Since neither the USA nor most developing countries offers adequate public health care at affordable cost, infected individuals and their families will face massive out-of-pocket costs for their health care. This is in addition to the consequences of unemployment and other forms of economic discrimination described above.

The scale of this problem in the developing countries is well illustrated by research done in Zaire which shows that the average cost of a hospitalisation for a child with AIDS was three times the average monthly income (equivalent to $30) of fathers of the children in the study.[29] Although such costs might be borne by employers, this is not the case for the self-employed or the unemployed (42 per cent of fathers in the study). The problem is made worse by the funeral expenses for family members who die. In the same study, these expenses amounted to the equivalent of 11 months' income.

Additional economic burdens are imposed on families through income lost by those who have to give up work to look after people with AIDS. Where a breadwinner has died, extended families may also face the costs of supporting dependents. This problem may be aggravated in Africa, where the high rate of death from HIV/AIDS among people of reproductive age is leaving substantial numbers of orphans. One study, conducted in 10 East and Central African countries, estimates that during the 1990s, 6–11 per cent of all children below the age of 25 will be orphaned by HIV/AIDS.[30]

There is also an increasing body of very useful and important research work examining the impact of AIDS on local economies. One particular example that has been well studied is the impact of the epidemic on subsistence farming systems.[31]

The Impact of HIV/AIDS on Specific Economic Sectors

One sector that has been the focus of particular attention in developed countries has been the insurance industry. While a full analysis of trends in this sector is beyond the scope of this report, it is noteworthy that, in the USA, almost all insurance companies refuse to sell life insurance to people with AIDS, and one study indicates that, in 1988, 91 per cent of insurance companies refused to sell insurance to HIV positives.[32] We have found no published research on this issue for developing countries (but see Chapter 11 for a study of Zimbabwe). As noted above, however, there is now an increasing focus on the impact of AIDS on specific sectors in developing countries, with a particular concentration on highly labour-intensive areas of economic activity which will be most susceptible to AIDS-induced mortality.

Research on the Economic Implications of HIV/AIDS in South Africa

At the time of writing, research on the economic implications of the HIV/AIDS epidemic in South Africa remains limited and, for the most part, superficial. Available research has involved some attempts at estimating the direct medical care costs per case, and for the country as a whole, and some analyses of the potential impact of the epidemic on specific economic sectors, as well as on the economy as a whole. Aside from the research presented elsewhere in this book,[33] there has thus far been no attempt at estimating the indirect costs of HIV/AIDS in South Africa. The results of existing research work, and some significant problems in these analyses, are reviewed here.

The Direct Costs of HIV/AIDS in South Africa

Two fundamental problems which research in South Africa shares with international efforts are the very limited scope of the research, and the variability of the resulting estimates. With one very limited exception,[34] all direct cost estimates have concentrated exclusively on medical care costs, omitting all other direct costs. These cost estimates have covered only the costs of hospitalisation and, in some cases, the costs of AZT, but have excluded all other direct medical care costs. In addition, all estimates have been limited to the AIDS phase, with no attempt being made at estimating the costs of asymptomatic HIV infection, or of HIV-associated TB. There has also been no attempt to distinguish between public and private sector utilisation of resources, or to model differential use of public sector resources such as economically imposed limits on hospital admissions), or the development of community care arrangements.

The variability of results is demonstrated in Table 3.4, which summarises the available estimates for direct costs of treating AIDS patients in South Africa. The variability in the estimates of costs per year is largely the result of the widely varying methodologies employed. Only one estimate (van Niekerk's) is based on retrospective utilisation analysis and, in this case, only 25 cases at the very early stage of the epidemic were analysed. The remaining estimates are based on hypothetical models of resource utilisation and most of these are very superficial, based on unsupported assumptions. Spier simply cites 'authorities calculations'. Van der Merwe uses a very high estimate of hospital usage (168 days per case) imported from one of the early studies in the USA, and multiplies this by an average cost per public sector hospital day. Whiteside borrows van der Merwe's figure of R15 000 per case without defending this. Only Taylor's figures are based on a detailed hypothetical model of resource usage to which accurate costs are attached and, in this case the estimates apply only to the private sector.

The reliability of these estimates is thus undermined both by their variability and, more importantly, by the faulty or unsupported assumptions which underpin them. This problem is more serious in the estimates of total direct costs to the country. As shown in Table

Table 3.4 Review of estimates of direct costs of AIDS in South Africa

Source	Year of estimate	Cost per case per year (R) (no AZT)	Cost per case per year (R) (with AZT)	Year concerned	Total direct cost (R)
Spier	1990		55 000	2000	7.5 bn
van der Merwe	1988	15 692	31 692	1995	197m–9.6 bn
van Niekerk	1988	20 160	44 460		
Taylor	1991		36 666		
Osborne	1990		80–100 000	2000	90 bn
Whiteside	1990	15 000		1995	537m–2.97 bn
				2000	6bn–15 bn

Sources A. Spier, 'Medical Aid', *Aids Analysis Africa*, 1, 1 (June/July 1990), p. 5; J.A. van der Merwe, 'AIDS', unpublished paper, SANLAM, 1988; W.A. Niekerk, Minister of National Health and Population Development, November 1988, cited in Retrovir slide presentation, undated; G. Taylor, personal communication, calculation of 'best care' hypothetical model for a patient in the private sector, 1991; E. Osborne. 'AIDS – what if?' in *Nedbank Guide to the Economy* (Johannesburg, undated); A. Whiteside, 'AIDS in Southern Africa', a position paper for the Development Bank of Southern Africa (Durban: Economic Research Unit, University of Natal, 1990).

3.4, these vary even more widely than with estimates of costs per case. For 1995, the range is R537 million to R4.8 billion, and for the year 2000, the range is R6 billion to R90 billion. The obvious explanation here is the widely varying estimates of total case load generated by the different projection models used by these authors. Many of these models are highly problematic, and almost certainly unreliable.

All of these estimates are thus likely to be inaccurate; the costs per case are not well supported, the numbers of cases generated by most of the models are also likely to be inaccurate, and there is no account taken of the very likely reality that only a small proportion of all AIDS cases will actually receive the package of care being postulated by all models. This is so because not all cases will actually gain access to the health services and, more importantly, because the health services are likely to be unable to cope with the case load so that large numbers of cases will be offered cheaper alternative care settings, or no care at all. The high cost estimates (R75–90 billion in the year 2000) are thus likely to be a gross overestimate of the total direct cost of HIV/AIDS, even taking into account the omission of the pre-AIDS phases and TB care.

There are several problems with this kind of superficial research. The wide variation in results undermines the trustworthiness of this and of any subsequent data, for policy-makers and planners at all levels. In addition, the extremely high estimates generated by some models for total costs creates a sense of helplessness in the face of overwhelming and unmanageable costs. This further undermines efforts to combat the disease, and to find cost-effective care options for those who are ill.

THE IMPACT OF HIV/AIDS ON OVERALL ECONOMIC DEVELOPMENT IN SOUTH AFRICA

Published work on the overall economic development impact of HIV/AIDS in South Africa is once again scanty, speculative and superficial. It is generally argued that the epidemic is likely to have devastating consequences for overall economic development in South Africa, and that these consequences are likely to be felt in the first decade of the next century, as the demographic impact of the disease begins to have an effect.[35]

Two major mechanisms are postulated to have a negative impact on economic growth. The first is the impact of HIV/AIDS on the labour market. Here the argument is that disability and deaths from AIDS will result in serious shortages of skilled, semi-skilled and perhaps even unskilled labour. This in turn is predicted to drive up wages, as labour shortages and the premium on skills take effect. These developments are then argued to result in higher cost structures in the economy, an increasing mechanisation drive, and the possibility of serious losses in the productive and competitive capacity of the economy.

The second mechanism is the shrinking of both domestic and international markets for consumption of South African goods. It is suggested that the negative demographic impact in South Africa will have a dramatic effect on local markets, although Osborne recognises that this effect might be offset by the effects of higher average wages, and increased wage dispersion.[36] It is also argued that the potential collapse of the economies of several African countries will have a detrimental impact on the demand for South African exports.

None of these speculative analyses is accompanied by any attempt at quantification. As noted earlier, there has as yet been no attempt to quantify the indirect costs of the HIV/AIDS epidemic in South

Africa. There has thus been no effort to link the disability and mortality impact of the disease to levels of unemployment, or to the distribution of skill levels in the economy.

The absence of these linkages renders speculation about the effects of the disease on both the labour market and on demand highly suspect. For example, in a situation of substantial unemployment it is likely that a significant proportion of the employed labour force who die from HIV/AIDS will be replaceable from among the unemployed. This is clearly true for the unskilled but may also be true for more highly-skilled categories, although some training and hiring costs are likely to be incurred. High unemployment, or very low wages among many of those formally or informally employed, also means that the effect of domestic demand will be far less than the simple demographic impact suggests.

Similarly, the speculation that the economies of several African countries which import goods from South Africa will collapse is not substantiated. Unemployment is high in all these countries; it is also not clear how seriously the relatively small formal economies that account for imports of South African goods will be affected by HIV/AIDS, and there has not been any attempt to assess the potential of international economic aid to assist in the maintenance of these economies, and thus of their capacity to import.

This is not to argue that these overall economic effects will not be felt in South Africa. It is clear that HIV/AIDS will have an impact on economic development, and that the mechanisms suggested here are those likely to mediate the effects of the epidemic. However, in the absence of detailed analysis and quantification of the labour market and demand effects of the disease, speculation about the size and nature of overall economic impact is unhelpful.

Much of the research quoted here might fall into the category of scenario analysis. While it is recognised that such analysis may well have some role to play in preparing decision-makers to cope with the HIV/AIDS epidemic, this should not replace the more detailed analyses that are now required.

While it is possible that several industries and economic sectors have conducted in-depth internal analyses of the impact of HIV/AIDS, the published literature once again is characterised by speculative and probably inaccurate assessments of the effects of the epidemic on a wide variety of economic sectors.

One common trend is simply to extrapolate projections, and the overall economic impact speculations for the country as a whole (which, as noted above, may be very inaccurate) to a particular sector. One example of this is the extrapolation of speculated 25 per cent or 50 per cent seropositivity rates to the labour force of the sugar-growing industry.[37] These extrapolations are then used to argue that there are likely to be major labour supply shortages, affecting production. There is also speculation about the impact on demand for sugar. In this instance, the fact that sugar is a basic commodity is taken to suggest that demand will not be seriously affected.

Similar speculative work has been done for the building industry.[38] Here it is suggested that serious skills shortages (aggravated by the fact that the industry is an employer of last resort) will push up prices, thus reducing demand, and that demand will be even more seriously affected by the decline in actual and potential homeowners as people die, lose jobs or are forced to vacate homes (or abandon plans to purchase due to heavy medical expenses). The net effect of all of this is a prediction that the end of the decade could see the decline of the construction sector.

In the case of the impact on the stockmarket, Bell[39] argues that the epidemic may adversely affect the demand for both equities and bonds as well as the exchange rate, resulting in a flight to currency hedges that earn income outside the country. This will occur as a result of decreasing demand affecting the performance of companies, as increased mortality rates affect cash flow from large institutions, and as the government is forced to adopt a lax fiscal policy and an accommodating monetary policy to cope with increased social spending needs.

Spier analyses the impact of HIV/AIDS on tourism, and argues that tourism will be adversely affected by overseas perceptions of the spread of the disease, by declining service standards in the tourism industry due to skills shortages, and by declining numbers of 'shoppers' from neighbouring states as the effects of the epidemic take hold there.[40]

A more sober analysis is available for the insurance sector, although the publicly available work is again lacking in detail.[41] The major points of note here are that insurers – in particular, life insurers – are exposed to increased liabilities on existing policies. However, current evidence suggests that the degree of exposure will not be sufficient to constitute a threat to the viability of insurance companies, especially in view of their substantial reserves.

Perhaps the major issue facing insurers is how to limit future liabilities. At present two approaches seem to have emerged: the first is to offer full cover provided HIV infection is excluded, and the second is to offer cover without HIV testing, but to exclude from cover HIV/AIDS-related death or disability. We have not come across an analysis which suggests which of these two is currently the dominant pattern. However, it is likely that, as has happened in the USA, people with HIV infection will increasingly find themselves uninsurable.[42]

The problems with all these analyses are obvious. None of them is accompanied by, or supported by, detailed sectoral impact analysis. Instead, they simply extrapolate existing case load projections or existing views on the macro-economic effects of HIV/AIDS directly to the sector concerned. The difficulties and inherent dangers of projection models for HIV/AIDS have already been stressed. These problems are amplified when these models are extended to micro-sectors of the economy without alteration or adaptation. The effect is to generate crude and almost certainly inaccurate assessments of the effects of AIDS in different sectors. These assessments are also remarkably homogenous. Their basic message is this: 'AIDS will affect your industry seriously. It will do this by altering labour supply and demand. These effects cannot be quantified at present, but they will be large (or devastating), and the industry should begin to prepare now.'

There is again no doubt that all economic sectors will be affected in important ways by the HIV/AIDS epidemic. The message that these effects should be predicted and planned for is also an important one. However, this message should be communicated by detailed analysis of the situation of each sector, rather than by the rote application of a crude formula in the guise of sophisticated economic assessment. In the absence of accurate assessments, attempts at sectoral analysis should probably be avoided. The danger of these crude assessments is not only that they are inaccurate, but also that they allow the propagation of extreme, alarmist predictions. As argued earlier, the effect of these is more likely to paralyse than to galvanise society into action.

References

1. M.F. Drummond, 'Priority setting for Aids and other health care programmes', in M.F. Drummond and L.M. Davies *AIDS: The Challenge*

for Economic Analysis (University of Birmingham, AIDS European Regional Programme, 1990), pp. 106–11.
2. D.E. Bloom and G. Carliner, 'The economic impact of AIDS in the US', *Science*, 239 (1988), pp. 604–9.
3. J.E. Sisk, 'The costs of AIDS: a review of the estimates', *Health Affairs*, (Summer 1987), pp. 5–21.
4. M.F. Drummond and L.M. Davies, 'Treating AIDS: the economic issues', *Health Policy*, 10 (1988), pp. 1–19.
5. M. Over, S. Bertozzi, J. Chin, B. N'Galy and K. Nyanunyekung'e, 'The direct and indirect costs of HIV infection in developing countries: the cases of Zaire and Tanzania', in A.F. Fleming, M. Carballo, D.W. FitzSimons, M.R. Bailey and J. Mann, *The Global Impact of AIDS* (New York: Alan R. Liss, 1988), pp. 123–35.
6. A.A. Scitovsky and M. Over, 'AIDS: cost of care in the developed and developing world, 1988', *AIDS*, 2 (1988), suppl. 1, s. 71–81.
7. See n. 2.
8. A.A. Scitovsky and D.P. Rice, 'Estimates of the direct and indirect costs of acquired immunodeficiency syndrome in the United States, 1985, 1986, and 1991, *Public Health Reports*, 102, 1 (1987).
9. See n. 5.
10. A. Griffiths, 'Implications of the medical and scientific aspects of HIV and AIDS for economic resourcing', in Fleming *et al.*, *The Global Impact*, pp. 111–17.
11. See n. 5.
12. See n. 6.
13. See n. 5.
14. See n. 5.
15. A.A. Scitovsky 'Studying the costs of HIV related illness: reflections on the moving target', *The Millbank Quarterly*, 67, 2 (1989), pp. 318–45.
16. M. Rees, 'Methodological and practical issues in estimating the direct cost of AIDS/HIV: England and Wales', in Drummond and Davies *AIDS: The Challenge*, pp. 69–74.
17. A.M. Hardy *et al.*, 'The economic impact of the first 10 000 cases of Acquired Immunodeficiency Syndrome in the U.S.', *Journal of American Medical Association*, 255 (1986), pp. 209–11; see also n. 6.
18. See n. 5.
19. see n. 5 and n. 8.
20. See n. 5.
21. M.F. Drummond, 'The economic impact of AIDS', paper prepared for the Montreal Summary edition of *AIDScare*.
22. Ibid.
23. J.E. Sisk, 'Trends in the prevention, diagnosis and treatment of HIV and their economic implications', in Drummond and Davies, *AIDS: The Challenge*, pp. 8–15.
24. M.F. Drummond and L.M. Davies, 'Topics for economic analysis', in *AIDS: The Challenge*, pp. 1–7.
25. See n. 23.
26. See n. 15 and n. 21.
27. See n. 23.

28. Ibid.
29. F. Davachi, P. Baudoux, K. Ndoko, B. N'Galy and J. Mann, 'The economic impact on families of children with AIDS in Kinshasa, Zaire', in Fleming *et al.*, *The Global Impact*, pp. 167–9.
30. E.A. Preble, 'Impact of HIV/AIDS on African children', *Social Science and Medicine*, 31, 6 (1990), pp. 671–80.
31. S. Gillespie, 'Potential impact of AIDS on farming systems. A case study from Rwanda', *Land Use Policy*, 1, 4 (1989), pp. 301–12; N. Abel, A. Barnett, S. Bell, P. Blaikie and S. Cross, 'The impact of AIDS on food production systems in East and Central Africa over the next ten years: a programmatic paper', in Fleming *et al.*, *The Global Impact*.
32. See n. 2.
33. See Chapter 8 of this volume.
34. J.A. van der Merwe, 'AIDS', unpublished paper (Suid Afrikaanse Nasionale Lewens Assuransic Maatskappy). 1988.
35. E. Osborne, A. Whiteside and J.A. van der Merwe have all written about the overall economic impact of HIV/AIDS.
36. See n. 35.
37. Ibid.
38. T. Hosking, 'The effects of AIDS on the building and construction industry', *Aids Analysis Africa*, 1, 1 (June/July 1990), p. 4.
39. G. Bell, 'AIDS and strategies for the stock market', *AIDS Analysis Africa*, 1, 4 (1991), p. 4.
40. A. Spier, 'AIDS and the future of tourism', *AIDS Analysis Africa*, 1, 3 (1990), p. 3.
41. D.B. Kier, 'AIDS and group insurance', *AIDS Analysis Africa*, 1, 3 (1990), p. 8.
42. D.B. Kier, 'AIDS and the insurance industry: the problem', *AIDS Analysis Africa*, 1, 1 (1990), p. 3.

Part II

Modelling the AIDS Impact in South Africa

4 South African Trends and Projections of HIV Infection
Hilary Southall

INTRODUCTION

Modelling the course of AIDs and its impact on society has proved no simple task. Even the collection of basic information is problematic for, as Bailey has noted,[1] the accumulation of data renders the situation more complex rather than less, and 'the paradox is that we shall be able to do the work properly only when it is too late to be useful'. In the meantime, he continues, Ministers of Health around the world have no alternative but to make policy decisions which will have far-reaching consequences on the basis of inadequate if not erroneous information.

In South Africa, AIDS emerged far later than in many other countries. This should mean that we should be able to learn from these others' experience and benefit from the knowledge that has now been accumulated. However, South Africa is an extraordinarily complex society. It is not only a mix of cultures and traditions, but also a mixture of First and Third Worlds which exist alongside, largely separate, but smack up against each other. Consequently, while the health care system is in many ways remarkably sophisticated, it co-exists with rates of, for instance, TB which are comparable with the rest of Africa. Although South Africa is rich in AIDS data in comparison with most parts of the developing world, and whilst its research capabilities should place it at the forefront of AIDS research and surveillance throughout the continent, its health-care providers are viewed with widespread distrust by perhaps the majority of the population. The country is also simultaneously isolated from the accumulated wisdom and experience of such bodies as the WHO. For all that this global isolation may diminish in the years ahead, South Africa will continue to face not only the generic problems of understanding AIDS, but also the ramifications resulting from the peculiar complexities of its society. South Africa may as a result add a unique dimension to the epidemiological pattern of AIDS.

In South Africa, as elsewhere, forecasts of the numbers of AIDS cases and their impact vary widely. Some estimates are frankly irresponsibly apocalyptic. This chapter will attempt to present an overview of the particular South African context in which the spread of AIDS must be considered and of the evidence accumulated so far, and then offer comments upon some of the projections that have been put forward. The assessment will be based on the credibility of the underlying assumptions of each model and projection, and in the light of the information obtained from the first national HIV survey carried out at the end of 1990. The argument will be that exaggeratedly gloomy projections can be as harmful as overly optimistic scenarios, and need to be clearly exposed as such.

AIDS CASES AND DEATHS:
WHAT CAN THE DATA TELL US?

AIDS cases and deaths are reported to the South African Institute of Medical Research, which in turn provides this data to the Department of National Health and Population Development (DNHPD). The figures arrived at almost certainly underestimate the actual prevalence of the disease. For a start, they rely on voluntary, not compulsory, reporting by doctors. Second, the difficulty of diagnosis means that the actual incidence of AIDS is obscured by its manifestation as other opportunistic infections, such as TB. Third, South African data artificially excludes reported cases in the 'independent' homelands. Meanwhile, on the plus side, there is no suggestion, as yet, that information concerning AIDS is being deliberately withheld, as it is by the authorities in some countries which fear the impact of the truth on such economic sectors as the tourist industry. The extent of underreporting of AIDS in South Africa would therefore seem to lie between (i) the 90 per cent rate of underreporting which the WHO estimates to be the case in some parts of Africa;[2] and (ii) the estimated 41 per cent in the USA.[3]

The annual numbers of cases reported in South Africa by mode of transmission are shown in Figure 4.1. Since it can take up to ten years or more for an HIV-positive case to develop into full-blown AIDS, these figures reflect the spread of the epidemic over the last ten years

Cases

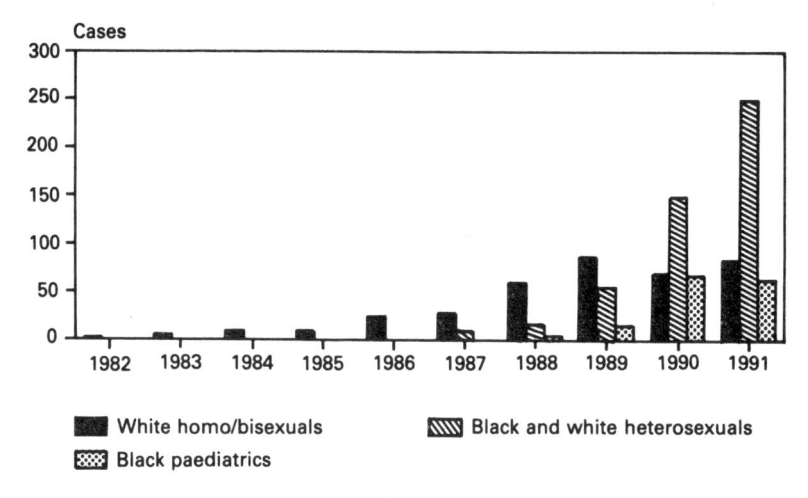

Figure 4.1 AIDS cases in South Africa by year and transmission

■ White homo/bisexuals
▨ Black and white heterosexuals
▩ Black paediatrics

(that is, each annual figure includes cases which might have become infected at any time over the previous ten years).

From the available data, it becomes apparent that two distinct epidemics of AIDS are manifest in South Africa. Pattern I transmission, which is typical of industrialised countries in North America, Australasia, Western Europe and urban areas of Latin America, occurred first. This affects predominantly homosexual and bisexual males. Overall population seroprevalence is estimated to be less than 1 per cent, but has been measured to be over 50 per cent in some groups practising high-risk behaviour.[4] It occurs in South Africa amongst whites and, to a lesser degree, among the coloured community. Today, the number of new cases appears to be levelling off and even falling slightly, as is the case in the UK and the USA.[5]

Within the last four or five years, a different AIDS epidemic has also become apparent in South Africa.[6] This Pattern II transmission occurs among heterosexuals: the male to female rate is approximately 1:1 and mother-to-infant transmission is common. It is the predominant mode of transmission in Africa, where in certain urban areas some 30 per cent of the sexually active group is infected.[7] In South Africa it is seen mainly amongst black (as opposed to white, coloured and Asian) men, women and children. The number of cases reported is increasing very rapidly, both of adults and of children. Indeed, by

1990 more heterosexual than homosexual cases were being reported.

Meanwhile, the South African Asian community follows Pattern III behaviour, with only small numbers of AIDS cases having been reported. This pattern is otherwise found in areas of eastern Europe, North Africa, Asia and the Middle East.[8]

All this must be kept in perspective. The total number of AIDS *cases reported* in South Africa to September 1991 is 893, of whom 353 have died.[9] This compares with some 350 000 reported cases worldwide, over 50 per cent of which have been in the Americas. Estimated *actual* figures are more than a million adult cases, and over half a million paediatric cases of whom 90 per cent have been in Africa.[10] We can therefore (cautiously) conclude that South Africa has so far escaped the major impact of AIDS which other countries have experienced. The good news is that the initial epidemic mainly among white male homosexuals appears to have settled down. The bad news is that a new epidemic among black heterosexuals, of far greater proportions than the first, is taking off.

As a consequence of the long incubation period the number of *HIV infected persons*, in contrast to the number of actual AIDS cases, is much greater. The WHO estimates that by April 1991 there were around 8–10 million adults and one million children infected worldwide. Of these, some 6 million are in Africa. About 70 per cent of all global HIV infections are thought to have been spread by heterosexual intercourse.[11] These figures are more informative than AIDS case data, and give far greater cause for concern. A better understanding of the future will be afforded by considering these other forms of data.

WHAT IS AN EPIDEMIC AND WHY DOES IT STOP?

An epidemic occurs when a number of 'infective' people in a population each spread an infection to a number of 'susceptibles'. In simple terms, each of the latter then infects a number of others (x), and then they too each infect a similar number, and so on. The total number of cases per thousand population (prevalence) initially builds up very quickly. In the early stages of the epidemic the prevalence of the infection in fact increases exponentially.

If we assume individuals leave the infective group at a rate y to play no further part in the epidemic, the prevalence of the infection will nonetheless increase exponentially initially, as long as x exceeds y.

(Whether such leavers are recovered but immune, have been isolated or withdrawn from the population, or are dead, is irrelevant to the mathematics.) The 'doubling time' of the epidemic, the time taken for the number of infectives to double, will equal $ln2/(x - y)$ in the *initial exponential* stages of the epidemic.[12]

However, this rate of increase is bound to slow down. The epidemic will spread fastest initially when it is spreading in high-risk groups and when there is the most scope for new cases. In time, though, some contacts will begin to duplicate among people already infected (or in diseases from which recovery is possible, among people who have recovered and obtained immunity), the susceptible population will 'shrink' and therefore the number of *new cases* becoming infected will start to fall. Eventually there will begin to be a shortage of candidates for infection. The infection cannot sustain itself unless each old case infects at least one new case on average. In a closed population the epidemic will therefore eventually die out. Alternatively, in a limited community, prevalence will level out at an endemic rate (in which x roughly equals y) until a sufficient number of new susceptibles is available to allow a new epidemic to occur. Measles, for instance, typically follows this pattern where epidemics erupt with great regularity.

What does this tell us about the spread of AIDS in South Africa? First, the rate of growth of the epidemic will be fastest initially when the prevalence is lowest. Exponential growth cannot be sustained indefinitely. Doubling times do not remain constant but will lengthen over time. This is an important point which requires emphasis. A doubling time calculated early on in the course of an epidemic does not remain valid for years to come. The intuitive evidence for this assertion presented above can be substantiated by fairly simple mathematics.

Second, the formula for exponential growth calculated early on in an epidemic and based on the parameter x is anyway only applicable to the population risk group from which x was calculated. Such a formula cannot be applied to another population or group of individuals whose behaviour does not allow infection to spread at such a rate. In other words, the AIDS epidemic in South Africa might spread extremely rapidly initially among people who exhibit high-risk behaviour (such as homosexuals and prostitutes), but there is no way this growth could be sustained among the wider population which has lower rates of partner acquisition, and neither could it continue at all among those who exhibit no risk behaviour.

Third, even if the rate of addition of new cases were to continue, because of the extremely long incubation period for AIDS the prevalence of HIV-positive cases in the community will accumulate and peak before the effect of deaths begins to reduce it again. An endemic level of infections and disease due to HIV will eventually be established in which the number of new infections at any one time is approximately equal to the number of AIDS-related deaths. How high or low this level will be will depend on the effectiveness of AIDS prevention and education programmes.[13]

USING HIV DATA

Data on the extent of HIV infection as determined by seroprevalence studies give a far better view of the HIV epidemic than does AIDS data. Quite apart from the underreporting of AIDS cases, changes in diagnostic criteria that occur from time to time may significantly affect AIDS statistics, and the relevance of AIDS data may lead to over- and undervaluing the extent of the epidemic in high/low risk populations.[14] Most importantly, the AIDS cases seen today originate from infections that occurred at some point in the last ten years, this point depending on the distribution of the incubation period about which there is little South African data. The only data to reflect what is now happening are HIV data.

A number of sources for seroprevalence studies have been used in South Africa. All use samples of blood that are routinely collected for some other purpose. The groups tested include blood donors nationwide, and attenders at STD clinics, family planning clinics and antenatal care clinics. Schoub et al.[15] argue that the concept of using a family of HIV serosurveillance studies on various sentinel populations has the major advantage that information on HIV infection within selected populations can be monitored at reasonable cost and provides useful information on the epidemiological characteristics of the country as a whole. A disadvantage is that the sample will not necessarily represent the complete population. Blood donors, for instance, may significantly underrepresent the true extent of infection because of self-exclusion of high-risk individuals from becoming donors and removal of seropositive persons from donor panels. Schoub et al. also argue that in addition to these sentinel studies, which are required to quantify the magnitude of infection in high-risk reservoirs, a nationwide screening programme is needed to assess the extent of HIV penetration amongst the general population.

The first South African national HIV survey was carried out on women attenders at antenatal clinics in October and November 1990. The various projections that have been made in the past can, therefore, to some extent, now be assessed against its results.

THE FIRST NATIONAL HIV SURVEY: WHAT DOES IT TELL US?

The results of this survey of over 14 000 women attending antenatal clinics suggest that there are indeed marked differences in HIV point prevalence rates in different geographical areas of the country and between population groups.[16] The overall prevalence rate was calculated at 0.76 per cent.

Of the four provinces, Natal (including KwaZulu) had the highest rate, at 1.6. The Orange Free State (including QwaQwa) and the Transvaal (which was taken to include KaNgwane, KwaNdebele, Gazankulu and Lebowa) had similar rates of 0.58 and 0.53 per cent. The Cape was much lower, with a figure of 0.16. The three urban areas specifically included gave rates for Johannesburg of 0.83 per cent, Durban 0.7 per cent and Cape Town 0.02 per cent. The population group-specific results indicate that black women had a higher prevalence rate of HIV infection (0.89 per cent) than either coloured (0.16 per cent) or white women (0.06 per cent), the final sample containing only a small number of Asian women. A very provisional result was that it appeared that younger women are more affected than older women.

Under the assumptions that the prevalence rate for all women aged 15–49 (and for those aged 15–34) is equal to the rate for all pregnant women, that the rate for all pregnant women is the same as that for ANC clinic attenders, that for every infected woman there is a man, and that 30 per cent of babies born to HIV-positive women are infected, the number of HIV-infected persons in South Africa at the end of 1990 was estimated to be between 74 000 and 102 000.

Several points about this survey should be noted.

1. Antenatal clinic attenders are a sexually active group.
2. The estimated total number of HIV-infected persons includes all population groups, whereas some estimates by other sources apply only to blacks.

3. The estimated total could be an overestimate in that the number of male cases is assumed to equal the number of female cases. Schoub et al.[17] report a male:female ratio of 1:1.17 among blood donors in 1989 and a ratio of 0.8:1 in 1988. On the other hand, because male homosexuals have been excluded from the survey, the number of male cases may be underestimated. (This underscores the need to conduct sentinel studies to complement the national survey.)
4. The age distribution of pregnant women differs from that of all women of child-bearing age. In the absence of age-specific prevalence rates, it was first assumed that women aged 15–49, and then, those aged 15–34 had the same prevalence rate as pregnant women. This led to the two estimates of 74 000 and 102 000, but both could be overestimates, depending on the gradient with age of HIV positivity.
5. Sexually active women who intend never to become pregnant and pregnancy terminations will be missed.[18]
6. Women who attend antenatal clinics are not entirely representative of all pregnant women. At one end of the social spectrum (mainly white) women who attend private antenatal clinics would be excluded. Pregnant women who do not attend antenatal clinics at all will also be excluded from the survey. They will tend to be drawn from the opposite (black) end of the social class gradient and their low socio-economic status will be conducive to a high rate of all infectious diseases, including HIV and AIDS.
7. The survey did not attempt to correct for different racial compositions in the various geographical areas reported.

These considerations have led to some criticism of the national survey and its findings. While it is undoubtedly a most useful further item of information, the possibility of its under- or overestimating national seroprevalence must nevertheless be borne in mind. The differences in racial and geographical seroprevalence rates indicated by the survey underscore the risk involved in generalising from sentinel studies based on limited groups only. It is intended to conduct the survey annually, and so more evidence will emerge in time. Since the biases may not vary much over time, inferences about rates of change can be made with more certainty.

WHY IS SOUTH AFRICA SPECIAL?

The Environment

The social, political and environmental conditions to which the vast majority of black people in South Africa are subject are precisely those in which ill health will generally flourish, and disease (including the STDs of which AIDS is one) is rife. There is no reason to suppose that the effects of AIDS in the townships in this country should be any less severe than in the slums of Kampala or Blantyre where the conditions in which people live and work are very similar.

The realisation that the health of individuals is determined to a great extent by the circumstances in which they live is not new. Individual behaviour and health services *per se* have relatively little impact,[19] and yet the response to the AIDS epidemic worldwide has mainly concentrated on the need for education programmes aimed at changing the sexual behaviour of individuals rather than on the determinants of the disease and identifying high-risk situations of populations.

Packard and Epstein argue that the perceived importance of sexual promiscuity in Africa has arisen out of the desire to explain the different pattern of African transmission of HIV from that of Western experience by focusing on peculiarities of African behaviour.[20] Previously, similar reasoning had been used with TB and syphilis. However, this approach loses sight of the fact that background levels of infection and malnutrition, and associated problems of poverty and maldevelopment, may be as important in the heterotransmission of HIV as the frequency of sexual contacts.

In contrast, Zwi and Cabral examine the range of social, economic and political forces that place groups at particularly high risk of HIV infection.[21] They conclude that the explosion among commercial sex workers and injecting drug users in Asia was entirely predictable once the virus had been introduced there. They go on to say: 'Epidemics in populations of migrant workers, in rapidly urbanising populations, and among the indigenous populations of the world much affected by sexually transmitted diseases and alcohol use, are likely next targets.' A description of the black population in South Africa could scarcely be more apt.

The migrant labour system is seen as a particularly high-risk situation.[22] Large numbers of men are drawn to industrial and mining centres. They almost always leave their families behind, seeing them infrequently, and are themselves housed in single-sex hostels. These men seek companionship with women living near their place of work. This context poses a high risk for the spread of STDs and HIV infection.[23]

De Beer argues further that not only is people's health related to their environment, but that this is, in turn, determined by the position that people hold in the political and economic structures of the society in which they live.[24] He emphasises that ill health is directly related to exploitation and oppression. In this respect, too, the black population of South Africa would seem totally vulnerable to the spread of HIV and AIDS.

In South Africa this important dimension is recognised by influential commentators.[25] Schoub says: 'HIV infection in the heterosexual population is unequivocally consequent on the social, economic and political factors that produce the poverty, squalor, inadequacy of facilities and destruction of family life so characteristic of the rapid urbanisation of blacks in South Africa.' But this recognition has not been translated into suggestions for appropriate action, and policies have not been structured with these considerations in mind. Perhaps the problem is knowing *what* to do. One would not want to do anything except work for, and wait for, social change. Zwi and Cabral argue for considering the structural dimensions in each setting and using individuals drawn from a similar high-risk background who might be the most acceptable and effective in promoting health. Ivan Toms is not optimistic at present. He maintains, 'Generally, however, the state health department remains wedded to the notion that AIDS is the result of profligate sexual behaviour and the best remedy is celibacy.'[26]

The Dual Society

Despite the relative wealth of South Africa and its well-developed infrastructure, black people would in many ways be better off if there were no First World society existing in parallel to theirs. For a start, 'black' South Africa has suffered no less than numerous Third World countries from the inappropriate imposition of high cost, low coverage, low impact, Western 'scientific' medicine. But whereas other African countries have, since independence, been adopting a PHC approach, South Africa's isolation from the influence of the WHO and other international organisations has meant that, in contrast,

PHC is still in its infancy. The WHO's AIDS Control Programmes which are mounted through PHC networks have also been excluded.

Second, the 'separateness' of racial groups permits a lack of concern for health problems in townships and squatter areas on the part of urban decision-makers, many of them white, who should be the very ones most able to rectify the situation. Without the First World in authority over them, those affected would be in a better position to help themselves. De Beer describes the initial hysterical coverage from the establishment press in the early 1980s when cholera came to South Africa.[27] However, publicity soon dwindled when early fears that it might spread to the privileged urban white population proved groundless. It is by no means inconceivable that AIDS could in time come to be treated in the same way. In a society riddled with racial paranoia, once whites realise that the major impact of the disease will be in the townships and peri-urban areas rather than in their suburbs, they could choose to ignore the massive pain and suffering, and AIDS prevention and treatment might not receive the attention or resources they deserve. Barnett and Blaikie in Chapter 12 comment on a similar opinion in Europe and North America that AIDS can now be seen as 'just' another tropical disease – like malaria – against which people in the West can protect themselves by means of simple precautionary measures.

Even more extreme is the view that since AIDS will fall largely on the black community, that community should somehow summon up the resources to cope with the problem. Edelston, for instance, proclaims that 'In South Africa, white taxpayers will, as always, fund costs resulting from large numbers of infected blacks . . . Truly will white taxpayers then be justified in saying "never . . . has so much been owed, by so many, to so few".'[28]

These viewpoints are entirely in keeping with a society based on segmented actions lacking any sense of overall community, and one in which ill health, especially amongst blacks, is commonly regarded as the patient's own fault. In South Africa, illness is often seen as nature's revenge on people who live unhygienically and who do not observe proper rules of cleanliness.[29] This could be further reinforced by the isolation suffered by people with HIV/AIDS who tend to be feared, stigmatised and rejected.[30]

Finally, there is a significant minority who hold the extreme view that AIDS will have the beneficial effect of solving the 'overpopulation' problem.[31]

Health Education and Behaviour Change

Health education programmes worldwide have by and large met with limited success unless they coincide with other aspects of social change.[32] For instance, the massive amounts spent on family planning programmes in India have been singularly unsuccessful except in places where there have also been significant improvements in living standards and in the role of women.[33]

Skrabanek and McCormick argue that the fact that diseases such as AIDS are not prevented is not the result of ignorance but of a failure to translate knowledge into appropriate action.[34] Education programmes may succeed in disseminating information, but they are far less successful in bringing about behavioural change. People often know *what* they should do but are less willing, or unable, to do it. In general, we do not understand what makes people decide to change their behaviour even when they have that option.

Political, social and economic factors often create conditions which make it extremely difficult for people to change their sexual lifestyles. Women struggling to feed themselves and their families may have no option but to turn to prostitution. The ability to practise safer sex may be impaired by the use of alcohol and other addictive drugs, as well as a lack of information, resources and power. Commercial sex workers may be aware of the necessity to protect their health but may be unable to ensure that their paying and non-paying partners use condoms.[35] Fleming (see Chapter 13) argues that the lower perceived value of women than of men leads to females in Africa being exposed to HIV and other STDs more often and at an earlier age through being forced into prostitution, through being allowed to drift into a life of casual sexuality for trivial reward or through rape.

In addition to these general problems, South Africa faces specific difficulties in health education just as she does in other areas. Surveys of children of primary school age have shown no infection whatsoever in this age group. If health education could successfully target them it would be possible to keep a cohort free of HIV.[36] But a hurdle in South Africa is the reluctance to educate children in some schools about sex and HIV infection.

The relative underdevelopment of PHC in South Africa is coupled with the distrust of authorities which makes it doubly difficult for the latter to play a role in changing the sexual behaviour of those it has traditionally oppressed. For years government health services have discouraged condom use in family planning clinics in favour of more effective methods of birth control. No wonder clients are suspicious of advice now that they should insist their partners use them. Some blacks even view AIDS as a disease introduced by whites to reduce the black population. Others distrust prevention programmes, seeing talk of AIDS as an empty scare tactic to lower sexual activity and therefore population growth.

If health education programmes are to succeed, the routes through PHC and community health organisations are likely to be the most successful. In South Africa, communities have been broken up and massive forced population removals have deliberately destroyed traditional communities and family groupings. Social networks have been smashed so that organised opposition to the apartheid state was more difficult. But perhaps a hope for the future lies precisely in the strength of community structures established for political opposition. There is the possibility for exploiting the *political* unity of the people in health prevention and strategies to fight AIDS. It must be recognised, however, that many communities, although politically mobilised, are simultaneously divided along class, ideological, ethnic and other lines. The African National Congress made a commitment in the Maputo Declaration in 1990 to develop a progressive response to AIDS in South Africa through the National Progressive Primary Health Care Network, but may well have more immediate goals in mind than AIDS education.

Rural Prevalence Rates

Until recently, seroprevalence rates in rural parts of South Africa have remained low, as earlier studies indicated for rural areas in other African countries.[37] It would also appear that prevalence rates in rural areas elsewhere in Africa can be extremely 'patchy', differing widely from community to community.[38] In other words, once HIV infection is introduced into a community, it can spread very rapidly.[39] A particular pattern to this patchiness between communities has recently been reported by Wawer *et al*.[40] in which seroprevalence in rural Uganda was found to be highest in main-road trading centres, intermediate in rural trading villages on secondary roads, and lowest in rural agricultural villages, suggesting a definite route for transmission.

In South Africa, the high level of movement of migrant workseekers between rural and urban areas may mean that seroprevalence rates in rural areas may become as great as in urban settings. In 1949

Kark reported a similar finding for the spread of syphilis to rural areas of South Africa.[41] This could mean that even if South Africa has a similar urban rate of infection to those of urban areas in Central Africa, the rates for the country as a whole could be higher.

AIDS and TB

More than 12 million people in South Africa are thought to have latent TB infections. If they become infected with HIV, TB can quickly develop.[42] In addition, it is thought that the presence of TB, as well as of other infectious diseases, malnutrition and other STDs, may accelerate the seroconversion of HIV to full-blown AIDS.[43] The very high incidence of active TB among HIV positives is likely to contribute significantly to the overall burden of morbidity and mortality of HIV/AIDS (see Chapter 8).

STDs

The presence of an STD increases the probability of transmission of HIV per contact, particularly among those causing ulceration of surfaces.[44] The very high rates of STD prevalence in South Africa will almost certainly play a major role in the spread of AIDS.

Health Care Availability

The relative sophistication of the health care system in South Africa could act to prolong the incubation period before full-blown AIDS develops, or to prolong the AIDS sick time. If sexual contacts are continued during this period, the number of people drawn into the epidemic will increase. It has been suggested, for instance, that the use of the drug zidovudine, while extending the life of an individual already infected with HIV, might actually reduce the life expectancy of a whole population cohort by leading to a greater number of people being infected.[45]

The Plus Side

South Africa has embarked on wide-ranging epidemiological surveys and data collection exercises and now has the benefit of meaningful HIV data. It also has considerable research expertise to assess the situation as it develops and to act upon it. South Africa can learn from the experience of other countries further advanced with the epidemic. Broomberg *et al.* point in Chapter 8 to the collaborative research efforts that are taking place between different groups. The need to evaluate the effectiveness of AIDS prevention policies has been recognised.[46]

Blood testing was introduced at an early stage in South Africa so that a virtually completely safe blood supply is now assured. And even though the economy is in a poor state compared with formerly, the resources available for intervention are huge compared with those available in most parts of Africa. In addition, South Africa has a substantial infrastructure compared to the rest of the continent, even though it is imposed on Third World squalor of appalling conditions.

PROJECTIONS OF THE FUTURE OF THE HIV/AIDS EPIDEMIC

Every serious projection seems to agree that the impact of HIV and AIDS in South Africa will be substantial. Beyond that they differ widely. Some of the significant forecasts are as follows.

Doomsday Projections

The most alarming and sensational forecasts have been made by Keith Edelston of the AIDS Economic Research Unit.[47] He has been quoted as saying that between 22 and 70 per cent of the sexually active black population will be dead, HIV-positive, or dying of AIDS by 1996. In Durban, he maintains – the worst affected region in the country – between 50 and 70 per cent of the sexually active blacks will be HIV positive in the year 2000 (*Sunday Star*, 11 November 1990). He then goes on to conclude that, as a result of the AIDS epidemic, industry will face a shortage of labour as from the mid-1990s, and there will be excessive black housing stock in ten years time.

Edelston's projections have been roundly criticised by the scientific community in South Africa. In an editorial in the *South African Medical Journal* in November 1990,[48] Schall and Padayachee point out that such sensational forecasting in the media may create public interest but it is likely to be superficial and short lived, and will therefore probably hinder rather than help public education. Prevention becomes seen as a hopeless task. They point out that if efforts to create jobs, housing and social services are decreased, the resulting shortages in South Africa would constitute another, self-made catastrophe compounding the effects of AIDS.

What is disturbing is that these doomsday projections are believed. For instance, Volkskas Bank is said to base its projections on Edelston's model[49] and has proceeded to outline alarming recessionary and depressive scenarios.[50] Furthermore, although people may be reluctant to accept the outcomes he is predicting, they do not feel able to challenge his mathematics. Hence, for instance, Vincent Brett, a labour adviser to the South African Chamber of Business, is quoted as observing that although Edelston's figures may be mathematically correct, 'things don't work out that way' (*The Citizen*, 20 February 1990). Yet the point is precisely that Edelston's mathematics are *not* correct. His figures are a myth that must be exposed as such once and for all, for he bases his predictions on a *fixed* doubling time for the proportion of people infected, extrapolating this assumption forward over long time intervals. However, as demonstrated above, this technique is completely mathematically incorrect. What is more, he extrapolates the figures to include the *whole* population, whereas – again, as discussed above – not everyone is at equal risk or susceptibility.

On a note of caution, we may note that individuals or bodies with a vested interest in these doomsday projections might try to confirm them by quoting data from high-risk sentinel groups. High figures obtained for, say, STD clinic attenders in an urban area in Central Africa cannot be used to confirm misleading projections about the South African population.

Other High Projections

Several other high projections have been proposed. For instance, Prentice of Old Mutual has predicted 110 000 HIV-positive cases in 1990 (which is not unreasonable) but rising to 11.6 million by the year 2000 (Table 4.1). He projected 1000 AIDS deaths would occur in 1990 and 321 000 in 2000 (non-cumulative).[51]

Other high projections would seem to use a constant doubling time uncritically. The Population Research Institute, an American monitor of global population trends, reports Newbury's estimates of 1.6 million people infected by the end of 1993, rising to 12.8 million by the end of 1995. Newbury says, 'AIDS will almost certainly depopulate this country and probably reduce our population to less than one quarter of its present size by the year 2010' (*Eastern Province Herald*, 31 October 1991).

Table 4.1 Estimated prevalence rates, present and projected

Source	Date	Seroprevalence rate (%)	Number of HIV positives
National HIV survey	End 1990	0.76 (all races)	74–102 000
Edelston	1996	22–70 and 50–70	
Old Mutual	1990		110 000
	1998	40	
	2000		11 600 000
Newbury	1993		1 600 000
	1995		12 800 000
Padayachee and Schall	1990		119–168 000 (blacks)
	1991		317–446 000 (blacks)
Shapiro	End 1989	1.5	
	End 1990	6.0	
Doyle	Jan. 1991		97 000
	2000–5	18 peak, adults (behaviour change)	4 800 000
	2010	27 peak, adults (no behaviour change)	
Schall	2000–5	30 (black urban) 30–40 (absolute maximum)	

Sources H. Kustner, 'First national HIV survey of women attending antenatal clinics, South Africa, October/November 1990', *Epidemiological Comments*, 18, 2 (1991), pp. 35–45; K. Edelston, *Countdown to Doomsday* (Johannesburg: Media House, 1988); G. Prentice, 'South African Mutual Life Assurance Society: AIDS Information Report', mimeo, 21 May 1990; G.N. Padayachee and R. Schall, 'Short-term predictions of the prevalence of human immunodeficiency virus infection among the black population in South Africa', *South African Medical Journal*, 77 (1990), pp. 329–33; M. Shapiro, R.L. Crookes and E. O'Sullivan, 'Screening antenatal blood samples for anti-human immunodeficiency virus antibodies by a large-pool enzyme-linked immunosorbent assay system', *South African Medical Journal*, 76 (1989), pp. 245–7; P.R. Doyle, 'The impact of AIDS in the South African population', in *AIDS in South Africa: The Demographic and Economic Implications* (Johannesburg: Centre for Health Policy, 1991); R. Schall, 'On the maximum size of the AIDS epidemic among the heterosexual black population in South Africa', *South African Medical Journal*, 78 (1990), pp. 507–10.

Projections released to the public by life insurance companies, medical aid schemes and other private fiscal bodies might be expected to be 'conservative'. Indeed, upon making an enquiry from one insurance company as to whether they had produced AIDS projections, they said that details of how the projections were arrived at could not be released since 'the models we produce serve the industry interest and not the actual medical predictions'.

These considerations add further credibility to Peter Doyle's estimates, made on behalf of Metropolitan Life, for these are amongst the lowest projections of AIDS cases and deaths currently on offer. His model will be discussed below.

Short-Term Medical Forecasts

Several short-term forecasts have been proposed, based on the *careful* extrapolation of fixed doubling time for an acceptable short time interval only. Most notably, in April 1990, Padayachee and Schall reviewed the various forecasting techniques available.[52] They used seven sets of longitudinal sentinel serosurveillance data for extrapolation: (i) antenatal clinic attenders from Johannesburg,[53] augmented by data from Baragwanath Hospital; (ii) and (iii) blood donors from the South African Blood Transfusion Services, stratified into male and female donors; (iv) attenders of family planning clinics in the greater Johannesburg area; (v) attenders at STD clinics for miners; and (vi) and (vii) attenders at STD clinics in the greater Johannesburg area, stratified into males and females. The researchers found that, with the exception of the female STD data, the data sets fitted an exponential growth curve rather well. Furthermore, the doubling times were remarkably similar. A common model using the six similar sets of data yielded a doubling time of 8.5 months.

Using data on relative levels of HIV infection in the different parts of South Africa as determined by data on new blood donors, and taking account, too, of urban/rural differences, they estimated that there were between 44 763 and 63 076 HIV-positive individuals in the black population of South Africa aged 15–49 years by the end of 1989.

Based on these estimates and a doubling time of 8.5 months, they projected 119 069–167 782 HIV-positive individuals by the end of 1990, and 316 725–446 300 by the end of 1991, assuming no change in the pattern of infection (see Table 4.1). They noted, however, that there were indications that this doubling time may have been increasing. A second set of estimates based on assumed incubation distributions and using the back calculation method gave relatively good agreement with these estimates.

In 1989 Shapiro, Crookes and O'Sullivan reported a 0.22 per cent incidence of confirmed anti-HIV positivity among pregnant black women resident in the southern Transvaal. These investigators estimated an approximate six-month doubling time and projected a 1.5 per cent rate by the end of 1989 rising to 6 per cent at the end of 1990.

Estimates quoted from other sources such as WHO (*Business Day*, 27 April 1990) and the DNHPD (*Business Day*, 22 January 1991) would appear to rely on the Padayachee and Schall estimates rather than having made them independently.

These short-term predictions for HIV prevalence in 1990 made by medical researchers in a correct and cautious way nevertheless might seem to be on the high side as compared to the results of the national HIV survey (which reports a seroprevalence rate of 0.76 per cent and a point prevalence at the end of 1990 of between 74 000 and 102 000). However, given the number of factors which might have caused the latter to underestimate the true prevalence, and also given that Padayachee and Schall themselves caution that the doubling time may have been increasing, this projection is in good agreement with the national survey. It must be stressed, however, that the doubling time was only carried forward over an extremely short time period, and even this was recognised as perhaps being too long.

Demographic Cohort Models

A rather different approach to modelling the course of the AIDS epidemic lies in using a macro-simulation model based on an actuarial-type demographic cohort model. Bongaarts[54] and Doyle and Millar[55] of Metropolitan Life use the similar approach of dividing a community into a number of sub-groups, or risk groups, so that sexual behaviour within each stratum is of a homogeneous nature. The pattern of the epidemic is determined by age- and duration-specific mortality factors, rather than by assuming the shape of an epidemic curve as many models do. An advantage over other actuarial models is that Doyle's model runs on the more reliable HIV rather than AIDS data.

This model has captured the salient demographic and behavioural features of the epidemic very elegantly, while using very few variables and parameters. It is difficult for insurance companies to collect certain information, such as their clients' sexual behaviour, and in this model empirical evidence is used to calibrate the parameters so that projected scenarios fit known HIV-prevalence data. As new data becomes available, projections are adjusted accordingly.

For the public health planner it is possible to alter one variable at a time in this model (such as condom use) in order to evaluate the possible impact of various public health strategies. Indeed, the variables in the model have been chosen in such a way that they directly relate to possible intervention strategies. For instance, Doyle has produced high and low scenarios based on the assumptions of (i) no eventual change in sexual behaviour or (ii) considerable change following educational programmes. The resulting high and low peak estimates are 27 and 18 per cent of the adult population occurring in years 2010 and 2000–5 respectively.[56]

The Doyle model results for January 1991[57] are very close to those found by the national HIV survey. This model is described in more detail in Chapter 5.

Maximum Epidemic Size

Also using a macro-simulation model, Schall has estimated the maximum size of the AIDS epidemic among the heterosexual black population over the next 30 years.[58] He recognises that data on many variables are rather scant and his model therefore makes no attempt at a long-term forecast as such; instead he employs 'worst-case' scenarios to assess the maximum size of the epidemic. Schall's results suggest that it is most unlikely that the impact of AIDS will be such that the size of the black population will be substantially reduced during the next three decades. A realistic 'worst-case' scenario is that population growth could cease but at a population level substantially higher (at about 40 million) than the present one. A further result is that it is most unlikely that peak infection levels among the sexually active population will exceed 30–40 per cent. However, infection levels of 30 per cent could be reached within the next 10–15 years, particularly in urban populations. The realistic 'worst-case' scenario also suggests that the number of HIV-infected individuals will peak at about 7.5 million around 2005.

This study, specific to South Africa, confirms previous more general findings that the total size of a population is unlikely to actually drop.[59]

WHICH MODEL? WHICH PROJECTION?

Modelling is not simply a neutral, technocratic matter of plugging numbers in and getting numbers out. In the context of AIDS, for instance, Doyle has noted very different dynamics of the spread of HIV infection between countries.[60] That there are many distinctive features in South Africa which could lead to a unique pattern has been discussed. A model which assumes a fixed mathematical form (such as Edelston's constant doubling time) is therefore unlikely to be as successful as one tailor-made to the South African situation employing local South African variables, as does Doyle's, and Padayachee and Schall's. Doyle's model has the additional advantage that, since it continually self-calibrates to the most recent accumulated data, the difficulties of unreliable assumptions and data can to some extent be corrected for.

Since there are choices open to us about the future, a model producing a range of scenarios is more reasonable. A model producing only a single projection implicitly assumes that the epidemic will run its course regardless of any interventions. Here, the Doyle and Schall models score.

Several of the projections shown in Table 4.1 are consistent with each other and can be assessed against objective measures. At the lower end of the range, at the beginning of the period, both Doyle's January 1991 projection and that of Padayachee and Schall for 1990 are reasonably consistent with the first national survey (given its possible inaccuracies).

Similarly, at the top end of the range, at the other end of the period, data from other African countries can be used as a yardstick. The Doyle projection which assumes no behavioural change (27 per cent) is close to that of Schall (30 per cent) and both are not unrealistic in relation to data that has already been observed elsewhere in Africa. For instance, infection levels of 30 per cent have been observed among antenatal clinic attenders and blood donors in urban areas elsewhere in Africa.[61] In other African countries these rates have been observed among urban groups, while rural rates remain lower. Since the rural rate in South Africa can be expected to catch up to the urban rate eventually, rates of 25–30 per cent for the whole country could be a realistic projection.

In other words, the analysis presented by Padayachee and Schall for the short-term and Schall's maximum size considerations are consistent with the Doyle model and its results, which in turn are consistent with the first national survey and considerations from elsewhere in Africa. The assumptions on which the Doyle model was based and the way it was constructed also add to its credibility.

In contrast, the projections by Edelston, while consistent with other very high forecasts produced for South Africa, are completely out of line with experience from other African countries where evidence suggests that peak prevalence is unlikely to exceed 30–40 per cent. They take no account of South African variables, are poorly justified and mathematically are totally implausible.

CONCLUSION

Despite the uncertainties surrounding the spread of HIV infection and AIDS, nonetheless there are conclusions we can draw from these epidemiological trends. The very different approaches to modelling the AIDS epidemic in South Africa have resulted in substantially different projections. However, although these estimates appear to differ widely, they can mainly be grouped into two categories. The first, the 'doomsday' forecasts of economic collapse and large-scale labour shortages, are unlikely to materialise.

The second group converge to a consensus view that if we continue as at present, with no significant interventions being made to alter the course of the epidemic, there is no reason to suppose the impact in South Africa will be any less severe than in the worse-hit African countries. The effect could even be slightly worse. Population growth could level off, but it is unlikely that the population total will actually fall. The situation in South Africa is not hopeless but, make no mistake, it *is* potentially very serious indeed; just as it is in other tropical African countries.

South Africa is fortunate in having such sophisticated modelling tools available for planning, which are matched by data of reasonably good quality. However, it would be irresponsible not to caution that all forecasts must be treated with circumspection and that the unpredictability of the AIDS virus as well as unforeseen events could prove these South African analysts wrong, in either direction.

South Africa is also extremely fortunate in being at an early stage in the spread of HIV infection and AIDS. Lessons can be learnt from elsewhere and interventions made which would convert these gloomy projections of the status quo into more optimistic predictions for what the future could hold. Options to reduce the spread of AIDS, and hence reduce pain and suffering, are available if society chooses to pursue them.

An examination of the underlying political and economic structures in South Africa, and the prevailing racial attitudes, do not give rise to much hope that these options to reduce the impact of AIDS will be pursued. The political will to avoid an AIDS catastrophe appears to be lacking. One hope for the future would seem to lie in the PHC network which is firmly rooted in community action.

South Africa is a unique society, not least because of the disconnected existence of the First and Third Worlds within it, but also because of its diverse cultures, traditions and structural racial inequalities. AIDS will therefore have a unique impact. There is thus an urgent need to analyse the peculiarities of the South African situation and to devise strategies for preventing and controlling AIDS that are uniquely appropriate for its society. The energy and success with which such strategies are devised and pursued will determine the future South African trends and the resulting projections.

Acknowledgement

Malcolm Steinberg, Director of the Medical Research Council's Programme on AIDS, provided me with invaluable assistance and insights in my early thinking about AIDS. I am greatly indebted to him.

References

1. N.T.J. Bailey,'Simplified modelling of the population dynamics of HIV/AIDS', *Journal of the Royal Statistical Society A*, 151 (1988), pp. 31–43.
2. J. Chin and J.M. Mann, 'Global patterns and prevalence of AIDS and HIV infection', *AIDS*, 2 (1988), suppl. 1, s.247–52.
3. US General Accounting Office, *AIDS Forecasting: Undercount of Cases and Lack of Key Data Weaken Existing Estimates* (Washington, DC, 1989), pp. 21–33.
4. Chin and Mann, 'Global patterns'.
5. B.D. Schoub, A.N. Smith, S. Johnson, D.J. Martin, S.F. Lyons, G.N. Padayachee and H.S. Hurwitz, 'Considerations on the further expansion of the AIDS epidemic in South Africa', *South African Medical Journal*, 77 (1990), pp. 613–18.
6. R. Sher, 'HIV infection in South Africa, 1982–1988 – a review', *South African Medical Journal*, 76 (1989), pp. 314–18.
7. WHO, *Projection of HIV/AIDS in Sub-Saharan Africa using an Epidemiologically Based Modelling Approach* (Geneva: WHO, 1989); WHO, *The Epidemiology and Projected Mortality of AIDS in Sub-Saharan Africa* (Geneva: WHO, 1989).
8. Chin and Mann, 'Global patterns'.
9. Department of National Health and Population Development, 'AIDS in

South Africa since 1982 – as on 16 September 1991', *Epidemiological Comments*, 18, 9 (1991), p. 210.
10. WHO, 'UPDATE: AIDS cases reported to surveillance, forecasting and impact assessment unit, 30 April 1991', *Weekly Epidemiological Record*, 66, 18 (1991), pp. 125–6.
11. WHO, Press release no. 74, 1991.
12. V. Isham, 'Mathematical modelling of the transmission dynamics of HIV infection and AIDS: a review', *Journal of the Royal Statistical Society A*, 151 (1988), pp. 5–30.
13. Chin and Mann, 'Global patterns'.
14. Schoub *et al.*, 'Considerations'.
15. Ibid.
16. H. Kustner, 'First national HIV survey of women attending antenatal clinics, South Africa, October/November 1990', *Epidemiological Comments*, 18, 2 (1991), pp. 35–45.
17. Schoub *et al.*, 'Considerations'.
18. Editorial, 'Anonymous HIV testing', *Lancet* 1 (1990), pp. 575–6.
19. T. McKeown and C.R. Lowe, *An Introduction to Social Medicine* (Oxford: Blackwell Scientific, 1966).
20. R.M. Packard and P. Epstein, 'Epidemiologists, social scientists, and the structure of medical research on AIDS in Africa', *Social Science and Medicine*, 33, 7 (1991), pp. 771–94.
21. A.B. Zwi and A.J.R. Cabral, 'Identifying "high-risk situations" for preventing AIDS', *British Medical Journal*, 303 (1991), pp. 1527–9.
22. C.W. Hunt, 'Migrant labour and sexually transmitted disease: AIDS in Africa', *Journal of Health and Social Behaviour*, 30 (1989), pp. 353–73.
23. K. Jochelson, M. Mothibeli and J.P. Leger, 'Human immunodeficiency virus and migrant labour in South Africa', *International Journal of Health Services*, 21 (1991), pp. 157–73.
24. C. de Beer, *The South African Disease: Apartheid Health and Health Services* (London: Catholic Institute for International Relations, 1986).
25. N. Padayachee and C. Evian, 'A relook at AIDS prevention in South Africa', *AIDS Scan*, 3, 2 (1991), p. 3; B.D. Schoub, 'The AIDS epidemic in South Africa – perceptions and realities', *South African Medical Journal*, 77 (1990), pp. 607–8.
26. I. Toms, 'AIDS in South Africa: potential decimation on the eve of liberation', *Progress*, Fall/Winter 1990, pp. 13–16.
27. De Beer, *The South African Disease*.
28. K. Edelston, *Countdown to Doomsday* (Johannesburg: Media House, 1988).
29. De Beer, *The South African Disease*.
30. S.Y. Friedman and B.A. Robertson, 'Human immunodeficiency virus infection in children – prevalence and psychosocial impact', *South African Medical Journal*, 78 (1990), pp. 528–32; C. Mathews, L. Kuhn, C.A. Metcalf, G. Joubert and N.A. Cameron, 'Knowledge, attitudes and beliefs about AIDS in township school students in Cape Town', *South African Medical Journal*, 78 (1990), pp. 511–16.
31. S. Robertson, 'Doomsday – chimera or reality?', *South African Medical Journal*, 79 (1991), pp. 566–7.

32. N. Freudenberg, 'Health education for social change: a strategy for public health in the US', *International Journal of Health Education*, 24 (1981), pp. 1–8.
33. D. Sanders with R. Carver, *The Struggle for Health: Medicine and the Politics of Underdevelopment* (London: Macmillan, 1985).
34. P. Skrabanek and J. McCormick, *Follies and Fallacies in Medicine* (Glasgow: Tarragon, 1989).
35. Zwi and Cabral, 'Identifying "high risk situations"'.
36. J.W. Carswell, 'AIDS in Africa', *Epidemiological Comments*, 18, 2 (1991), pp. 46–50.
37. Schoub *et al.*, 'Considerations'.
38. P.O. Way and K. Stanecki, 'How bad will it be? Modelling the AIDS epidemic in Eastern Africa', paper prepared for the Annual Meeting of the American Association for the Advancement of Science, Washington, February 1991.
39. F. de Lalla, G. Rizzardini, D. Santoro and M. Galli, 'Rapid spread of HIV infection in a rural district in Central Africa', *AIDS*, 2 (1988), p. 317.
40. M.J. Wawer, D. Serwadda, S.D. Musgrave, J.K. Koude-Lule, M. Musagara and N.K. Sewankambo, 'Dynamics of spread of HIV-1 infection in a rural district of Uganda', *British Medical Journal*, 303 (1991), pp. 1303–6.
41. S.L. Kark, 'The social pathology of syphilis in Africans', *South African Medical Journal*, 23 (1949), pp. 77–84.
42. WHO, 'Global programme on AIDS tuberculosis programme', *Weekly Epidemiological Record*, 64 (1989), pp. 125–31.
43. P.R. Doyle, 'How AIDS could affect the economically active and reduce the educated and skilled in the workplace', paper presented to the Annual Conference of the Insurance Institute of South Africa, 1991.
44. A.A. Hoosen, J. Moodley, D.J. Pudifin, J. Duursma, K.D. Coetzee and A.B.M. Kharsany. 'Sexually transmitted pathogens and colposcopic findings in asymptomatic HIV-1 antibody-positive blood donors', *South African Medical Journal*, 77 (1990), pp. 626–7; N. O'Farrell, I. Windsor and P. Becker, 'HIV-1 infection among heterosexual attenders at a sexually transmitted diseases clinic in Durban', *South African Medical Journal*, 80 (1991), pp. 17–20
45. R.M. Anderson and R.M. May, 'Immunisation and herd immunity', *Lancet*, 335 (1990), pp. 641–5.
46. C.R. Evian, M. de Beer, M. Crewe, G.N. Padayachee and H.S. Hurwitz, 'Evaluation of an AIDS awareness campaign using city buses in Johannesburg', *South African Medical Journal*, 80 (1991), pp. 343–6; G.N. Padayachee, 'Evaluation of AIDS prevention programmes – the key to success', *South African Medical Journal*, 80 (1991), pp. 310–11.
47. Edelston, *Countdown*.
48. R. Schall and G.N. Padayachee, 'Doomsday forecasts of the AIDS epidemic', *South African Medical Journal*, 78 (1990), p. 503.
49. R. Hamilton, Social and Economic Update 14: Special Issue on AIDS (Johannesburg: South African Institute of Race Relations, 1991).
50. Volkskas Bank, *Economic Spotlight*, August 1990.

51. G. Prentice, 'South African Mutual Life Assurance Society: AIDS Information Report', mimeo, 21 May 1990.
52. G.N. Padayachee and R. Schall, 'Short-term predictions of the prevalence of human immunodeficiency virus infection among the black population in South Africa', *South African Medical Journal*, 77 (1990), pp. 329–33.
53. M. Shapiro, R.L. Crookes and E. O'Sullivan, 'Screening antenatal blood samples for anti-human immunodeficiency virus antibodies by a large-pool enzyme-linked immunosorbent assay system', *South African Medical Journal*, 76 (1989), pp. 245–7.
54. J. Bongaarts, 'A model of the spread of HIV infection and the demographic impact of AIDS', *Statistics in Medicine*, 8 (1989), pp. 103–20.
55. P.R. Doyle and D.B. Millar, 'Modelling the AIDS epidemic in South Africa', Metropolitan Life, mimeo, November 1990; P.R. Doyle and D.B. Millar, 'A general description of an actuarial model applicable to the HIV epidemic in South Africa', paper presented to the AIDS seminar of the Actuarial Society of South Africa, mimeo, 8 November 1990.
56. P.R. Doyle, 'The impact of AIDS on the South African population', in *AIDS in South Africa: The Demographic and Economic Implications* (Johannesburg: The Centre for Health Policy, 1991).
57. Doyle, 'How AIDS could affect the economically active'.
58. R. Schall, 'On the maximum size of the AIDS epidemic among the heterosexual black population in South Africa', *South African Medical Journal*, 78 (1990), pp. 507–10.
59. Bongaarts, 'A model'; Way and Stanecki, 'How bad will it be?'
60. Doyle, 'The impact of AIDS'.
61. WHO, *Projection of HIV/AIDS*; WHO, *The Epidemiology and Projected Mortality of AIDS*.

5 The Demographic Impact of AIDS on the South African Population
Peter Doyle

INTRODUCTION

This chapter presents a general description of an actuarial model that has been developed as a means of predicting the future spread of the HIV/AIDS epidemic in South Africa, and to estimate the demographic impact of that epidemic. It provides a detailed description of the fundamental approach to the model, its structure, and the key assumptions used in building the model. In addition, this chapter aims to illustrate the application of the model in developing scenarios for the HIV epidemic in South Africa. Two specific scenarios are presented, and are used to illustrate certain issues of fundamental importance in understanding the dynamics of the HIV/AIDS epidemic in South Africa.

BACKGROUND TO DEVELOPMENT OF THE MODEL

Any attempt to forecast the course of the HIV epidemic is fraught with many difficulties and uncertainties. These relate primarily to the large number of assumptions that must be made in building forecasting models, often with data that is not completely reliable. The results of models should therefore be treated with caution, and must be used responsibly. Uncertainty, however, should not deter ongoing attempts at developing realistic scenarios for the future course of the HIV/AIDS epidemic, since these are essential if we are to understand the possible impact of this disease on our society, and to plan accordingly.

The model described here was developed to meet the actuarial needs of a life insurance company.[1] At the time that initial work on the model was begun there was no other model that seemed suitable for use in South Africa, since it was clear that heterosexual transmission of HIV would constitute the major pattern of spread of the epidemic.

The other major actuarial models, for example those of Wilkie (Institute of Actuaries) and Cowell and Hoskins (Society of Actuaries) use one small homogenous risk group and use statistical probability distribution formulae or sets of differential equations to model the spread of infection through that single risk group. This is useful for the so-called Pattern I epidemic (the epidemic occurring mainly among male homosexuals) but it is clearly inappropriate to use this type of model for South Africa by simply assuming that a very large percentage of the population falls into one risk group. An extensive review of the literature available on modelling the epidemic is given by Haberman.[2]

A further reason for developing a model was our view that reporting of AIDS cases and deaths in South Africa would be unreliable for some time. Therefore it would be necessary to develop a model to utilise HIV prevalence data, since that would be significantly more accurate in the medium term. Again we found that most of the other actuarial models available at the time (early 1989) were designed to calibrate against AIDS case data rather than against HIV data. It is also obvious that HIV infections are the leading indicator of future AIDS cases.

For all these reasons, it was felt that a locally developed model that could more accurately predict the dynamics of the HIV epidemic in the South African context was required. In the next sections the structure of the model and the assumptions underlying it are described in some detail.

STRUCTURE AND BASIC PRINCIPLES OF THE MODEL

Many methods have been used worldwide to model the HIV epidemic. These methods include direct measurement of HIV seroprevalence in the population, extrapolation and back calculation methods, as well as macro- and micro-level forecasting models. These major methods and their applicability have been described in some detail by Padayachee and Schall.[3]

The method we have used is largely that of *macro-simulation forecasting*, since key assumptions are made about the epidemic at the society-wide or macro level. The model does, however, make certain assumptions at the individual risk level, or micro level. For

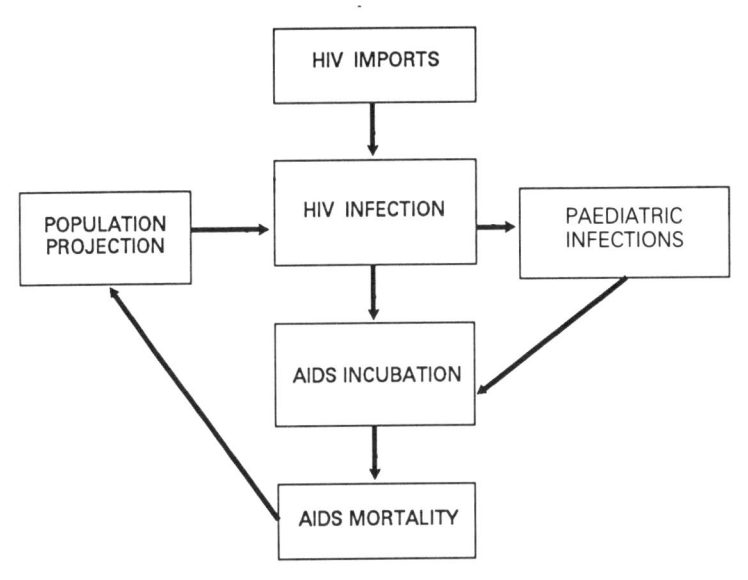

```
           ┌─────────────┐
           │ HIV IMPORTS │
           └──────┬──────┘
                  ▼
┌────────────┐  ┌───────────────┐  ┌──────────────┐
│ POPULATION │─▶│ HIV INFECTION │─▶│  PAEDIATRIC  │
│ PROJECTION │  │               │  │  INFECTIONS  │
└────────────┘  └───────┬───────┘  └──────┬───────┘
      ▲                 ▼                 │
      │         ┌───────────────┐         │
      │         │ AIDS INCUBATION│◀────────┘
      │         └───────┬───────┘
      │                 ▼
      │         ┌───────────────┐
      └─────────│ AIDS MORTALITY│
                └───────────────┘
```

Figure 5.1 Schematic view of model

example, assumptions are made about the risk behaviour of individuals within specified risk groups in the population.

The model is also an actuarial model, since it focuses on developing age and duration specific mortality factors, allowing also for select and ultimate experience. It consists of a number of discrete sections which are shown schematically Figure 5.1, and are described in more detail below.

The model is premised on certain basic assumptions.

1. HIV infection in Africa is transmitted predominantly via heterosexual contact.
2. There will be no cure or treatment for AIDS over the period for which the scenarios are developed.
3. There will only be significant changes in sexual behaviour once large numbers of persons in the community are sick and dying from AIDS.

The model attempts to simulate empirically-observed HIV infection. HIV infection data from the whole of Africa (including South Africa) were collected and used as inputs to the modelling process. Wherever possible, only well documented data sources were used. The three cardinal features of the model are its use of different risk groups, its modelling of the spread of HIV infection, and its use of the concept of 'imports' in the model. These features are described in the following sections.

Risk Groups

The spread of the HIV epidemic in any country is not uniform. Rather, the epidemic is stratified according to a range of risk behaviour and also according to a gradual geographic spread of infection.[4] The key assumption in this model is therefore that a community can be stratified into four homogenous risk groups. Sexual behaviour is, of course, not homogenous, but each group is defined and used so that it represents a cluster of individuals with an associated average HIV prevalence and infection rate. The approach of using risk groups has also been followed by other authors, notably Bongaarts[5] and Lorper.[6]

The four risk groups used here are shown schematically in Figure 5.2, and are defined as shown below.

PRO: Persons characterised by sexual mobility or promiscuity (for example, prostitutes and their frequent clients).
STD: Persons characterised by a high prevalence of STD. This indicates a high susceptibility to being infected by HIV, both because the presence of other STDs increases the probability of transmission of HIV per contact, and because the presence of an STD may suggest a relatively high number of new sexual partners per year.

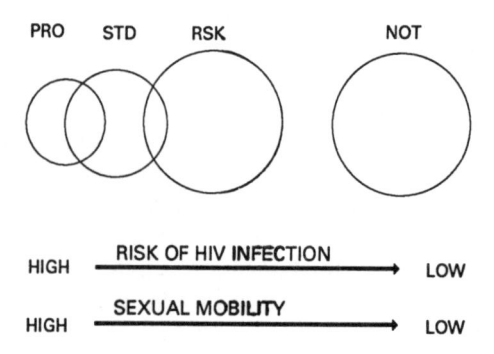

Figure 5.2   Interaction of risk groups in spread of HIV infection

Table 5.1 Percentage incidence of sexually transmitted diseases by population group

Group	(%)
White	0.5
African	16.0–24.0
Coloured	15.0
Indian	1.0

RSK: Persons characterised by stable sexual relationships, but who are at risk of infection because they, or their partners, have more than one sexual relationship.

NOT: Persons characterised by either having no sexual contact, or by having long-term monogamous relationships, and who are therefore not at risk of HIV infection.

Each level of risk represents a group that can be related to observed categories of data. For the PRO group, HIV data from studies of prostitutes and other very high risk groups were used. Similarly, HIV data from studies of STD patients were used for the STD category, although the effect of members of the PRO group on this data was excluded. In the RSK group, data representing the general adult population was used; for example, data on women attending antenatal clinics (with adjustments for the effects of members of the STD and NOT groups on this data).

The relative sizes of the different risk groups are critical to the overall results, as are the parameters describing the sexual behaviour of each group. Extensive sensitivity analysis has indicated that the most important group is the STD group. The STD group, however, can be large and is also an important link with the larger risk (RSK) group. Data is available on the prevalence of other STDs in the population and has been used as an estimate of the size of the STD risk group. Table 5.1 gives an estimate of the percentage incidence of other STDs amongst different population groups in South Africa. The PRO group is important in the early stage of the epidemic, but marginal in terms of the total size of the epidemic. The division of the rest of the population into the RSK group and the not at risk (NOT) group is somewhat arbitrary, but only has an effect on the theoretical maximum size of the epidemic.

A pattern of contact is assumed both within and between risk groups according to the assumed number of partners in each risk group. Some allowance is also made for variations in sexual activity according to age and gender. The groups are categorised according to behaviour during the peak sexually active years and so subsequent experience can be monitored using a risk group as a cohort; that is, persons are assumed not to change risk groups but to change behaviour within the risk group as they age.

The model can be applied to both homosexual and heterosexual transmission of the HIV virus and also allows for mother-to-child transmission. It runs in a yearly cycle and the population ages, generates births, normal deaths, new HIV infections, new AIDS sick and AIDS deaths. It can be applied to a specific 'community' where the following are examples of a community: male homosexual; white heterosexuals; African heterosexuals in Natal; rural African heterosexuals; and so on. The use of imports (HIV infections from other communities) makes this approach feasible in the model. The application of the model to a specific community is only meaningful, however, if empirical data for relating to HIV prevalence and its spread are available for that community.

The projections for the total South African population given here are thus the aggregation of several communities as described in the following section.

HIV Infection

The projection of the level and spread of HIV infection is the key to the modelling process. The resultant shape of the infection curve overrides all other factors and, as a result, we have focused our analysis on HIV infection and prevalence.

An initial prevalence is assumed for each risk group for the initial year in which HIV infections are assumed to start spreading rapidly in the community. New HIV infections are calculated each year, for each risk group, according to a formula that has the form:

New HIV Pos = Neg * [1 − (1 − P1 * P2)^N]

Neg = the number of HIV negative persons in the risk group assumed to be sexually active
P1 = probability of infection if partner is HIV positive
P2 = probability that a new sexual partner is HIV positive
N = number of new partners per year

The model formulae are more complex than shown above because of the interrelationships between the various risk groups and the detailed calculations of the probability factors. A mathematical description of these formulae is beyond the scope of this paper.

Medical evidence suggests that an extremely wide variation in the probability of infection from sexual contact will be found in practice. The level of infectivity varies according to the stage of HIV infection of the HIV-positive partner, and according to the condition of health of the uninfected. There will also be wide variations in the behaviour of a single relationship, measured by the number of sexual contacts. Similarly empirical evidence has shown a wide range in social behaviour. No attempt has been made to allow for the above variability, beyond defining different parameters for the four risk groups. Each risk group is characterised by defining its level of sexual mobility according to the number of new partners per annum. Hence the behaviour within a risk group is described by average values. It is here that the model must be regarded as a macro model.

Once the number of new HIV infections have been calculated, they are distributed by gender and age according to empirical data available for that risk group. Individuals socialise between the risk groups as shown schematically in Figure 5.2. The epidemic, measured by the prevalence, grows exponentially in the early stages and then grows more slowly as the risk groups becomes saturated and age.

A typical HIV epidemic can thus be regarded as falling into three stages: the first, or *pre-epidemic*, stage is characterised by a low incidence and prevalence of infection, which occurs mainly in the high-risk groups. The *epidemic* stage is characterised by a situation in which the prevalence of HIV in the high-risk groups is well over 1 per cent, and the annual incidence of new infections increases rapidly, even outside the very high risk groups. In the *endemic* stage a plateau is reached since spread has slowed down due to saturation of the risk groups, but there remains a sufficiently high incidence of new infections to replace deaths.

This picture is often incorrectly attributed to behaviour change. Demographers must, however, clearly distinguish this natural pattern from actual behaviour change.

Imports

The concept of 'imports' was developed in a model by Groeneveld.[7] The need for imports can be clearly seen if one considers that the formula given above is dependent on the proportion of the population that is already infected. In practice there would not only have been one initial person infected to produce an epidemic, but rather a number of infections over a period of time that arose from contacts outside the community. This effect is material if the HIV prevalence in the community from whence the imports come is significantly higher than that of the community being modelled.

Another critical aspect of the epidemic which the use of imports can help to describe is the fact that the total epidemic consists of an aggregation of many physically and socially separate sub-epidemics. This is apparent if one considers the spread of infection from homosexuals to the heterosexual community, from countries to the north of South Africa to the heterosexual community, from region to region, and from urban to rural areas.

Imports are expressed as an additional number of HIV-positive individuals in contact with the community each year. The import parameters are adjusted each year to account for the change in prevalence of imports relative to their community of origin.

DETAILS OF THE MODEL STRUCTURE AND INPUTS

The model also requires a range of other parameters which are discussed in the following sections. Note that the specific parameters examined below relate to the particular scenarios described here.

Demographic Data

The model is a demographic projection, and therefore requires a range of demographic data as input: the community, distributed by age, gender, race and demographic area; fertility rates; normal population mortality rates and others. Population at the start of the epidemic is split according to age (5-year age groups) and gender.

The total population of South Africa (including the so-called TBVC states – Transkei, Bophutatswana, Venda and Ciskei) was estimated at 32.8 million in 1985.[8] In order to allow for the different progression amongst different racial and geographic communities, the total population was segmented as in Table 5.2. The estimated epidemic start year for the white population refers to the start of the heterosexual spread, since infections amongst white male homosexuals probably started in about 1980.

Table 5.2 South African population distribution

Group	Area	Size (million)	Epidemic start year
African	Natal	4.9	1985
African	other urban	7.5	1986
African	other semi-urban	10.2	1987
African	other rural	2.3	1988
White	all areas	5.6	1986
Coloured	all areas	1.5	1987
Indian	all areas	0.8	1987
Total		32.8	

Distribution of the Population into Risk Groups

The average distribution of the population into the four risk groups, in these scenarios, is as follows:

PRO	STD	RSK	NOT
2.5%	22.5%	45%	30%

The 2.5 per cent in the PRO group is a guess; it is obviously some small percentage of the population. The 22.5 per cent in the STD group is based on data that shows 15–26 per cent of sexually active Africans have a history or presence of an STD. The size of the RSK group was considered from two perspectives. The first was to assume a level of HIV prevalence that defines the group. Relative to an STD prevalence of 3.2 per cent, the RSK group was assumed to have an HIV prevalence of about 0.4 per cent. Therefore, by using HIV prevalence data for antenatals and assuming a mix of STD, RSK and NOT lives in the antenatal group, it is possible to solve for the RSK group. Second, it seemed reasonable that the NOT group is 25–33 per cent of the population. These two approaches led to values for the RSK group of 40–50 per cent of the population.

The Probability of Infection per Contact

The probability of infection formulae use parameters that are really in the realm of micro-modelling variables. We have used these variables as parameters to calibrate our results. It is nevertheless interesting to consider some values that we have used in the light of existing

Table 5.3 Probability of infection parameters

	RSK	STD	PRO
Probability of infection per contact (if partner is HIV+)	0.002	0.0065	0.0065
New partnerships per year	1	10	200

empirical data.[9] The model is presently calibrated using the data shown in Table 5.3.

The probability of infection per contact has been analysed in various empirical studies. Most suggest that this probability is less than 0.001 (that is, a 1 in 1000 chance). This is one-tenth of the values we have used. There is evidence, however, to suggest that the presence of other co-factors (such as STDs or other illnesses) will substantially increase the probability of infection per contact. The values may thus not be unreasonable in a community where the standard of health is already low. This is the main parameter that determines the observed time of infection.

The number of partners per year in a sense defines each group: for example, the RSK are those persons that have (or their partners have) an average of one new sexual partner per year. The value of 10 for the STD group is somewhat high compared to empirical data, but this might be explained by situations where the partnerships are short-term or irregular; perhaps weekend or monthly partners (which might be common, for example, amongst semi-urban workers). The value of 200 for the PRO is lower than the international data indicates, but prostitution is illegal in South Africa and we have assumed that other persons are included in that group.

Pattern of Sexual Contact with other Risk Groups

A pattern of contact between the risk groups is also assumed, and is based on the size of the groups and the number of new partners for each group. The total number of new partners and contacts in the community does not necessarily balance, but the point is rather to 'expose' the STD group to infection from the PRO group, and to 'expose' the RSK group to infection from the STD group. The assumed pattern of contact is rather pessimistic and probably overestimates the impact on the RSK group.

These infection factors do not consider specific male and female differences, which may be a short-coming of the model. One example is the fact that the probability of infection per contact is thought to be higher for women than for men. The fact that the model does not take into account of this difference suggests that the model may underestimate that differences in HIV prevalence between men and women. However, currently available data from some African countries (and from South Africa) indicates that the male to female HIV prevalence ratio is just over 1.1:1. This suggests that gender differences in probability of infection per contact are being balanced by other gender-specific factors. The fact that the model projects male to female ratios which are very similar to actual data indicates that the model parameters act to balance the effect of eliminating gender differences in probability of infection per contact.

Initial Number of HIV Positives and Annual Number of Imported HIV Infections

The initial HIV infections and the imports were set to arrive at the desired HIV prevalence levels for 1990, but bear some relation to the possible movement of persons, and thus also HIV-infected persons, between South Africa and other countries where the HIV prevalence is higher.

Age Distribution of New Infections

Since most HIV infections in South Africa are comparatively recent, and are increasingly at a very rapid rate, it is reasonable to use the age and sex distribution of those who have recently been identified as HIV positive, taking account of any bias inherent in the samples used.[10] After adjusting for some bias in the data, the distribution of new HIV infections according to age and gender can be calculated. Table 5.4 gives the distribution used in the model. A valid concern may be that this age pattern will change over the course of the epidemic.

Table 5.4 Age distribution of new HIV infections (%)

Gender	15–19	20–24	25–29	30–34	35–39	40–44	>44
Female	24	33	24	10	7	2	0
Male	5	24	33	20	12	6	0

The Incubation Period

The incubation period – that is, the time from initial HIV infection to AIDS – is a critical variable in any scenario of future AIDS cases. Although some data is available, much is still uncertain, and even current experience is changing as medications (such as AZT) and other interventions have an impact on the length of the incubation period. In addition there are virtually no data from elsewhere in Africa, but only speculation that the incubation period will be significantly shorter than in the more developed countries, mainly because of the existence of TB and many other infectious diseases, malnutrition and other STDs.

The more recent studies show an apparently longer incubation period than the early studies report for cases in San Francisco. The mean time to AIDS now appears to be at least 10 years.[11] It seems reasonable to suggest, however, that the state of health of the persons on whom the earliest cohorts of those infected in the developed countries studies were based was not dissimilar to the state of health of those currently being infected in Southern Africa. The only significant factor that has been observed to influence the incubation period is age: people infected at a younger age show a longer incubation period.

Taking all these factors into account, it seems that, for South Africa, a mean incubation period of about 8 years is still not unreasonable. The incubation period for HIV infected infants is, however, much shorter.[12] Table 5.5 illustrates the incubation periods used in the scenarios.

Mother-to-Child Transmission

The rate of transmission of HIV infection from mother to infant has been difficult to establish and rates of between 13 and 41 per cent have been observed.[13] There is nevertheless clear evidence of paediatric seroconversion and, in addition, a higher observed infant mortality rate among babies born to HIV-positive mothers. The model uses a 35 per cent mother-to-child transmission rate.

AIDS Mortality

More is known about the mortality of AIDS patients.[14] There has been some evidence that the AIDS mortality rate may be higher in

Table 5.5 Incubation period

Time since infection (years)	Cumulative AIDS sick Adults (%)	Infants (%)
0	0	10
1	0.2	20
2	3.2	40
3	9.0	60
4	16.3	80
5	24.7	100
6	32.2	
7	40.3	
8	47.5	
9	55.4	
10	62.1	
.	.	
.	.	
.	.	
20	92.5	

Africa than in the developed countries, although this may be influenced to some extent by late diagnoses. For both adults and infants, the model uses a mortality rate of 50 per cent in the first year and 100 per cent in the second year.

CALIBRATION OF THE MODEL

The model projections have been calibrated against over 300 data points reported from the whole of sub-Saharan Africa, including South Africa. This data originates from many sources and some references are given.[15] Only two major features of this calibration will be illustrated here.

The Geographic Spread of Infection

The most consistent and homogeneous HIV data observed in Africa is that from studies on antenatal clinic attenders. The model was calibrated so that the *projected* spread of HIV infection, for 1990, among females aged 16–35 (which should represent antenatal clinic attenders), matched the *reported* HIV prevalence for antenatal clinic

Table 5.6 Comparing projections to reported antenatal data

Model projections (females 16–35)		Reported antenatal data			
Mid year	HIV (%)	Location	HIV (%)	Year	Lag (yrs)
1985	0.015				−5
1986	0.05	SA: W. Cape	0.08	1990:Nov	−4
1987	0.13				−3
1988	0.32	SA: E. Cape	0.5	1990:Nov	−2
1989	0.7	SA: Soweto	0.6	1990	−1
1990	**1.3**	**SA: Natal**	**1.8**	**1990:Nov**	**0**
1991	2.4	Malawi	2.0	1984	+7
1992	4.1	Mali	4.1	1988	+4
1993	6.5	Kenya	6.0	1989	+4
1994	9.7	Tanzania	9.8	1989	+5
1995	13.5	Uganda	13.5	1986	+9
1996	17.5	Uganda	15.0	1987	+9
1997	21.3	Uganda	22.0	1989	+8
1998	24.4	Zambia	25.0	1990	+8
1999	27.0	Malawi	28.0	1990	+9
2000	29.0	–	–		–

SA = South Africa.

attenders in the African population in Natal in the corresponding year. Thus, in November 1990, actual reported data for Natal shows an HIV prevalence of 1.8 per cent, while the calibrated model for mid-1990 showed a similar projection of 1.3 per cent. This is shown in the bold line in Table 5.6.

Once the calibration had been performed, the resulting projections for each year could be compared to reported HIV prevalence data for other areas. When a correspondence between projected and reported data is found, the difference in years is a measure of the time difference in the spread of the epidemic between the particular area and Natal.

This process is illustrated in Table 5.6. The first two columns show the model's *projections* for each year. The last three columns show the location, year and *reported* prevalence rate for other areas. Thus the model projection for mid-1989 was 0.7 per cent. Actual data for Soweto in mid-1990 was very close to this at 0.6 per cent. This suggests that the epidemic in Soweto is 1 year behind that in Natal. Similarly, the Western Cape appears to be 4 years behind Natal, while data from Malawi suggests that it is 7 years ahead of Natal. Several other examples are given in the table.

The time lags in the spread of HIV infection illustrated in Table 5.6 are in fact compatible with the scenario of an epidemic spread by transport routes, and by the movement of people through Africa. There is no intention to imply from this data that infection started in any particular country. Rather, this exercise aims to illustrate the various stages of the epidemic in different countries, and to use that data to project the local epidemic more accurately.

One example is seen in the case of Malawi. The reported data for Malawi, for 1990, looks higher than what would have been expected from projections and from the data from other countries. From a geographical perspective, and from the reported data from Malawi in 1984, it seemed reasonable to assume that the epidemic in Malawi was one or two years behind that of Uganda. However, the 1990 data indicates that Malawi is currently at higher levels than Uganda was in 1989 (28 per cent as opposed to 22 per cent). This suggests very different dynamics of spread between countries. This is corroborated by evidence from other countries, notably Zaire, that the epidemic is levelling off at levels of infection lower than is the case in Malawi. This apparent difference is worthy of further research.

Spread of Infection by Risk Group

The model should also be able to reproduce the data reported for the different risk groups described earlier. This is illustrated in Table 5.7. As noted in the table, the model's projections for 1990 for the prevalence levels among the different risk groups is very similar to the reported data for these groups in Natal in the same year.

The previous exercise suggested that the epidemic in Tanzania appears to be five years ahead of that in Natal. Thus, the 1989 reported data for Tanzania is compared to projected data for Natal in 1994 for each risk group. Similarly, 1990 data for Zambia (8 years ahead) is compared to 1998 projections. As the table shows, in all these cases there is a remarkable correspondence between the reported data and the model projections.

The important point of these comparisons is that the scenarios being presented here are not unrealistic in relation to data that has already been observed elsewhere in Africa.

Table 5.7 Comparing projections to reported risk group data[16]

PROJECTED HIV+	1990 (%)	REPORTED NATAL HIV+	1990 (%)
Female 16–35	1.3	antenatal (Nov.)	1.8
STD	3.9	STD clinic	4.0
PRO	7.7	prostitutes	8.5
PROJECTED HIV+	1994 (%)	REPORTED TANZANIA HIV+ (5 years ahead)	1989 (%)
Female 16–35	9.7	antenatal	9.8
STD	27.1	STD clinic	25.8
PRO	43.6	prostitutes	39.0
PROJECTED HIV+	1998 (%)	REPORTED ZAMBIA HIV+ (8 years ahead)	1990 (%)
Female 16–35	24.4	antenatal	26.0
STD	60.4	STD clinic	52.5
PRO	–	prostitutes	–

SCENARIOS FOR SOUTH AFRICA

Two scenarios for the total South African population are described here, and are compared to the results that would have been expected if there were no HIV epidemic. The scenarios are as follows:

BASE   No HIV infection
SCEN60 HIV infection calibrated to data from other African countries
SCEN61 HIV infection as for SCEN60, but with the assumption of significant changes in sexual behaviour occurring 12 years into the epidemic.

The projected numbers of HIV positive individuals, AIDS sick, and AIDS death for each scenario are shown in Table 5.8. The figures in the table show clearly that changes in behaviour occur between 1995 and 2000, since that is when Scenario 60 and Scenario 61 start to diverge. It is also interesting to compare the projected figures for 1991 with an estimate that has been reported for South Africa. The projection for 97 000 HIV-infected persons at January 1991 compares to an estimate of 74 000 to 102 000 made by Kustner based on the

Table 5.8 Summary of model projections

	1991	1995	2000	2005
HIV-infected				
Scenario 60	97 000	970 000	4 112 000	6 410 000
Scenario 61	97 000	970 000	3 700 000	4 762 000
AIDS sick				
Scenario 60	1 190	25 000	259 000	743 000
Scenario 61	1 190	25 000	255 000	618 000
AIDS deaths				
Scenario 60	1 350	23 000	203 000	525 000
Scenario 61	1 350	23 000	197 000	429 000
Cumulative deaths				
Scenario 60	2 200	47 000	602 000	2 588 000
Scenario 61	2 200	47 000	594 000	2 321 000

Table 5.9 Heterosexual and paediatric AIDS cases: comparison of projected and reported cases

Year	(1) Projection (Scenario 60)	(2) Reported	(2)/(1)%
1985	18	2	11
1986	25	3	12
1987	58	11	19
1988	176	25	14
1989	501	80	16
1990	1289	221	17

national antenatal seroprevalence survey carried out in 1990.

Table 5.9 gives a comparison of the model's projected AIDS cases (up to 1990) and actual AIDS cases reported in South Africa (excluding cases reported for male homosexuals). If the projections are realistic, they imply that only approximately 20 per cent of heterosexual and paediatric AIDS cases are actually reported. This is not inconsistent with the estimate that only 10–50 per cent of AIDS cases are reported elsewhere in Africa, and with the fact that AIDS is not a notifiable disease in South Africa.

One could argue, however, that 20 per cent reporting is too low a figure for South Africa, and that closer to 50 per cent of cases would

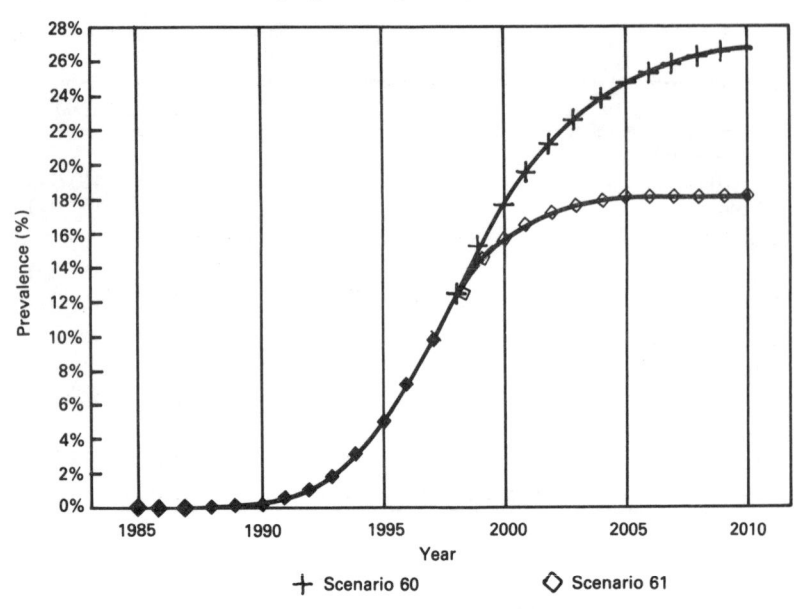

Figure 5.3 HIV prevalence: adults aged 15–49 years

be expected to be reported there. If this is the case, the discrepancy between the projections and reported data may be due to late diagnosis of AIDS in South Africa, and/or due to the fact that the mean incubation period of about 8 years used in the model is too rapid, and that the average incubation period is actually closer to 10 years. These issues clearly require further research.

Figure 5.3 shows the trends in HIV prevalence among the adult population (aged 15–49) to the year 2010 for the two scenarios. Both curves illustrate well the pre-epidemic, epidemic and endemic stages of HIV described earlier. As will be noted from the graph, South Africa is currently thought to be at an early point of the *epidemic* stage, so that very rapid spread of HIV is likely in the next few years.

For both scenarios, the increase in prevalence during the epidemic stage is very rapid, but the assumed change in sexual behaviour (Scenario 61) causes the endemic stage to occur sooner. As the figure shows, the epidemic is predicted to peak at a prevalence of approximately 27 per cent of the adult population by year 2010 in the absence of behaviour change. If we assume that such changes will occur, a peak prevalence is predicted or approximately 18 per cent, to be reached between 2000 and 2005.

There are a number of other African countries where this sort of

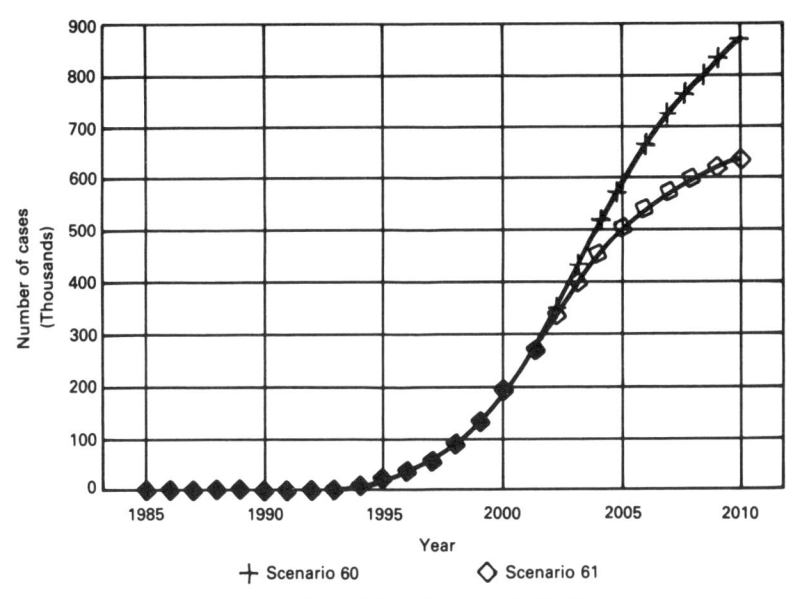

Figure 5.4 AIDS sick: adults aged 15–49 years

infection curve has already been observed in urban areas. In many of these countries, the prevalence is still significantly lower in the rural areas. This should not be expected in South Africa, however, because the efficient transport network and the high mobility of labour will probably mean that the epidemic in the rural areas will follow the urban epidemic more closely, but with a lag of a few years.

It is vital to note that the epidemic does not spread indefinitely within the population. As explained earlier, the *endemic* stage occurs when the risk groups in the population become saturated, and when the number of new infections at any one time is approximately equal to the number of AIDS-related deaths. The predictions of this model bear out the experience from other African countries, where evidence suggests that the peak prevalence is unlikely to exceed 30–40 per cent of the adult population.[17]

Figure 5.4 shows the number of people sick with AIDS-related illnesses over the projection period. The shape of this curve follows that of HIV prevalence, but with a time lag of a number of years because of the incubation period. This also illustrates the important point that even if new HIV infections were to stop immediately, there would still be a growth in AIDS cases for a number of years. This must be considered when monitoring the success of AIDS control programmes.

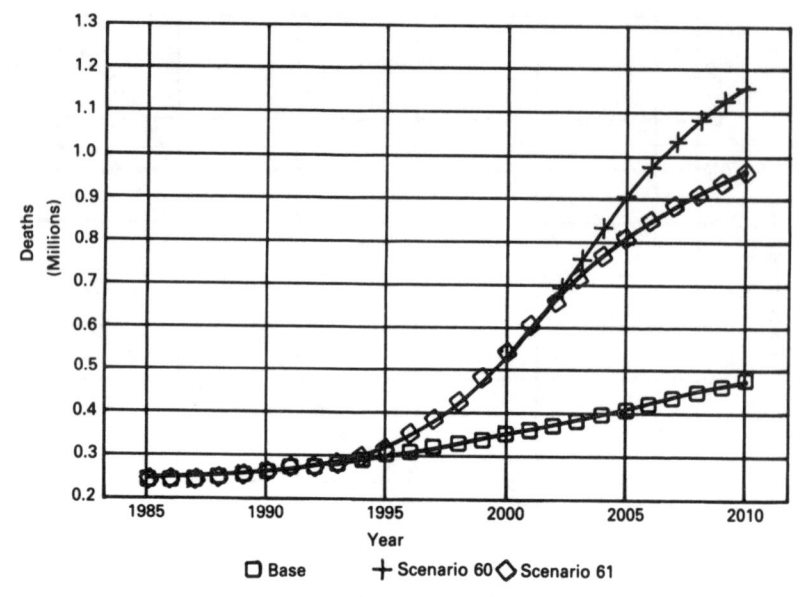

Figure 5.5 Total deaths for all ages

Figure 5.5 illustrates projected total deaths from AIDS, including paediatric AIDS. These projections clearly show the increasing impact of AIDS from the year 1995 in both scenarios. Once again, the curve here is very similar to that of the HIV prevalence curve but with a time lag, attributable on this occasion to the time from HIV infection to death.

Figure 5.6 shows the projected age-specific mortality rate for adults. This demonstrates the relatively greater impact on young adults because their normal expected mortality is relatively low at these ages.

Figure 5.7 gives the projected impact of AIDS on the total population over the projection period. The critical point to here is that at no stage does the AIDS epidemic generate a negative population growth rate. Instead, in both scenarios, population growth is predicted to slow down significantly. In Scenario 60 the rate is predicted to slow down to a minimum of 1.2 per cent, while in Scenario 61 the equivalent figure is 1.7 per cent per annum.

Sensitivity analysis indicates, however, that the fertility rate is the critical factor in determining the ultimate rate of population growth. The fertility rate may be subjected to several influences over the next decade, both related to AIDS and independent of it. Examples

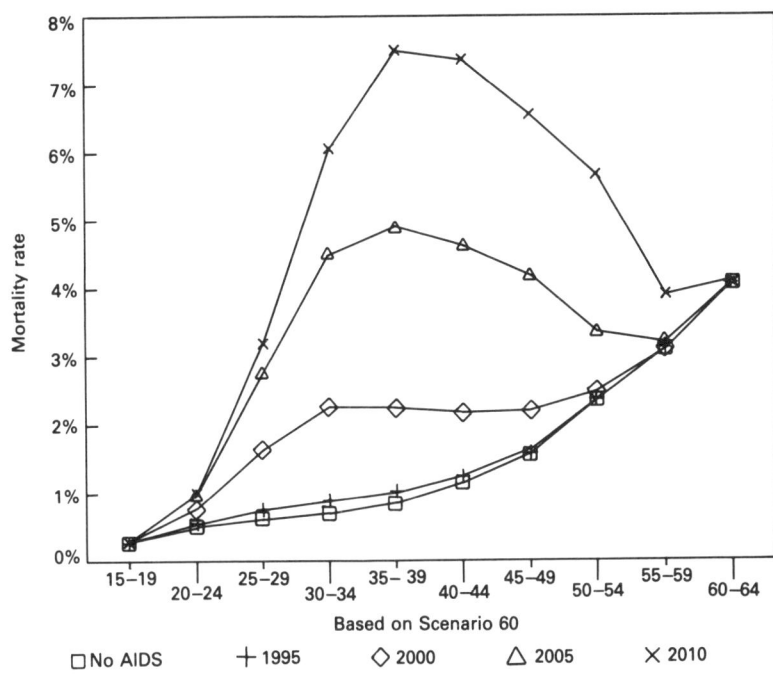

Figure 5.6 Mortality rate for male adults aged 15–64 years

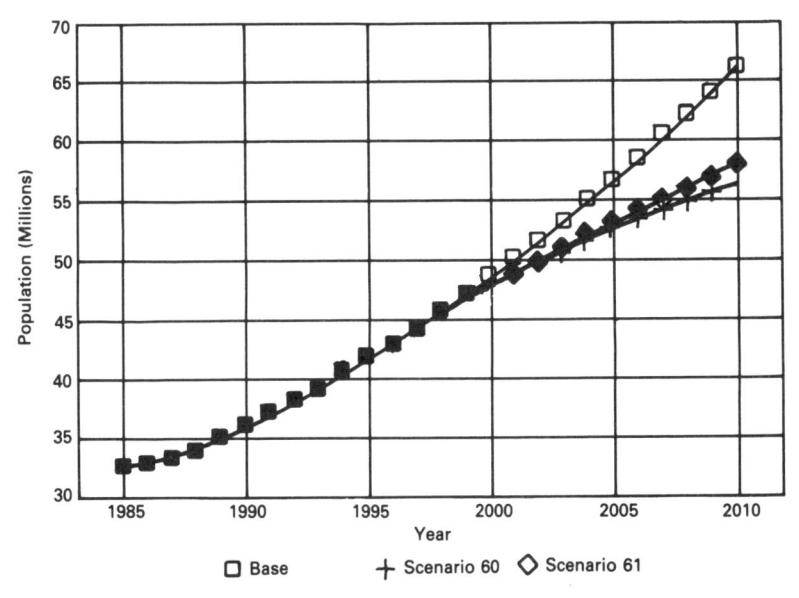

Figure 5.7 Total population, all ages

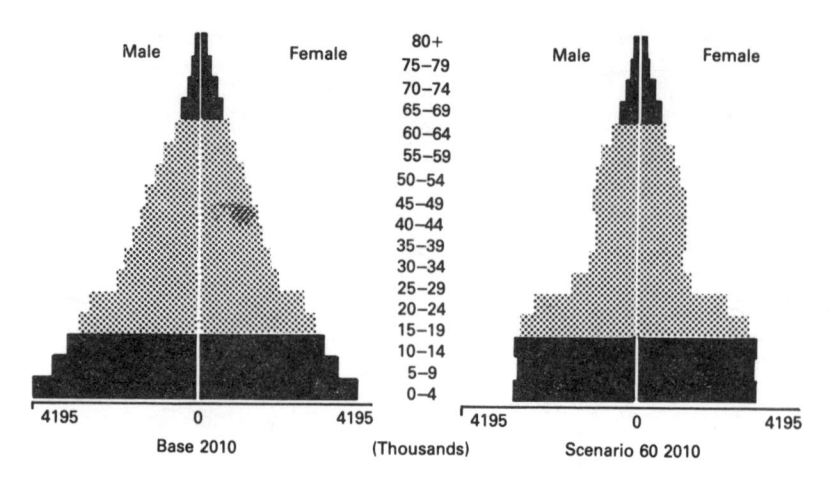

Figure 5.8 Age structure of the population

include a reduction in fertility rates due to increasing educational standards and AIDS control programmes. On the other hand, it is possible that infant AIDS deaths could exert upward pressure on fertility rates. It is thus hard to project the fertility rate with accuracy. These scenarios and the base projection have all assumed constant fertility rates over the projection period. Note that the fertility rate used in the model is age specific: it refers to the number of children born to women of a specific age per year. It is this age-specific fertility rate that is held constant in the model.

Figure 5.8 indicates the impact of AIDS on the age structure of the population by the year 2010. The most profound effects of the epidemic are seen in the 15–49 year age group, as well as in the 0–4 year age group, due to deaths from paediatric AIDS. The major impact that these deaths have on the population pyramid in both scenarios is well illustrated here.

These changes in the age structure of the population and the resulting disruption of family economic units could well prove to be the most damaging effect of the HIV epidemic on the population. There is not, however, projected to be a material change in the overall dependency ratio (the ratio of dependents to those of income-earning age in the population). This is because infant deaths offset, to some extent, the deaths in the economically active age groups. This observation of a constant dependency ratio, however, disguises the fact that there will be substantial numbers of orphans who will have lost one or both parents, and who will present an enormous burden to their communities.

CONCLUSION

Although there is an 'expanding funnel of doubt' for longer-term projections of the epidemic, there is now sufficient data and knowledge available to develop realistic scenarios of the potential impact of HIV infection on the population of South Africa. The predictions generated by the model described in this chapter correlate well with empirical observations from several other countries where the epidemic has been in progress for substantially longer than is the case in South Africa.

These observations suggest that the approach adopted in building this model, and the assumptions which underpin it, are reasonable. This implies that the model's current projections can be regarded as best guesses, and as realistic scenarios on which to base assessments of the impact of the epidemic and to plan for it. Clearly, the model will need to be updated and calibrated as more accurate and more recent data becomes available. In the interim, however, several important conclusions can be drawn. These can be summarised as shown below.

1. South Africa has the benefit of meaningful HIV prevalent data, and the opportunity of observing the longer HIV infection and AIDS sickness experience of many other countries. We can therefore develop realistic long-term scenarios on which long-term plans and the allocation of resources can be based.
2. The identification and treatment of other STDs in the community is the key factor in slowing down the early stage of the epidemic. Education and changes in sexual behaviour are also urgently required.
3. In the absence of significant behaviour change, the HIV epidemic is likely to peak at a prevalence rate below 30 per cent of the adult population, while with some change peak prevalence may be below 20 per cent.
4. It is unlikely that there will be a decline in the total South African population in the foreseeable future; however, the impact of the HIV epidemic could significantly reduce the rate of population

growth rate by the year 2005. An important factor is how AIDS and AIDS control programmes affect fertility rates.
5. The HIV epidemic will cause the sickness and death of many young adults in South Africa and could have the following critical effects; many of those affected will be skilled and educated persons in the workplace and this will affect productivity and training. It is likely that health-care facilities will be placed under severe pressure, and difficult policy decisions will be required about the treatment of persons with AIDS.
6. Many family units will be affected, creating large numbers of orphans and a noticeable change in the expected age structure of the population.
7. The spread of HIV infection throughout South Africa had the potential to be worse than in other African countries because of the efficient transport system and mobility of labour.
8. Any long-term scenarios of the potential impact of AIDS must be used responsibly in the context of the many uncertainties that still remain. Nevertheless, it is important to use realistic scenarios to provide a tangible base from which to plan.

Further research and debate on a range of these assumptions and approaches is also required. Some priority areas for research are defined by the following questions: how can this model be used to test the sensitivity of HIV transmission in South Africa to specific interventions and behavioural changes? What is the real extent of other STDs in South Africa, and what is their effect on the transmission of HIV? What is the expected incubation period for AIDS in South Africa? What factors are most crucial in the spread of HIV, and where should AIDS control interventions be directed? What are the long-term plans and short-term actions required of the health care sector in coping with AIDS?

In addition to assessments of the overall demographic impact of AIDS, more detailed assessments of the impact of AIDS on specific communities and economic sectors/industries is now required. The structure of this model means that it can be used for these purposes as well.

Acknowledgements

I wish to thank the following: my colleagues at Metropolitan Life, particularly Donald Millar who developed the computer model; also

Russel Lok, Jose de Nobrega, Tjaart Esterhuyse and Janine Toerien; members of the Actuarial Society Aids Sub-Committee, particularly Douglas Kier, for their advice and guidance; Jonny Broomberg, who assisted in extensive editing of early drafts of this chapter; and to the numerous other persons who gave me access to their ideas, data and time.

References

1. P.R. Doyle and D.B. Millar, 'A general description of an actuarial model applicable to the HIV epidemic in South Africa', paper presented to the AIDS Seminar of the Actuarial Society of South Africa on 8 November 1990, mimeo.
2. S. Haberman, 'Actuarial review of models for describing and predicting the spread of HIV infection and AIDS', *Journal of the Institute of Actuaries*, II (1990).
3. G.N. Padayachee and R. Schall, 'Short-term predictions of the prevalence of human immunodeficiency virus infection among the black population in South Africa', *South African Medical Journal*, 77 (1990), pp. 329–33.
4. B.D. Schoub, 'Epidemiological consideration of the present status and future growth of the acquired immunodeficiency syndrome epidemic in South Africa', *South African Medical Journal*, 77 (1990).
5. J. Bongaarts, 'A model of the spread of HIV infection and the demographic impact of AIDS', *Statistics in Medicine*, 8 (1989), pp. 103–20.
6. J. Lorper, 'Projecting the spread of AIDS into the general population – application to life assurance', *Journal of the Institute of Actuaries*, 116 (1989).
7. H. Groeneveld, 'A stochastic micro-simulation model of the HIV epidemic', Medical Research Council lecture, 23 March 1990.
8. J.L. Sadie, 'A reconstruction and projection of demographic movements in the RSA and TBVC countries', Bureau of Market Research, University of South Africa, Research Report no. 148, 1988.
9. M. van der Graaf and R. Diepersloot, 'Routes, efficiency, cofactors and prevention. A survey of the literature', *Infection*, 17, 4 (1989).
10. C.R.B. Prior and G.C. Buckle, 'Blood donors with antibody to the human immunodeficiency virus – the Natal experience', *South African Medical Journal*, 77 (1990), pp. 623–5; B.D. Schoub, A.N. Smith, S. Johnson, D.J. Martin, S.F. Lyons, G.N. Padayachee and H.S. Thurwitz, 'Considerations on the further expansion of the AIDS epidemic in South Africa – 1990', *South African Medical Journal*, 77 (1990), pp. 613–18 and personal communication.
11. P. Bachetti and A.R. Moss, 'Incubation period of AIDS in San Francisco', *Nature*, 338 (1989); R.J. Bigger *et al.*, 'AIDS incubation in 1 891 seroconverters from different exposure groups', *AIDS*, 4, 11 (1990).

12. European Collaborative Study, 'Mother to child transmission of HIV infection', *Lancet*, 2 (1988), p. 1039.
13. Ibid., S.K. Hira *et al.*, 'Perinatal transmission of HIV-I in Zambia', *British Medical Journal*, 299 (1989).
14. G. Marasca and M. McEvoy, 'Length of survival of patients with acquired immune deficiency syndrome in the UK', *British Medical Journal*, 292 (1986), p. 1727.
15. H.G.V. Kustner, 'National antenatal surveillance results', *Epidemiological Comments*, 18, 2 (1991), pp. 35–45; N. Clumeck *et al.*, 'Seroepidemiological studies of HTLV-III antibody prevalence among selected groups of heterosexual Africans', *Journal of American Medical Association*, 254, 18 (1985); N. Melbye *et al.*, 'Evidence for heterosexual transmission and clinical manifestation of human immunodeficiency virus infection and related condition in Lusaka, Zambia', *Lancet* (November 1986); J. Carswell, 'HIV infection in healthy persons in Uganda', *AIDS*, 1, 4 (1987); P. Piot *et al.*, 'Retrospective seroepidemiology of AIDS virus infection in Nairobi populations', *Journal of Infectious Diseases*, 155, 6 (1987); R.W. Goodgame, 'AIDS in Uganda – Clinical and Social Features', *The New England Journal of Medicine*, 323, 6 (1990), pp. 383–9; Robert W. Ryder *et al.*, 'Heterosexual transmission of HIV-1 among employees and their spouses at two large businesses in Zaire', *AIDS* 4, 8 (1990), pp. 725–32; Datafile. WorldAIDS, July 1990; Information drawn from *World AIDS* (No. 10, July 1990, Datafile Section 8, Panos Institute, London). M.O. Santos-Ferreira *et al.*, 'A study of seroprevalence of HIV-1 and HIV-2 in six provinces of people's Republic of Angola: clues to the spread of HIV infection', *Journal of Acquired Immune Deficiency Syndrome*, 3, 8 (1990); Fifth International Conference on AIDS in Africa Abstracts: Kinshasa, Zaire, October 1990; Sixth International Conference on AIDS, San Francisco, 1990; J. Chin *et al.*, AIDSTECH workshop on modelling the AIDS epidemic, Harare, May 1991; US Bureau of the Census, 'Recent HIV seroprevalence levels by country', *Research Notes*, 3, February 1991; US Bureau of the Census, 'Recent HIV Seroprevalence levels'.
16. I.M. Windsor, 'AIDS – The Current Picture', *Proceedings of the 7th Annual Congress of the National Medical and Dental Association*, Durban, Oct. 1990.
17. See Chin *et al.*, AIDSTECH workshop.

6 Modelling the Demographic Impact of AIDS: Potential Effects on the Black Population in South Africa
Gwenda Brophy

INTRODUCTION

HIV infection levels are now rising rapidly in South Africa. In an initial stage of the AIDS epidemic in the country where the first cases of AIDS were seen among homosexuals in 1982, the pattern of AIDS resembled that initially seen in the USA and Europe. That phase now appears to have been superseded by a new one. Whilst the rate of increase amongst male homosexuals may even be showing some signs of levelling off, according to some reports,[1] this second phase, one in which the disease is primarily heterosexually transmitted and which appears to be predominant among the black heterosexual population, is showing indications of gaining momentum. The first reported black heterosexual cases were seen in December 1987; 1988 saw paediatric cases being reported, and relatively recently around 100 cases of vertical transmission had been reported in the black population.[2]

This new phase gives concern for at least two reasons; first, because of the size of the black population as a proportion of the overall population size in South Africa and, second, because of the rapid rate with which the virus has apparently spread among this group, at least as recorded among specific sub-groups of the population and in particular geographical areas.[3]

Since reported HIV infections tend to represent but a fraction of the true pool of infected individuals, and given that information tends to accrue first for particular groups who may not be representative of the broader population as a whole, the actual number of HIV infections in South Africa is an unknown quantity. However, estimates can, frequently are and need to be made, not least since such estimates can indicate the 'momentum' of HIV infection embedded in the population, a proportion of which will likely demonstrate itself as subsequent AIDS cases within a given time period, whose boundary can now be at least roughly drawn given increasing (albeit still inadequate) information relating to the course of the disease.

Estimates of current HIV infections and AIDS cases in the future are, however, not sufficient for the purposes of many planners and analysts. There is increasingly a need to establish what implications such rates could have when absorbed into the existing population fabric and are subsequently reflected in various demographic indicators, such as levels of crude death rates, infant mortality rates and life expectancy levels, as well as on the overall population size and its rate of natural increase.

The following analysis uses a large-scale simulation model to consider the potential demographic effects of AIDS in South Africa. The chapter is constructed as follows: first the nature of the model used in this analysis, and the type of inputs – demographic, behavioural and epidemiological – that it requires will be outlined. The inputs and assumptions relating to these three areas that are used in the subsequent projections for South Africa are then discussed. The results of utilising those inputs in the model are presented next, and their implications discussed. Finally, we note some pertinent areas in which we are currently lacking vital information that would facilitate the modelling of the impact of AIDS, specifically in the area of behavioural factors related to sexual activity, although we note that such information is as problematic to obtain as it is vital.

MODELLING THE DEMOGRAPHIC IMPACT OF AIDS

There are a number of ways in which the future trend of HIV infections in a given context may be estimated, which have been succinctly summarised by Padayachee and Schall.[4] At one end of the spectrum probably the simplest method is that of extrapolation from initial growth rates of HIV infection over time; however, while this may be a useful device at the beginning of an epidemic, it tends to become increasingly inappropriate after a while since the AIDS virus has typically spread more rapidly first among those whose behaviour is conducive to a faster dissemination, and less so as the remaining population is increasingly composed of those whose behaviour renders them less susceptible to acquiring it. In other words, the infection rate may not grow linearly. In addition, progression of the AIDS virus within a population tends to be a complex matter, so that the actual 'shape' of the curve representing the increase in HIV infection can vary empirically, reflecting the net result of the complex interactions in the prevailing profile of behavioural, epidemiological and other variables and co-factors that both facilitate and hinder its spread in a given context.

More sophisticated models that can incorporate a range of relevant variables and mathematically track their effects are therefore required. Several models have been developed. Possibly the most complex are the highly mathematical models developed by Anderson, May and McLean in the UK.[5] Other models that have been developed include that of Bongaarts[6] and, in a similar vein but developed to a more advanced stage, those of the Centre for International Research at the US Census Office: the iwgAIDS model[7] and the PRAY AIDS model developed at the World Bank.[8]

These models essentially seek to assess the effects of HIV infection in terms of AIDS cases and demographic indicators on a population that is stratified into various risk groups – for example, heterosexual males, blood product recipients, and so on – in which the risk groups in turn are distributed according to their variation relating to factors relevant to that risk group, such as numbers of new partners per year or propensity to receive blood transfusions. Essentially these latter models take the form of a standard cohort component-projection population package[9] that works in conjunction with an epidemiological and behavioural component.

In this analysis we have adopted the World Bank PRAY model, which permits the inclusion of a wide range of variables believed to be of key import in the spread of HIV; it can also be used, with some data manipulation, on a PC, and its output is readily usable in terms of recognised demographic indicators. The model is constructed to require the input of population data, and assumptions relating to epidemiological and behavioural parameters for the context in which it is to be used. For the population section, data in the form of a population structure by five-year age intervals and sex for a chosen base year (ideally from a census of some accuracy) is required. Total fertility rates (the average number of lifetime births per woman according to cross-sectional age rates, or TFRs), the age pattern of fertility, and mortality levels for males and females – typically represented by life expectancy from birth levels – for the base year and subsequent periods also need to be specified. It is these rates that, when used in what may be termed a 'without AIDS' projection, give the demographic profile for future periods that would prevail in the absence of the AIDS epidemic, and which acts as a reference for comparison with the demographic profile that results under the impact of AIDS.

The model considers the population formed by the following partly overlapping groups: individuals subject to blood transfusions, individuals subject to injections, heterosexual females, heterosexual males and bisexual males. If blood transfusion and injections are viewed as playing a minor role in the transmission of the AIDS virus (as we assume for the South African case below), sexual transmission plays a relatively more important role. Since populations are rarely homogeneous in terms of sexual activity the heterosexual males and females, homosexual and bisexual males are distributed to a greater or lesser degree of homogeneity/heterogeneity in terms of the average number of new sexual contacts they have each year, together with the average coital frequency per relationship. Information relating to this area is, as may be expected, not plentiful, and assumptions therefore have to be made. The model also permits different activity groups to vary according to other factors related to sexual activity, in particular the prevalence of genital ulcers and level of condom use.

Regarding epidemiological parameters relating to the progression and transmission of HIV, there remains some uncertainty among analysts – for example, the conversion distribution (from seroprevalence to AIDS) over time demonstrates a high variance – although information has increased for many of the epidemiological parameters. For instance, in terms of the interval from exposure to the virus to the development of specific antibodies, we now know that periods of more than 6 months are quite unusual.[10] Regarding other parameters, there is less concrete evidence; for example, as Anderson and Medley have noted, 'with the exception of the perinatally infected child, knowledge of the incubation period of AIDS in the major risk groups will continue to accumulate slowly. It will be a decade or more before we fully understand what fraction of those infected will develop AIDS and on what time scale.'[11] The model assumes an interval of 6–8 years for the period between time of infection and the development of AIDS for sexually-active adults and, in terms of the interval between the onset of AIDS and death, an average of 11 months.[12]

A further significant area in modelling the effects of HIV infection on ultimate demographic impact, and which appears to demonstrate variation according to a variety of factors, is infectivity. The infectiousness of a partner appears to be a function of, *inter alia*, gender, co-factors (such as the presence of STD) and the stage of disease in the individual, as well as behavioural factors such as the use of condoms. Male-to-female transmission appears to be relatively more efficient than vice versa. Given that the presence of genital ulcers in the female has been associated with increased frequency of acquiring the AIDS virus, a high prevalence of genital ulcers may be one of the reasons that explains the high male to female ratio of transmission in Africa.[13] HIV seropositivity appears to be correlated with the presence of other STDs. While the acquisition of both STDs and the AIDS virus may result from a common cause, a further link is plausible: open lesions may facilitate susceptibility to acquiring the virus.

The question of how infectiousness changes throughout the incubation period remains a speculative one. One hypothesis suggests that there may be two periods of peak infectiousness, one shortly after infection and a second one as individuals progress towards the latter component part of the time-span between infection and AIDS proper.[14]

As in the case for other epidemiological factors, however, '(I)t is unlikely that knowledge will accumulate rapidly in this area, and hence current estimates of the probability of transmission, either defined per partner contact . . . or per sex act . . . must be regarded as tentative.'[15]

THE INPUT DATA FOR SOUTH AFRICA

The demographic input for South Africa makes use of a 'reconstructed' population structure by age and sex from the 1985 Census.[16] Initial runs of the model to include back projection periods to the year 1975 (using other published sources for the 1985 population structure unadjusted for underreporting) indicated that there had been serious problems with the accuracy of the population profile, particularly at the youngest age.[17] In terms of the assumed levels of fertility and mortality for future periods, we adopted those rates given in the University of South Africa's Bureau of Market Research's report, which assumes a steady and consistent decline in average fertility levels for the black population in the period 1985–

Table 6.1 Assumptions for levels of male and female life expectancy levels, and for the total fertility rate, South African black population, 1985–2010

Period	1985–90	1990–5	1995–2000	2000–5	2005–10
Male	56.9	58.9	60.9	63.0	64.0
Female	64.0	65.9	67.7	69.3	70.0
TFR	5.12	4.86	4.60	4.32	4.10

Source 1985–2005, Bureau of Market Research, University of South Africa; 2005–10 figures author's assumptions.

2005, and improving mortality levels over the same period. Since we wished to extend the period of projection slightly further, to 2010, we took levels of fertility and mortality that continued this trend for five-year period not covered by the Bureau. The levels adopted are shown in Table 6.1.

While there have been cases traced to the source of contaminated blood products in South Africa this route of transmission has played a relatively minor role in the country, and all donated blood has been screened since 1985. We have therefore assumed for this analysis that blood is screened and that neither blood products nor infection from injection is a cause of HIV transmission.

Given the lacuna of data relating to sexual behaviour, the input regarding this area has had to be set arbitrarily, with assumptions being made regarding the relative proportions in different subgroups, the average number of sexual partners per year, and the average coital frequency per new contact per year among these groups.

While we have attempted to use figures that may be considered plausible, it must be emphasised that without supporting information they remain 'guestimates'. Table 6.2 shows the assumptions relating to sub-groups, numbers of new sexual partners and coital frequency per new contact.

The scenario shown in the table thus assumes a proportion of the population to demonstrate a low level of sexual activity – for example, 20 per cent of heterosexual females and 15 per cent of the heterosexual males are assumed to have only 0.02 new sexual contacts per year – with only one new sexual contact therefore over a lifetime. An intermediate group has a higher rate of 0.05. Almost 40 per cent of both females and males are assumed to have two and

Table 6.2 Assumptions relating to the distribution of adult heterosexual population according to sexual activity group size, average number of new contacts per year, and average coital frequency per new sexual contact

	\multicolumn{5}{c}{Sexual activity group distribution}
	1	2	3	4	5
Heterosexual females	0.2	0.3	0.399	0.1	0.001
Heterosexual males	0.15	0.2	0.4	0.2	0.05
Average number of new sexual contacts per year					
Heterosexual females	0.02	0.05	2	4	145
Heterosexual males	0.02	0.05	3	6	15
Average coital frequency per new sexual contact per year					
Heterosexual females	75	104	14	6	1
Heterosexual males	75	104	14	6	1

Notes Homosexual and bisexual men are assumed to form a negligible component of the black South African adult population at 0.01 per cent.

Scenario 2 assumes males in sexual activity groups 3 and 4 have 5 and 8 partners respectively, and Scenario 3 that females in activity groups 3 and 4 have 3 and 5 partners respectively, males 4 and 7.

three new sexual contacts per year respectively, with an average coital frequency of 14 per partnership, while a higher activity group comprised of 10 and 20 per cent of women and men are more sexually active (in terms of partners) with 4 and 6 new partners per year and a coital frequency of 6 per partnership. A fraction of women are very active with around three new partners per week of one sexual contact each, while some 5 per cent of men are very sexually mobile with 15 new contacts per year of one sexual contact each. The parameters in Table 6.2 above represent 'AIDS Scenario I'.

AIDS Scenario II is constructed by varying the numbers of partners (but not the average coital frequency) for males in the third and fourth risk groups, which increase from 3 and 6 to 5 and 8 respectively. AIDS Scenario III is represented by the third and fourth activity groups of both females and males all increasing their average numbers of new partners a year by one, to 3 and 5 respectively for women and to 4 and 7 for males.

The decision was made to vary partner numbers in this analysis for the following reasons. We know that estimates of average coital frequencies per sexual contact are more uncertain than sexual contact numbers. Second, in terms of policy implications, the number of new sexual partners per year is a more meaningful unit to consider than average coital frequency per partnership.

In this analysis we assume a greater efficiency of transmission from male to female than vice versa, and that there are two peaks of infectiousness, with the highest infectivity at the stage of immediately prior to outright AIDS. The rates adopted in the successive infectivity periods are 0.0036, 0.0029, 0.0016, 0.0022, 0.0034 and 0.0051 for infected male-to-female transmission, and 0.0018, 0.0015, 0.0008, 0.0010, 0.0017 and 0.0025 for infected female-to-male transmission.[18] In the absence of other information we have assumed a low level of condom use: zero use for the two lowest activity groups, and 1 per cent among the three highest sexual activity risk groups. Genital ulcers are assumed to be prevalent among all groups, but increasing with the sexual activity group, and with increasing activity measured by new partners per year. Furthermore, we assume that condom use reduces the probability of HIV transmission on average by 70 per cent,[19] and that a negative relationship exists between condom use and presence of genital ulcers of 80 per cent.

In terms of levels of HIV infection, we took a level of HIV within the band 119 000–168 000 estimated by Padayachee and Schall in their 'direct' estimates for the year 1990 in a recent analysis.[20] Stressing the lack of adequate data[21] but using existing case data, they estimate the likely numbers of HIV-infected black South Africans at between 45 000 and 63 000 at the end of 1989; between 119 000 and 168 000 by the end of 1990; and 317 000–446 000 by the end of 1991. These figures, if correct, very much serve to put the relatively low number of reported AIDS cases to date into perspective.[22]

For the projections we ran the model iteratively until we obtained levels of HIV infection for adults in South Africa for 1990 approximately in the mid-band of Padayachee and Schall's estimates (that is, in the region of 140 000).

PROJECTION RESULTS

First we projected the South African black population in 1985 through the year 2010, representing the 'without AIDS' scenario. Then the model was re-run for the same period, this time incorporating the assumptions regarding the various parameters outlined above.

Using the parameters outlined in Table 6.2 for Scenario I the

Table 6.3 Numbers of HIV cases in the adult black population, 1990–2009, under the three AIDS scenarios (000s)

Year	Scenario I	Scenario II	Scenario III
1990	144	149	141
1991	198	222	221
1992	268	319	336
1993	351	438	490
1994	449	571	680
1995	556	719	894
1996	674	879	1119
1997	792	1042	1340
1998	914	1201	1542
1999	1036	1352	1729
2000	1156	1491	1898
2001	1275	1621	2055
2002	1386	1731	2195
2003	1490	1833	2319
2004	1585	1928	2429
2005	1671	2004	2528
2006	1751	2079	2620
2007	1824	2153	2706
2008	1890	2214	2785
2009	1950	2278	2861
2010	2007	2344	2934

number of HIV adult cases in 1990 is 144 000, for Scenario II 149 000 and for Scenario III 141 000. In order to adopt the number of partners for the three scenarios and keep other variables constant it was necessary to allow slightly different levels of HIV prevalence to prevail in 1990. However, while the three scenarios represent levels of HIV infection of increasing severity, this nevertheless cannot be explained simply by different levels at this date; the Scenario III level of HIV infection is the lowest – 141 000 – in 1990, but exceeds the other two scenarios at an early stage. If the 1990 level for Scenario III matched either Scenarios I or II, then the differential between Scenario III and the other two would be even more exaggerated.

Table 6.3 and Figure 6.1 show the rates of HIV prevalence among the adult population for the period up to 2010 as calculated by the model. All three show a steady rise, with Scenario III showing the steepest and strongest increase. At each successive quinquennium, assuming no interventions, the difference in the estimated number of HIV infections between Scenario I and Scenario III widens, from

```
         3000
         2500
         2000
Thousands
         1500
         1000
          500
            0
            1990      1995      2000      2005      2010
                              Year
```

+ AIDS Scenario 1   □ AIDS Scenario 2   × AIDS Scenario 3

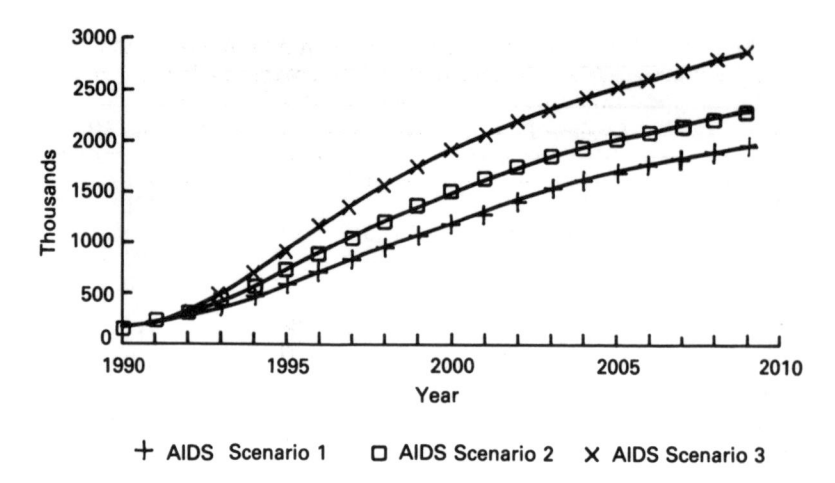

Figure 6.1 Simulated numbers of HIV
infections in the adult South African black
population 1990–2010: three scenarios

338 000 in 1995 to 742 000 in the year 2000, 857 000 by 2005 and 927 000 in the year 2010. This additional number of cases represents a large additional momentum whose demographic effects would not be seen until after the end of our projection period.

Table 6.4 and Figure 6.2 show these numbers of HIV cases as proportions of the population aged 15 and over. These increase for Scenario I from 0.9 per cent of this age group in 1990 to a peak of close to 7 per cent. For Scenario II a peak of just over 8 per cent is observed, while for Scenario III the peak rises above 10 per cent. In all three cases, there has been some levelling off from the 2005 period. Two points need to be made: these numbers of HIV infections consist of a high percentage of the 15–45 age group. Since older age groups are less at risk of infection it may be useful to consider the percentages if a narrower group is considered; this results in 9.48 per cent of the adult population aged 15–45 being HIV positive by the end of our projection period for Scenario I, 11.11 per cent for Scenario II and 14.07 per cent for Scenario III (Table 6.4). Second, it must be emphasised that these results hold only for the conditions specified.

When we examine demographic indicators, it is clear that they are affected in all projections, with Scenario III causing more serious

Table 6.4 Percentage of the adult black South African population HIV positive under three AIDS scenarios as a percentage of all adults aged 15 and over, and as a percentage of 15–45 year olds

	Scenario I	Scenario II	Scenario III
1990			
All adults	0.90	0.94	0.89
15–45	1.18	1.22	1.16
1995			
All adults	3.0	3.88	4.83
15–45	3.94	5.09	6.33
2000			
All adults	5.39	6.96	8.87
15–45	7.14	9.19	11.71
2005			
All adults	6.74	8.13	10.30
15–45	8.97	10.79	13.67
2010			
All adults	7.11	8.39	10.65
15–45	9.48	11.14	14.07

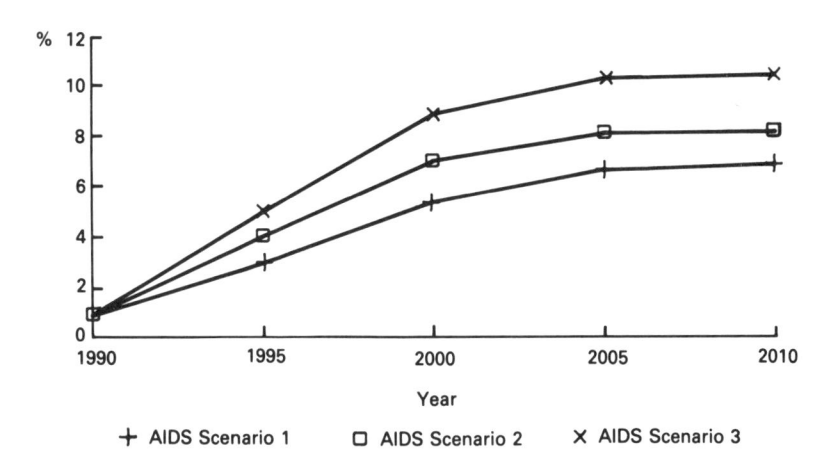

Figure 6.2 Pecentage of the adult black South African population HIV positive, 1990–2010, under three scenarios

Table 6.5 Demographic indicators under 'without AIDS' and three AIDS scenarios

	1985–90	1990–5	1995–2000	2000–5	2005–10
CDRs (per thousand)					
'Without AIDs'	9.4	8.2	7.3	6.5	6.2
Scenario I	9.4	8.6	8.6	9.2	10.1
Scenario II	9.4	8.6	8.9	10.0	11.1
Scenario III	9.4	8.6	9.9	10.9	12.6
Infant mortality rates (per thousand)					
'Without AIDs'	70	61.0	52.7	43.9	41.3
Scenario I	70	62.2	56.5	50.9	48.9
Scenario II	70	62.3	57.6	52.8	50.9
Scenario III	70	62.5	58.9	55.3	54.2
Life expectancy (male) in year					
'Without AIDs'	56.9	58.9	60.9	63.0	64
Scenario I	56.8	58.1	58.0	57.1	55.5
Scenario II	56.8	58.1	57.4	55.4	53.7
Scenario III	56.8	58.1	56.9	53.9	51.4
Life expectancy (female) in year					
'Without AIDs'	64.0	65.9	67.7	69.8	70
Scenario I	64.0	65.0	64.3	62.5	60.4
Scenario II	64.0	64.9	63.5	60.8	58.0
Scenario III	64.0	64.8	62.6	58.4	54.9

deviations from the 'without AIDS' scenario. Table 6.5 and Figure 6.3 show the trend in crude death rates (CDRs) 'without AIDS' and under the three scenarios. Without AIDS CDRs were projected to decline smoothly over the period. In contrast, with all scenarios this anticipated decline is halted and reversed from the 1990–5 period. By the end of the projection period all three scenarios show a wide differential from the 'without AIDS' rate, with Scenario I resulting in death rates reaching 10.1 per thousand by the end of the period, Scenario II 11.1 per thousand, and Scenario III resulting in the greatest differential, CDRs in this scenario reaching 12.6 per thousand (double the 6.2 per thousand for the 'without AIDS' rate).

Levels of infant mortality, assumed 'without AIDS' to fall consistently throughout the projection period to reach a low of 41.3 per thousand by the end of the projection period, under the AIDS

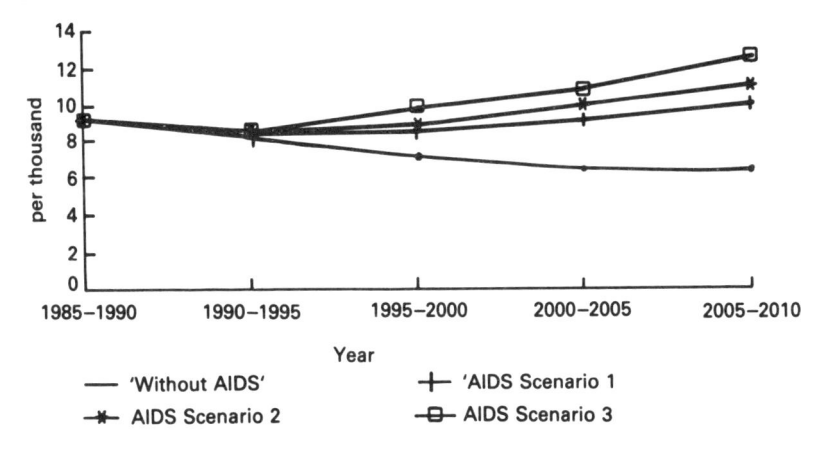

Figure 6.3 Death rates, South African black population, 1985–2010, 'without AIDS' and under three scenarios

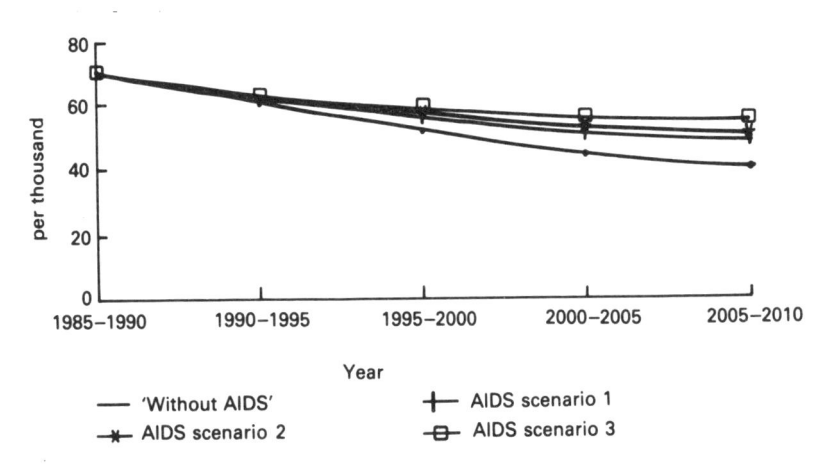

Figure 6.4 Infant mortality rates, South African black population, 1985–2010, 'without AIDS' and under three scenarios

scenarios experience a stemming of that decline (Table 6.5 and Figure 6.4). The rates for the three scenarios indicate rates of 48.9, 50.9 and 54.2 respectively. Levels of infant mortality probably underestimate the effects of the AIDS epidemic at very young ages since they exclude those deaths which occur in early childhood but which take place after infancy (the first year of life).

```
  70
  60
  50
  40
  30
  20
  10
   0
```

Number of years

1985–1990 1990–1995 1995–2000 2000–2005 2005–2010

Year

— Without AIDS   + AIDS scenario 1
✳ AIDS scenario 2   ▣ AIDS scenario 3

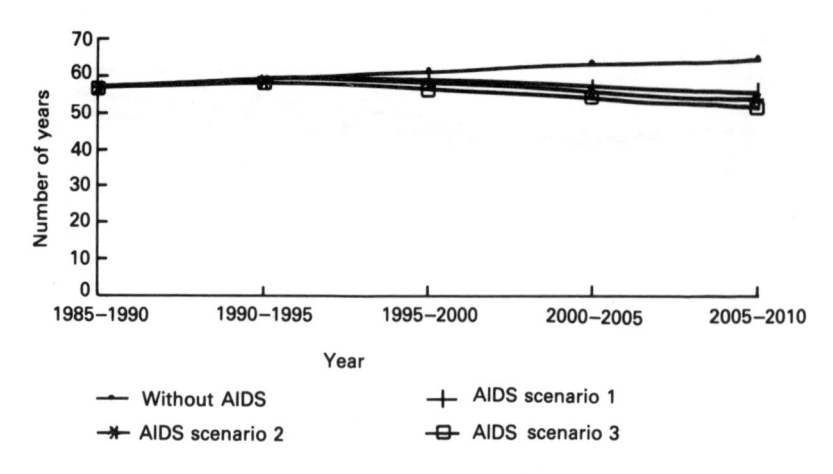

Figure 6.5   Life expectancy for South African
male black population, 1985–2010,
'without AIDS' and under three scenarios

The potential effects on levels of life expectancy are increasingly pronounced as the projection period progresses for all three scenarios (see Table 6.5 and Figures 6.5 and 6.6). For the 'without AIDS' scenario the life expectancy levels of both males and females were assumed to be set to increase steadily over the period, for males rising from 56.9 years in the 1985–90 period to 63 in the period 2000–5. For females a rise from 64 years to 69.8 in the same period was anticipated, giving around seven years of 'female excess'. All three AIDS scenarios alter that trend. By the end of the projection male life expectancy is estimated at only 55.5 for Scenario I, 53 for Scenario II and 51.4 years for Scenario III, a differential of between 8.5 and 12.6 years for Scenarios I and III respectively, compared with the 'without AIDS' scenario. In the case of females the differential ranges from 9.6 years (Scenario I) to 15.1 (Scenario III) compared with the 'without AIDS' scenario. It is also of note that over the projection period the male–female differential narrows substantially, at the end of the projection period dropping to 4.9 years, 4.3 years, and 3.5 years respectively for Scenarios I, II and III.

In terms of population size, by the end of the projection period effects are still modest; focusing on the broad key working age group of those aged 15–45 the shortfall between the 'without AIDS' scenario and the three AIDS scenarios are 538 000, 670 000 and 842 000 respectively (see Table 6.6). These are not insignificant numbers, but neither are they catastrophic. These more moderate effects on

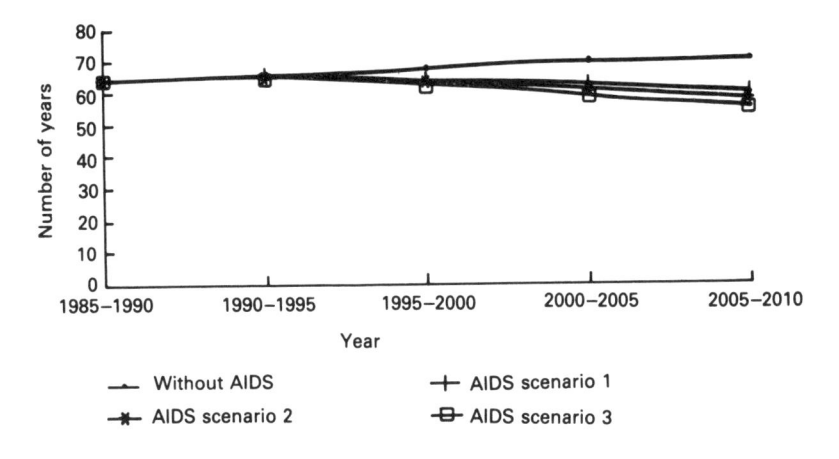

Figure 6.6 Life Expectancy, South African female black population, 1985–2010, 'without AIDS' and under three scenarios

Table 6.6 Population (000s) aged 15–45 'without AIDS' and under three AIDS scenarios

Scenario	2000	2005	2010
'Without AIDS'	16 349	18 903	21 702
Scenario I	16 250	18 368	21 164
Scenario II	16 231	18 573	21 032
Scenario III	16 215	18 499	20 860

population size and growth rates even in the face of a reasonably serious AIDS epidemic are not unique; other studies have reported similar results.[23] However, there are two important qualifications to that remark: first, it must be reiterated that these results hold only under the assumptions given and, second, the above figures for HIV infection suggest a large momentum within the population figures co-existing simultaneously with the shortfall figures that obtain up to the year 2010.

In terms of the rate of natural increase of the population, while the rates are reduced, they remain positive (Table 6.7 and Figure 6.7). For the period of the projections a rate of natural increase (RNI) which was close to 3 per cent in 1985 was gradually reduced to 2.57 by the end of the projection period under the 'without AIDS' scenario. Under the various AIDS scenarios, these rates are lower and the differential widens as the projection period progresses. By the year

Table 6.7 Rate of natural increase, 'without AIDS' and under three AIDS scenarios (%)

Scenario	1990–5	1995–2000	2000–5	2005–10
'Without AIDS'	2.85	2.77	2.67	2.57
Scenario I	2.85	2.68	2.42	2.22
Scenario II	2.85	2.68	2.34	2.13
Scenario III	2.85	2.58	2.25	2.00

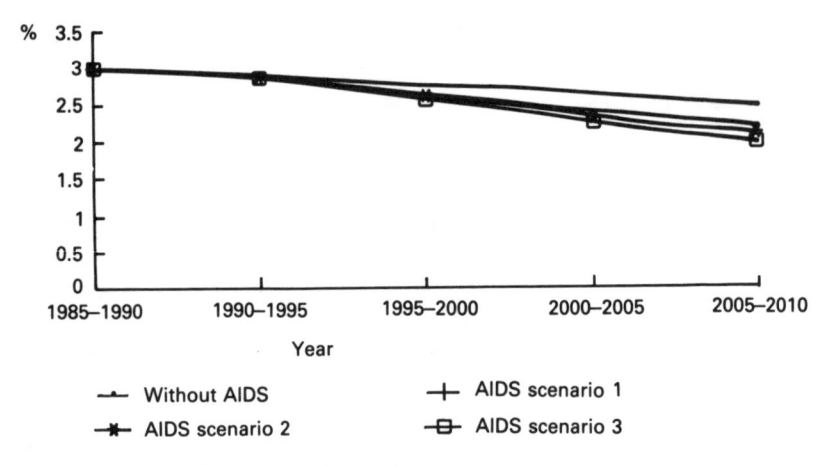

Figure 6.7 Rate of natural increase of the South African black population, 1985–2010, 'without AIDS' and under three scenarios

2000, for example, the RNI is around 2.6 for all three scenarios compared with 2.77 per cent for the 'without AIDS' scenario. Similarly, in the following quinquennia, the rate would have been 2.67 per cent but is reduced to 2.42, 2.34 and 2.25 per cent respectively. By the end of the projection the differential between the 'without AIDS' and the worst case scenario is in the order of some 0.57 per cent. The rate of natural increase of the population is, then, reduced but not eradicated, at least under these assumptions.

DISCUSSION

Outside the male homosexual group South Africa experienced a relatively late onset of HIV infection, but the second phase, which potentially can affect a very large proportion of the population, now appears to be clearly embedded. Projections provide some indications of what the effects of given levels of HIV in the population may be.

What we can say in the light of the many caveats and qualifications given above is that, even using what we consider to be fairly conservative assumptions (Scenario I), and a level of HIV infection of around 144 000 in 1990, there could be profound impacts on major demographic indicators. On the basis of more liberal assumptions, particularly relating to average numbers of new sexual partners a year, the impact worsens sharply, creating a large momentum of HIV cases which will exert their effects after our projection period. To put the effects on one of the indicators in the context, the levels of life expectancy for men obtained in Scenario III – in the low to mid-fifties – are comparable to those currently prevailing in countries such as Tanzania and Zambia.[24]

Our conclusion regarding the percentage of the adult population that could be HIV positive during the projection period is more conservative than some other estimates,[25] illustrating the significance of the assumptions underpinning each analysis. Different analyses do offer a range of estimates of the trajectory which, with our current information, we believe the AIDS pandemic may follow; but there remains a wide margin of error. For example, there is a particular need for information on sexual networking, an area much neglected in the past not just in the South African context, and not least because of the difficulties of obtaining accurate and meaningful data.[26] Good quality information would enhance our understanding of the main mode by which HIV is transmitted in South Africa.[27] The problems of collecting data on such sensitive and delicate topics cannot be overestimated.[28]

Specific areas that merit attention are the relative sizes of the different sexual activity groups; the rate of partner change between different groups and observed patterns of behaviour regarding serial and simultaneous sexual mobility; information relating to coital frequency in different relationships (marital and non-formal union types, prostitution, casual and other liasons); the extent to which prostitutes and more sexually mobile males have repeated sexual contact with the same individual; the typical 'combinations' of casual and other types of sexual relationships among those individuals who are more sexually mobile, and how simultaneously engaging in more than one sexual relationship affects the coital frequency in each of them. Data on sexual behaviour also needs to be carefully acquired with reference to specific time-periods over which behaviour takes place.[29]

There are particular features of the South African context that particularly merit attention. One such is the phenomenon of migrant labour:[30] the extent to which mine-workers are a high-risk group (or at least at higher risk than other groups of males) appears to be a matter of some debate.[31]

An additional aspect of sexual networking that would appear to merit particular attention in the South African context is the intergenerational nature of relationships, sexual behaviour between adolescents, and between them and older groups. A male preference for younger females, note Anderson, May and McLean,[32] could have important implications for the potential demographic impact of AIDS in developing countries, where the primary route is through heterosexual activity.

In addition, qualitative data relating to sexual behaviour – how decisions relating to sexual behaviour are formulated, gender power relations and the degree to which women can exercise control over the conditions under which sexual activity occurs, particularly in relation to exposure to unsafe or unwanted sexual activity – would provide important contextual information. Moreover, building up a body of information relating to sexual networking in conjunction with timely, accurate and nationally representative HIV prevalence data would greatly assist in characterising the nature of the AIDS epidemic in South Africa as well as its pace and progress.

In this analysis we have not considered the effects of behavioural change in terms of condom use. It is possible to use models such as the one we have to assess what the effects of changes in this parameter may have. Analyses have typically shown, not surprisingly, that increased condom use can alter the course of the epidemic and reduce its impact.[33] While it is easy to incorporate such changes into the model, two important points need to be made. First, the likelihood of achieving the levels of condom use that can make an impact on the epidemic must be assessed realistically, given the plethora of constraints on both the demand and supply side. From what we currently know of the South African context, increasing the level of condom use is not likely to be easy,[34] and it may be more realistic to estimate what ultimate effects only small increases in condom use may have. Second, changes in attitudes to condom use may occur, but may happen as part of other changes in sexual behaviour. There may, for example, be increased condom use and yet no alteration in numbers of sexual contacts, or no change in condom use but a reduction in numbers of sexual contacts, or a reduction in contacts and increased condom use. Quite simply, at this stage we know too little about current patterns of sexual networking in South Africa to speculate about in what ways sexual behaviour, sexual networking and condom use among different groups will change.

What we do know, however, is that HIV is present and growing in the South African population; that demographic effects are unlikely to be negligible; and certainly that further research now may prove of great benefit for the future.

Acknowledgements

The author acknowledges the assistance of Rodolfo Bulatao and Eduard Bos of the Population and Human Resources Department at the World Bank, Washington, in making available the 'PRAY' AIDS model.

References

1. Grania Christie, 'AIDS in South Africa', undated paper, AIDS Centre, South African Institute for Medical Research, Johannesburg.
2. Ibid.
3. The apparently rapid spread of HIV is reflected in the reported doubling times of male and female STD attenders. Figures of 10.7 and 9.8 months respectively, and 6.6 months for female family planning attenders have been given. Among these three groups the HIV infection rate was 1.56 per cent, 1.37 per cent and 1.91 per cent, respectively. These samples were, however, small and, as with much of the data on doubling times, relate to specific geographical areas (in this case, predominantly the Witwatersrand area). Nevertheless, these and other figures from around the country indicate a continuing silent spread of the disease. See 'Considerations on the further expansion of the AIDS epidemic in SA, 1990', *SA Medical Journal*, by five Wits Watersrand University Virology Department professors and two Johannesburg City Health Department doctors, and reported in *Business Day*, 19 June 1990. See also Alan Whiteside, 'AIDS in Southern Africa: a position paper for the Development Bank of Southern Africa', Economic Research Unit, University of Natal and Development Bank of Southern Africa, 1990.
4. G.N. Padayachee and R. Schall, 'Short-term predictions of the prevalence of human immunodeficiency virus infection among the black population of South Africa', *South African Medical Journal*, 77 (1990), pp. 329–33. They consider various forecasting models according to five

categories: extrapolation, the direct method, back projection, macro-level, and micro-level models.
5. R.M. Anderson, R.M. May and R.R. McLean, 'Possible demographic consequences of AIDS in developing countries', *Nature*, 332, pp. 228–32. See also R.M. Anderson, 'The impact of the spread of HIV on population growth and age structure in developing countries', in Alan F. Fleming, Manuel Carballo, David W. FitzSimons, Michael R. Bailey and Jonathan Mann. *The Global Impact of AIDS* (New York: Alan R. Liss, 1988), pp. 95–106.
6. John Bongaarts, 'Modelling the spread of HIV and the demographic impact of AIDS in Africa', The Population Council, Center for Policy Studies Working Papers, No. 140, October 1988.
7. Peter O. Way and Karen Stanecki, 'The demographic impact of an AIDS epidemic on an African country: application of the iwgAIDS model', US Bureau of the Census, Center for International Research, Staff Paper No. 58, 1991.
8. Developed by Rodolfo Bulatao and Eduard Bos, Population and Human Resources Division, The World Bank. See *PRAY: Projecting the Demographic Impact of AIDS* (Washington, DC: The World Bank, 1991). Rodolfo A. Bulatao, 'Projecting the demographic impact of the HIV epidemic using standard parameters', unpublished paper, The World Bank, Washington, DC, 1988.
9. Kenneth Hill, 'PROJ3S – a computer program for population projections', The Johns Hopkins University, School of Hygiene and Public Health, 1990.
10. Peter D. Glasner and Richard A. Kaslow, 'The epidemiology of human immunodeficiency virus infection', *Journal of Consulting and Clinical Psychology*, 58 (1990), pp. 13–21.
11. Roy Anderson and Graham F. Medley, 'Epidemiology of HIV infection and AIDS: incubation and infectious periods, survival and vertical transmission', *AIDS*, 2, suppl. 1 (1988), pp. 57–63.

    In transfusion-infected patients estimates of the mean latency period have ranged from 4.5–15 years, the most recent of which showed a mean of 8 years for those in the 5–59 age group; see Glasner and Kaslow, 'The Epidemiology'.
12. A summary of estimates of median survival times of AIDS patients reported by Anderson and Medley, 'Epidemiology', indicated a range of 9–13 months.
13. Glasner and Kaslow, 'The Epidemiology'.
14. Anderson and Medley, 'Epidemiology'.
15. Ibid.
16. J.L. Sadie, 'A reconstruction and projection of demographic movement in the RSA and TBVC countries', Bureau of Market Research, University of South Africa, Research Report no. 148, 1988.
17. For example, the demographic projection model estimates the level of TFRs that would have been prevailing in the five-year period prior to the base year according to the numbers in the 0–4 age group, in conjunction with assumed infant mortality rates. The calculated TFR was significantly lower than what would be anticipated and also lower than the level

assumed to be prevailing in 1985. This indicated a substantial underreporting of those in the 0–4 age group and, one may speculate, of the 0–1 age group in particular since this group has, in many contexts, a tendency to be underreported.
18. Transmission rates from a mother to her infant are assumed to be 0.64, 0.52, 0.28, 0.40, 0.60, 0.90 and 0.90 over successive infectivity periods. These rates are also those adopted in some World Bank runs of the PRAY model for other sub-Saharan African countries.
19. The degree to which condom use can assist in reducing the probability of transmission depends, of course, on a range of factors including, *inter alia*, the quality of the condom and the extent to which it is used in the correct manner through all the aspects of its utilisation (the latter aspect is obviously difficult to measure).
20. Padayachee and Schall, 'Short-term predictions'.
21. R. Schall, G.N. Padayachee and D. Yach, 'The case for HIV surveillance in South Africa', *South African Medical Journal*, 77 (1990), pp. 324–5.
22. The reported cumulative number of cases of AIDS in South Africa are as follows: 84 reported cases in 1987, 170 in 1988, 305 in 1989 and 554 to 1 November 1990. The WHO's estimates for the equivalent years are 1800, 31 000, 4900, and 7150.
23. Peter O. Way and Karen Stanecki, 'How bad will it be? Modelling the AIDS epidemic in Eastern Africa', paper prepared for the Annual Meeting of the American Association for Advancement of Science, Washington, DC, February 1991.
24. *Population Data Sheet, 1990* (Population Reference Bureau, Washington, DC).
25. A figure of 27 per cent of the black population, mainly in the 25–40 age group, infected by 2005 has been suggested by a Metropolitan Life study, reported in the *Financial Mail*, 24 May 1991. Other estimates – for example, by Padayachee – suggest 20–25 per cent of the population aged between 15 and 62 years could be HIV positive by 1999. See also Dr Jack van Niftrik , 'South African Consensus on Modelling', *AID Analysis Africa*, 2, 2 (August/September 1991).
26. It is of note that the WHO has initiated a new research initiative on sexual behaviour and reproductive health worldwide: see 'New research initiative on sexual behaviour and reproductive health', WHO Special Programme of Research, Development and Research Training in Human Reproduction, Task Force for Social Science Research on Reproductive Health.

Although these studies will be small-scale or exploratory studies rather than large-scale or national ones, they do focus on areas pertinent in the spread of AIDS.

A collection of studies on sexual networking is also presented in T. Dyson (ed.), *Sexual Behaviour and Networking: Anthropological and Socio-Cultural Studies on the Transmission of HIV*, forthcoming early 1992, International Union for Scientific Study of Population, Liège, Belgium.
27. In the South African context the author knows of one study of sexual

networking in the environs of a mine, but of no others at present.
28. See Wolf Bleek, 'Lying informants: a fieldwork experience in Ghana', *Population and Development Review*, 13, 2 (1987), pp. 314–22, for a pessimistic view on surveys relating to delicate issues.

   In his fieldwork in southern Ghana, Bleek noted the falsification of answers to survey questions asked by nurses, with the presentation of behaviour reported by respondents apparently conditioned by the desire to gain the nurse interviewer's respect, rather than by a willingness accurately to report actual behaviour patterns.
29. An example of a carefully executed study on this area is 'Sexual relationships, use and condoms, and perceptions of AIDS in an urban area of Guinea-Bissau with a high prevalence of HIV 2', in Dyson, *Sexual Behaviour*.
30. Karen Jochelson, Monyaola Mothibeli and Jean Leger, 'Restoring miners' family lives will help control AIDS', *Business Day*, 29 May 1991.
31. D.I. Foure, Medical Adviser, Chamber of Mines, has argued that the vast majority of mine workers do not have sexual behavioural patterns that place them at a greater risk for HIV than similar groups of males (Response to Jochelson, Mothibeli and Leger in *Business Day*, June 1991).
32. Roy Anderson, S. Gupta and W. Ng, 'The significance of sexual partner contact networks for the transmission dynamics of HIV', *Journal of Acquired Immuno-Deficiency Syndromes*, 3 (1990), pp. 417–29; and R.M. Anderson, R.M. May, M.C. Boily, G.P. Garnett and J.T. Rowley, 'The spread of HIV-1 in Africa: sexual contact patterns and the predicted demographic impact of AIDS', *Nature*, 352 (15 August 1991).
33. Rodolfo A. Bulatao and Eduard Bos, 'Implications of control measures for the spread of HIV infection', unpublished paper, The World Bank, Washington, DC, 1988.
34. Sharon Kingman, 'Sisters of the Revolution', *The Independent on Sunday*, 2 June 1991, reports on an AIDS counselling project in Soweto where the problems involved in attempting to increase condom use are pronounced; see also Anna Strebel, of the University of the Western Cape, Seminar on 'Women and AIDS in South Africa', London School of Hygiene, July 1991.

Part III

Economic Assessments for South Africa

7 A Socio-Economic Analysis of the Long-Run Effects of AIDS in South Africa
Sholto Cross

INTRODUCTION

The economic consequences of the AIDS epidemic in South Africa will be unique. While South Africa shares some of the characteristics of neighbouring countries in Africa (and indeed historic experience) in the matter of epidemics, the combination of the peculiar characteristics of AIDS with South Africa's highly specific economic and demographic state means that the course of this disease will be without parallel elsewhere.

This chapter addresses some of the most general considerations as to the broad nature of this impact. Detailed studies on the national labour force, and projections of mortality and morbidity due to AIDS, are addressed in Part II. Bringing together the data on projected demographic impact, and the scale and type of economic consequence, raises many profoundly difficult questions. How far down the chain of cause-and-effect is it possible (and reasonable) to go in considering this dimension of AIDS? To what extent can new modes of economic activity – perhaps less labour- and skill-intensive – which can be attributed to the loss by disease of significant economically active cohorts be anticipated, and quantified? Trotter demonstrates in Chapter 9 the very wide band of estimates to which an economic assessment of the AIDS impact, using the 'cost of human capital' approach, leads. Broomberg and his colleagues, in their attempt to sum the direct and indirect costs of AIDS, present in Chapter 8 an essentially financial (rather than economic) assessment of this issue, and argue for a direct cost range of R4–10 billion for the year 2000, with additional indirect costs up to three times this amount (declining in a ratio of 3.2:1 to 1.3:1 by 2000).

Moving beyond the direct costs, what can be said about the most general impact on socio-economic development of a change in mortality figures for certain sections of the population? And over what time periods is it possible to make any predictions?

In discussing issues arising from these questions, this chapter will concentrate on presenting an assessment of some of the less obviously quantifiable considerations. It will also attempt to bring into the picture some of the political dimensions which may arise from the differential impact of the disease on sections of the South African people.

The argument presented here surrounds a few related propositions. These concern, first, the nature of the South African economy and population structure, which presents a unique constellation of features for the impact of AIDS in relation to any economy and society in the 1990s.[1] While it is no longer the case (if this ever was a useful concept) that there is in any sense a dual economy, South Africa certainly has a dualistic population structure. This is likely to be undergoing very rapid change, predominantly as a consequence of urbanisation, but the skewing effects will persist for some time. The demographic context for the epidemic is accordingly wholly different from that of any other country.

Second, AIDS is likely to have a highly-differentiated impact on this population. Enormous variations in economic consequence will flow from the specific cohorts which do in fact suffer significantly higher than normal rates of morbidity and mortality.

Third, for each of these socio-economically defined cohorts or target groups it will then be important to assess the nature of the costs at different levels: that of the household, the economic sector and the national economy. Each level offers a different mix of factors for assessing the impact, and various balancing effects. There is useful comparative evidence in particular for the household level on these, and some indications from mono-sectoral economies on what very significant levels of AIDS mortality might imply. The South African case has such a different profile of household dependency ratios and income sources, sectoral substitution effects and manpower bottlenecks, and overall demographic structure that a unique model will have to be developed.

Fourth, this assessment needs to take into account further that the South African economy will be undergoing over the next two decades a multiple process of restructuring simultaneously with the expected major onslaught of AIDS, a process which in itself will present a variety of interactions whose overall consequences are so complex that assessment becomes highly speculative.

Fifth, this takes the argument to the macro level of the consideration between demographic shifts and economic growth. The global impact of AIDS has already opened a new chapter in the development of formal demographic theory and population policies; the case of South Africa will undoubtedly present a most important case-study in the elaboration of this theory. South Africa has its industrial cities with their economic hinterlands inextricably tied to rural labour reserves; a large migrant population based in rural areas for whom agricultural and even subsistence production provides only a small proportion of income; and a combined invasion of both Pattern I and Pattern II HIV infection. Moreover, as Byerley points out,[2] AIDS is likely to spread with a relatively high degree of uniformity throughout the country, which would be a very different pattern from either the rest of Africa or the high-income industrialised countries. In this, South Africa may well prove to be a forerunner of the diffusion pattern for Asian economies, where population densities and the urban–rural interplay suggest the disease may have a major impact.

Finally, the question must be asked what the linkage will be between the political mobilisation of communities concerned with health policies in general and the selective impact of AIDS in particular, and the ability of the state to allocate resources in a rational and sensible manner not just between areas of social spending and other budgetary items, but within the social sector between the competing demands of AIDS and the major areas for the construction of post-apartheid society: namely, education, housing, welfare and non-AIDS-related health matters.

In conclusion, it is argued that there will be an initial paradoxical economic impact of AIDS: over the short term at the macro level, and to some extent determined by the nature of the economic groups affected, the indicators suggest that the economy as a whole may benefit, even while a range of households are forced ever further into a state of unsustainability and poverty. Yet this will soon be followed by a second phase as the epidemic spreads where the direct costs of the loss of in particular skilled manpower are increased by the costs of health care; these costs will be powerfully pressure-group driven, given the peculiar political context of post-apartheid South Africa within which this scenario is likely to unfold. Certainly over the medium term the politically-induced cost will be very high, and perhaps will come to be the dominating issue in the politics of budgetary resource allocation early in the next century.

THE POPULATION STRUCTURE

It must be stated at the outset that it is more than somewhat ironic, indeed it is tragic, that the ethnic categorisations of the South African population should prove apposite for the initial point of departure of this discussion. However, the assumption that South Africa is displaying a combined AIDS epidemiology of Pattern II infection in the black population and Pattern I in the remainder appears to be supported by the preliminary indications of how the epidemic is moving. There is therefore a rational justification for using this statistical terminology although AIDS is a national problem, and population statistics specific to ethnic groups are used purely for functional purposes.

There are several related issues which may be addressed in considering the past, present and projected demographic picture. The first relates to the broad question of the basic relationship between population growth and economic development in South Africa, and in particular to the application of demographic transition theory. The second concerns the nature of dependency ratios, and the direction of movement of these in different sectors of the population which may have different risk profiles of exposure to AIDS.

The debate over the nature of the relationship – and direction of causality – between economic development and population growth is a continuing one. Within this broad debate, the question of the nature of the impact of AIDS on population growth rates is of particular significance.

It has been argued that rapid population growth is itself an engine for economic growth; and that the success in bringing down mortality rates has been a proximate cause in the explosive development of living standards across the international economy.[3] This position has been strongly contested by neo-Malthusian demographers who argue that rapid growth diminishes returns to land and capital, exacerbates income inequalities, and traps large proportions of rapid-growth societies in a vicious cycle of poverty. A particularly important point here is that the implications for economic development of rapid population growth vary considerably from country to country, depending on the nature of the resource base and a host of cultural factors. In the South African case, there is very strong evidence for the neo-Malthusian position: obscured as the situation has been by the social engineering policies of apartheid, nevertheless the intrinsically low levels of employment and the high reproduction rates – in association with a primary-resource based economy with no obvious possibilities for rural involution – mean that there is a strong correlation between high population growth rates and the entrapment in poverty of the majority.[4]

To the extent that AIDS will bring about an overall reduction in population growth rates, there is thus a prima facie case that the effect on economic growth – and of course on per capitum income, although this in itself is no very satisfactory indicator – will from one point of view be positive. Many studies, particularly for Africa, have sought to demonstrate the point that not only in per capitum terms, but also in absolute levels of GDP, declining population growth rates correlate positively with increased growth.[5] However, this level of generality needs to be treated with caution. Even if mortality rates are doubled by the impact of AIDS, this may not of itself necessarily imply very much change in the ratio of dependents to workers, as child mortality is likely to move *pari passu* with adult mortality;[6] and mortality itself does not really address the central issue of the propensity of a society to experience rapid population growth: namely, the fertility rate.

A major review of the arguments on the relationship between population growth and economic development prepared by the World Bank (1984) concluded that the decline in the TFR of a society (defined as the average number of births of women of child-bearing age) provides one of the strongest indicators for the general level of socio-economic development.[7] In a recent review of his path-breaking analysis of this relationship (made 25 years ago in respect of the Indian and Mexican economies), Coale presents the evidence for the way in which less developed countries which have achieved the transition to development have done so chiefly through a rapid and pervasive downward shift in their fertility rates.[8] Even where these have remained fairly high (for example, Mexico), he argues persuasively that they would have been very much higher had the TFR been significantly reduced.

The central point in analysing the demographic impact of AIDS from the macro-economic point of view therefore appears to be that significant and adverse shifts in the health and mortality rate of women of child-bearing age, which will have a direct downward pressure on TFR, should on the face of it be associated with both beneficial effects of increasing incomes and resource availability in per capitum terms, and higher overall growth rates. There is a difficulty with this argument, however. This arises from a closer examination of the causality links in the relationship, and the view that this effect is achieved because it principally reflects voluntaristic means, as potential mothers change their patterns of reproduction in deliberate expectation of enhanced welfare for themselves and their children, rather than as an adventitious and involuntary outcome of death and disease. The precise chain of linkages between declines in TFR and the onset of upward growth in socio-economic prosperity has defied even the most extensive analysis.[9]

In a useful recent examination of these issues for a range of African countries, Lesthaege argues that it is very difficult to generalise about voluntaristic fertility limitation as the evidence suggests that the maintenance of the high reproduction strategy, as an alternative to the Boserupian model of deliberate reduction in family size, varies greatly from region to region, with a host of variables of a highly local nature affecting the explanation.[10] On balance, the demographic situation in South Africa fits fairly closely in some respects with a number of the models addressed by Lesthaege (although it is fair to point out that his samples are ethnic groups). Accordingly, while this view needs to be treated with some caution, a decline in the South African TFR for whatever reason is likely, through various mechanisms referred to in the literature (see especially the World Bank Study of 1984), to have an initially positive effect on nationally aggregated socio-economic indicators.

However, the aggregated picture of the TFR for South Africa is not particularly informative: the figures which are presented in the recent World Development Report on Poverty for South Africa, for example, are hardly revealing in presenting TFR estimates of 6.1, 4.4 and 3.5 for the years 1965, 1988 and 2000, suggesting that South Africa is comfortably average for the upper middle income countries, and on course for population stability in 2020.[11] A more alarming picture emerges from a disaggregation.

Drawing on Coale and a recent demographic projection by Sadie,[12] it is clear that South Africa presents a strongly dualistic picture (see Table 7.1) in terms of demographic structure and economic growth paths. While the TFRs for the white, Asian and coloured population (currently some 25 per cent of the total population, but declining in terms of an AIDS-free projection to 20–22 per cent by the year 2000), are now in the 2.4–2.6 range, which is comparable to the average for high-income economies some 20 years ago, the black TFR at 5.1 (1985–90) is typical for the low end of the low-income economies.

Table 7.1 Age categories and dependency ratios of South African population groups

Period	Age 0–14	groups (%) 15–64	65 +	Dependency ratio
White				
1936	31.2	63.6	5.2	57
1960	32.1	61.2	6.7	63
1970	30.6	62.6	6.8	60
1985	25.2	66.3	8.5	51
2005	22.4	67.3	10.3	49
Asian				
1936	45.7	52.0	2.3	92
1960	45.3	52.7	2.0	90
1970	40.0	58.1	1.9	72
1985	34.1	63.1	2.8	58
2005	25.5	69.0	5.5	45
Coloured				
1936	40.7	55.6	3.7	80
1960	44.3	52.2	3.5	92
1970	45.4	51.4	3.2	95
1985	37.0	59.7	3.3	68
2005	28.6	67.1	4.3	49
Black				
1936	41.4	55.1	3.5	81
1960	43.5	53.0	3.5	89
1970	44.3	52.2	3.5	92
1985	42.9	54.1	3.0	85
2005	39.7	56.8	3.5	76

Source J. L. Sadie, 'A reconstruction and projection of demographic movement in the RSA and TBVC countries', Bureau of Market Research, University of South Africa, Research Report no. 148, 1988.

Global development indicators reveal that TFRs move systematically downwards as societies move on to a growth path (see Table 7.2): it is apparent that South Africa presents a staggered process in this respect. To the extent that AIDS forces a selective decline in black TFR, therefore, this should at the aggregate level be associated with more rapid progress overall up the national growth path.

The implications for the broad economic consequences of this bipolar demographic structure are perhaps more considerable when

Table 7.2 Reductions in the total fertility rate (TFR) for selected developing countries

Country	TFR I	Period I	TFR II	Period II	Reduction (%)
Low Income:					
China	5.9	1966–70	2.6	1977–81	56
India	6.2	1951–60	4.9	1979	21
Low/middle:					
Costa Rica	7.4	1960	3.8	1976	49
Turkey	6.8	1945–49	5.1	1970–74	25
Philippines	6.6	1960	5.1	1960	23
Tunisia	7.3	1965–66	5.9	1974–75	19
Indonesia	5.5	1968	5.0	1977	9
Upper/middle:					
Singapore	6.3	1959	1.9	1977	70
South Korea	6.0	1960	2.9	1976–80	52
Mexico	7.2	1965	4.2	1979	42
Malaysia	6.9	1957	4.3	1976	38
Brazil	6.2	1945–49	4.3	1975–79	31
Venezuela	6.8	1960–64	4.8	1975–79	29
South Africa:					
Coloured	6.4	1955–60	2.9	1985–90	55
Asian	5.2	1955–60	2.6	1985–90	50
White	3.5	1955–60	2.0	1985–90	43
Black	6.8	1951–60	5.1	1985–90	24
All	6.1	1960	4.4	1990–95	28

looking at dependency ratios, especially taking into account the potential impact of AIDS on that sector of the population with a continuing very high dependency ratio.

The dependency ratio profiles of whites, coloureds and Asians on the one hand, and blacks on the other, make this very clear. By the year 2000 (AIDS-free projections) the former population clusters will have more or less converged, with dependency ratios well under 50 per cent (non-working: working population), while the level for blacks – which peaked at over 90 per cent in the late 1970s – appears set to decline only very slowly to the 75–80 per cent bracket (see Table 7.1). Even these figures may well be understating the situation, as the age period for the black economically active population (15–64 years) is unrealistically high at the top end: a recalculation of the figures with the age of 54 as the cut-off point and a less conservative estimate for the share in the total black population of children under 15 years would push the overall dependency rates significantly higher. In comparison with global indicators (see Table 7.2) this staggered, or skewed, population process once again becomes apparent.

We also need to take into account here some of the dynamic processes at work, which suggest that the particular nature of the urbanisation process, and the rural–urban movement of people, has a critically important bearing on the interrelationship between the selective morbidity and mortality of the economically active cohort which will occur as AIDS spreads, and the specific nature of dependency relationships. For this it is necessary to move away from the aggregate picture.

DEPENDENCY RATIOS AT THE HOUSEHOLD LEVEL

The first feature to note is that the demographic structure of the black population in South Africa has been undergoing a major shift over at least the past three decades, and is reaching a moment of accelerated urbanisation during the 1990s just when the effects of the AIDS epidemic are starting to be fully visible. There has been a considerable debate over the nature of internal migration and urbanisation in South Africa, and this chapter will only touch on some of the key features. In general terms, it has been argued that the black population is essentially following a road pioneered by whites and others before them, tracing a path of migration from the dry to the wet rural areas, from rural areas to small towns and employment centres, and finally to a predominantly interurban form of migration.[13] The push–pull model of migration is no longer an accurate description of this process, as May convincingly argues,[14] since migration is now intimately linked to the prospects for survival and the chance to escape from poverty. The removal of artificial barriers to urbanisation will permit this traditional pattern of 'maintained' oscillation to change. However, while a massive influx to the towns can confidently be expected, the flow of workers, job-seekers and remittances between town and country is likely to continue for some time, and the point at which a new equilibrium will be reached is very hard to foresee. It is probable that, as in many parts of urbanising Africa, those within one generation of living in a rural community will wish at least to maintain links with the home area, while there will be substantial regional variation in the degree of maintenance and in the type of urban–rural linkages.

A large part of the unknown here is the extent to which the South African economy will be able to restructure and develop to offer expanding employment opportunities. Given that rural–urban movements are so critically related to the search for employment, the level of access to employment will be a crucial determinant in the survival prospects of rural households. This has been well recognised. Brand, for example, provides a powerful case for a policy direction of economic development which has the explicit aim in sight of increasing the disposable income available to black workers.[15] One must, however, take note of van den Berg's bleak warning that, in the absence of an exceptionally high rate of economic growth, the prospect for increasing incomes through rising wage rates will be sharply offset by declining employment opportunities; this picture is consonant not only with South Africa's recent economic history, but has many contemporary parallels.[16] As is apparent from a number of economic forecasting and scenario planning models,[17] the prospects for rising employment opportunities in South Africa largely depend on the potential for a shift towards manufacturing industry, combined with a breakthrough into major new export markets. This will not be attained in the short run, and the workforce is unlikely to be drawn from the current pool of the unemployed.

What is clear, however, is that rural households in South Africa, unlike those in other parts of Central and southern Africa, cannot be conceived of as peasant households, supplementing to a greater or lesser degree their family incomes with occasional forays into migrancy. The model is rather one of a nested set of relationships of dependency, in which rural households survive by virtue of their ability to build up a variety of income sources, of which production from the land may be only a small fraction. It is here that the broad picture of age dependency ratios for the black population meshes with the disaggregated level of internal forms of dependency of individual households.

Those households which do predominantly engage in agriculture are a very small proportion of all households resident outside cities and small towns: and even here, as Thormeyer and Ortmann have recently argued, for the large majority agriculture only provides a supplement to remitted wages and pensions, and hence the agricultural extension strategy which is required should paradoxically not be primarily concerned with agricultural activity at all.[18] The existence of such households within a community is, however, an important part of the survival strategy of households more obviously dependent on remitted incomes, as these provide a core of carers which enable labour-migrating households to cope better with the risks and uncertainties of the absence of bread-winners. Spiegel presents interesting evidence from the Transkei (Matatiele) of the fragility of these remitted incomes, and the role of settled households in sharing the burden of dependency.[19] Many households, of course, do not have regular incomes or pensions remitted, and the general picture tends to be of an opportunistic search for means of survival from a range of sources,[20] where the possibility of access to some forms of earnings – legal or otherwise – which the world of the shantytown offers can make the crucial difference for survival. More surveys of the type conducted by Seekings, Graaff and Joubert in Khayelitsha are needed to illustrate this process further, but their evidence drawn from 755 residents in four shack settlements provides a compelling picture of a particular type of dependency, tracing as they do the migration histories of households.[21]

Within this rural–urban framework of dependency relationships, women have a particularly difficult role, constrained both in agricultural and non-agricultural employment markets, and yet required to act as the main copers for survival strategies.[22] At the bottom of the survival ladder are the remnants of rural households – widows, orphans and the elderly without children – for whom the prospect is that of absolute poverty. In some areas, the process of impoverishment has extended so widely that the operation of safety nets provided by kin and neighbourhood groups is itself no longer functioning.[23]

While the Chayanovian model of the ability of a rural household to reproduce itself, based on its changing composition over time of adults and children, does not therefore apply in South Africa, there is another (not wholly unrelated) model of 'gleaners' and their dependants, with the gleaners moving between rural and urban worlds, spreading their income sources, sharing the burden of supporting dependents as far as possible, and hoping for establishment in a settled job, or else falling back down into destitution. The high levels of income variation within black South Africa reflect this process.

Rural households in South Africa are thus characterised by fragility and dependence of such magnitude that small reductions in the numbers of active gleaners will have large consequences. While it may be possible to forecast the expected decline through AIDS in the ranks of the gleaners, it is extraordinarily difficult to quantify the economic impact (concentrating on the economic, rather than the financial or direct medical, costs) of this in any meaningful sense. In an economy marked by exceptionally high levels of under- and unemployment, where the rural sector acts as a form of spatial sink, the long-run implications of the deaths of a significant proportion of remitters of wages are for widespread collapse of the rural economy altogether. Much of rural South Africa would be transformed explicitly into a vast refugee camp.

Can this be quantified? If so, over what time scale? The actuarial evaluation of the worth of a human life, which could possibly provide one measure of value, perhaps only has relevance from the perspective of policies of global relief on the assumption that the international aid community would experience a future cost of support. Alternatively, it is necessary to estimate the size of the informal economy and the role of the marginal rural household within it. Given that the informal economy extends ubiquitously throughout urban and rural South Africa, this is a task of some magnitude. Looking at the time scale, it might be possible to argue for a neo-Malthusian effect which will offset the implied costs of the destruction of rural households, given the existing pressure on economic resources in the rural areas. For certain areas – for example, Qwaqwa – the decline in the sustainability of households from agricultural sources of income is closely related to a relatively recent large rise in population, due particularly to the impact of farm mechanisation in commercial agriculture which served to displace large numbers of farm workers during the 1980s.[24] A restructuring of rural households in conjunction with interventionist programmes of rural development might be implementable if there is a major freeing up of land.

While it is not inconceivable, therefore, that AIDS may play the role of providing the impetus for a major change of direction in rural South Africa – as has often been the historic role of major epidemics in pre-modern societies[25] – the time scale over which this will take place is likely to be beyond the threshold of the concern of policy-makers in the near future. This perspective also ignores the intimate links between the urban and rural economies, and the massive trend towards urbanisation which now exists, and to which the remnants of collapsed rural households will inevitably turn. As has been well observed by Nattrass,[26] the dynamics of rural black poverty are intimately related to the nature of rural–urban linkages, and the prospects for stabilised living and occupational advancement within

South Africa's major conurbations. Accepting the hypothesis (as this chapter does) that the spread of AIDS is likely to be reasonably uniform across the country, it is therefore urban impact which is likely to have the most immediate and direct economic consequences, even though it has been argued that the human cost is likely to be highest in the rural areas.

PROJECTING URBAN EMPLOYMENT LEVELS

It has been argued that one explanation for the apparent paradox between the impact on economic growth of increasing levels of mortality and the increasing vulnerability of large numbers of households is that these processes operate on somewhat different time scales; the lifespan of a household is but a short moment from a demographic point of view. However, there is a more immediate approach to this problem, provided by a review of which sectors of the economy are likely to be most vulnerable to manpower losses. The picture is complicated by the absence of any precise data on the informal sector, estimated in some quarters to account for some 30 per cent of economic activity;[27] and it is not clear to what extent the data for the formal sector actually takes account of the wide range of self-employed people. Since the purpose of this review is to sketch in a broad trend, however, it may be sufficient to deal in somewhat imprecise terms.

A number of projections and analyses of the South African economy suggest that the high levels of unemployment which currently characterise it are likely to continue to rise. Bethlehem, for example, in a study of the impact of sanctions to the year 2000 (see Table 7.3), projects (on an AIDS-free, sanctions-free scenario basis) that unemployment will rise from 37.1 per cent (1985) to the 45–55 per cent range. While the employable population is increasing at an annual rate of some 3.5 per cent, the number of unemployed grows at 4.8 per cent per annum. Perhaps of greatest significance in these projections are the relative changes in the composition of the labour force: while high-level manpower grows proportionately with the increase in the economically active population, low-level manpower declines very significantly, and skilled artisan labour is at a premium, with demand growing at well over 10 per cent per annum in Bethlehem's 'best case' scenario. This transition in the structure of employment is typical of developing industrial countries as they mature, and South Africa in

Table 7.3 Indicative manpower requirements in South Africa

Category	1985 (million)	2000 (million)	Annual % change
Employable population	11.91	18.13	3.5
Professional & managerial	1.76	2.56	3.0
Service	1.17	1.89	4.1
Artisan	0.39	1.07	11.6
Semi-skilled	4.07	3.78	–0.5
Unskilled	0.45	0.32	–1.9
Other	0.85	1.26	3.2
Economically active population	8.69	12.61	3.0
Unemployed	3.22	5.52	4.8

Source Derived from Bethlehem, *Economics in a Revolutionary Society* (Cape: Donker, 1988), p. 217, Table 13.1.

the 1990s appears to resemble structurally fairly closely the USA of the 1890s. The implications here are obvious, and considerable. The South African economy is at its most vulnerable to the loss of economically active cohorts in the professional, managerial and skilled artisan areas.

Table 7.4, which summarises the record of black advancement in skilled occupations over 20 years, shows that the trend in black occupational advancement was fairly steady in the area of middle-level manpower, but is now somewhat stagnating at the higher skill level. Black middle-level occupations are well spread through the service sectors of the economy, with the exception of mining. It is notable that the black share of artisan and apprentice jobs has grown fairly rapidly over this period: from 11.5 to 23 to 28.5 per cent. Blacks occupy approximately one-third of high-level occupations, although this is largely made up of nurses, teachers and paramedical workers. In the professional and managerial bracket, black advancement appeared to halt in the mid-1980s, growing from 3 per cent of this group in 1965 to 6.9 per cent in 1975, and then declining slightly to 6.5 per cent in 1985.

The prospects for unskilled labour are, however, bleak: even with substantial growth levels (from 3 to 4.6 per cent), it has been estimated that the ratio of unemployed to employed unskilled workers

Table 7.4 Black (all other than white) occupational advancement in South Africa, 1965–85 (as % of all)

Occupational group	1965	1975	1985
Professional I	3.0	6.9	6.5
Managing directors	3.6	6.9	3.9
Other managers	1.7	9.3	6.0
Administrators	1.3	2.5	5.1
Other professional	5.5	8.8	11.1
Professional II	0.9	3.7	4.9
Engineers	0.0	0.5	0.1
Scientists	0.6	3.7	5.5
Lawyers	0.9	5.0	6.0
Medical doctors	2.0	5.7	8.1
Professional III	1.9	5.8	9.4
Technicians	5.4	11.7	17.8
Accountants	0.3	4.5	7.4
Architects	0.0	1.2	2.9
Professional IV	32.8	41.0	39.9
Educationists	56.2	61.2	63.0
Nurses	44.9	58.5	60.0
Paramedicals	6.0	6.0	20.0
Ministers	24.1	38.2	16.7
Total (high level)	24.7	30.4	31.0
Service & Trade I	5.8	11.5	14.3
Artisans	11.5	23.0	28.5
Mineworkers	0.0	0.0	0.1
Service & Trade II	15.1	24.4	34.2
Clerical	16.8	27.7	37.8
Sales	13.4	21.0	30.6
Service & Trade III	34.4	44.8	55.7
Transport	24.5	43.4	51.3
Supervisory	23.0	31.0	52.8
Service and domestic	55.6	60.1	63.0
Total (middle level)	20.1	30.7	40.1

Source Centre for Policy Studies, *South Africa at the End of the Eighties: Policy Perspectives* (Witwatersrand, 1989), p. 213, Table 18.

will range from 3:1 to 5:1.[28] Broomberg and his colleagues, in noting the unsatisfactory nature of the data generally, remark in Chapter 8 that: 'There are also no data as to the differential impact of AIDS on different economic sectors, such as the employed versus the unemployed, or different skill categories', and recognise that 'significant differences here would also have an important impact on these

Table 7.5 Socio-economic status of AIDS and STD patients

Socio-economic group	AIDS (1991)	STD (1989)	AIDS (%)	STD (%)
Managerial	102	10	8.0	1.7
Skilled	135	38	10.6	6.3
Semi-skilled	444	70	34.9	11.7
Other*	591	481	46.5	80.3
Total	1272	599		

* Unskilled, unemployed or informal sector.

measures'. However, it may be possible to get some indications of where the impact will be (apart from sectorally-specific information such as that provided by medical insurers, as Hore indicates in Chapter 11), using the proxy figures for the single most important AIDS co-factor – namely, that of STDs – where significant socio-economic information does exist.

Table 7.5 compares the socio-economic status of those expected to die from AIDS in 1991, allocated pro rata across the economy following the assumptions made by Trotter (see Table 9.13), with the socio-economic status of STD clinic attenders at the Alexandra Health Centre (Johannesburg) in 1991.[29] The most significant figure is that 80 per cent of STD attenders fell within the unskilled/ unemployed/informal group (representing 46 per cent of the population on a normal distribution). There must be a strong presumption from this that AIDS will be heavily skewed towards the unskilled and unemployed groups.

It is clear from this that, to the extent that AIDS is a disease of the poor and unskilled, its impact in terms of manpower economics – certainly for the formal sector – will not be great. However, this conclusion leads to a number of important caveats. While the existence of a labour surplus and ready substitutability break any obvious and direct linkage between economic impact and the status of this manpower sector, this group will presumably be benefiting in the post-apartheid decade from radically increased levels of social investment in housing, education, training and health provision. The stabilisation of the newly urbanised rural masses through low-cost housing and educational initiatives will be sorely jeopardised if a significant proportion of the adult beneficiaries are unable to make a return on this investment.

As a disease of the elite, the AIDS impact will be more difficult to determine. There are clear manpower bottlenecks at the upper ranges where substitutability from the large pool of the unemployed may be less effective. The demand for labour in these areas will also be crucially affected by the new directions which the economy takes during the post-apartheid reconstruction decade.

It is now clear that the labour-shedding which has been experienced in the agricultural sector during the 1980s will spread to the mining sector during the 1990s, as the South African economy attempts to restructure away from its dependency on the production of primary commodities towards that of a predominantly manufacturing industrial economy. The manpower constraints on this process – assuming a beneficial political climate – are likely to be concentrated in the skilled and artisan categories. This is where blacks have been making their most rapid advance, and where growth is projected to be the most rapid. Here the direct economic costs of manpower constraints will be much greater. Even so, with unemployment levels as substantial as they are, and prospects for growth set about with such uncertainties, it must be doubted whether there will, over the medium term (to, say, the year 2000), really be any significantly adverse economic impact from a decline in the numbers of this sector of the workforce. As has been argued above, the main cost over the short to medium term may be thought of as an indirect one – namely social investment with nil returns – rather than as arising from the direct constraints on manpower availability.

THE POLITICS OF HEALTH CARE

The tangible meaning for most South Africans of the ending of apartheid will lie in the enjoyment of economic opportunity and social welfare. The possession of the vote in the absence of a grounded belief that social upliftment is possible will not in itself count for much. What political empowerment will do is to provide legitimacy, organisational space and a set of issues surrounding the question of social provision which is likely to become one of the dominant themes of South African politics in the 1990s and beyond.

It is obvious to most analysts of the South African economy that it is not going to be able to provide sustainable employment for a large sector of the population. Leaving aside the demographic and economic issues addressed above, there remains a very considerable political problem to which heavy costs will be attached. It is already well established that major investment is required in the whole social infrastructure of black South Africa. In terms of demand, education and housing may be the expressed priorities, but health care is not far behind. There is a reality and immediacy to the need for health services which is perhaps more intensely experienced than any other social need. To the extent that the new generation of political leaders seeks to keep in touch with, and to remain legitimated by, popular sentiment, so will they be forced to attempt to mediate such demand into deliverable policies of health care.

Consideration also has to be given to the fact that South Africa has open land borders with its northern neighbours, and there is already substantial inward migration – by returning exiles, refugees and illicit population movement – from areas of high HIV infection. Concerns over the spread of the disease are likely to be compounded by competition for employment opportunities, leading to a potential deterioration of relations at a time when South Africa will be intent on building new bridges with the Southern African Development Coordination Conference (SADCC).

From the point of view of distinguishing between the investment and consumption aspects of spending on health, it is apparent that in the long run spending should be concentrated on prevention rather than cure, and on infrastructure rather than superstructure. The best economic returns on the curative side will be for the control of endemic sicknesses such as TB, malaria and nutrition-related illnesses, rather than necessarily for the care of preventable but possibly uncurable diseases.

Economically rational policies of spending in health also need to take account of the balance of spending in the social sector generally: directing relatively high levels of investment towards housing and education now may have a better outcome for overall levels of health in the long run than would a concentration of available resources on immediate health problems.

AIDS offers a number of complexities from this point of view. Campaigns which promote avoidance are likely to be cost-effective amongst the elite, who may be both relatively easily targetable and also prone to change their behaviour on the basis of an understanding of risks. Neither factor will operate particularly well amongst the poor, and consequently there is likely to be a considerable tussle between conflicting interests over the level of spending which can be afforded for the prevention of AIDS and the care of its sufferers. If it is indeed the case that Pattern II infection establishes itself specifically within the black population, then it is inconceivable that this debate will not also feed on and perpetuate historic interethnic grievances and rivalries.

CONCLUSIONS

The conclusions of this chapter are therefore not happy ones. The prospect ahead, it is argued, may be seen to fall into two broad phases. In the short term, the morbidity and mortality which may flow from the relatively regionally uniform spread of HIV infection through the South African population is unlikely to have a detrimental effect on the economy. There will, however, be a very substantial human cost, and it is possible that certain regions and household groups may experience a drastic deterioration and collapse of their social fabric.

Over the medium term, the economic impact will be determined by the combination of the extent to which South Africa is embarking on a rapid expansion of its industries, and requiring the services of increasingly skilled technicians and managers, and the inroads which AIDS may be making into these cohorts. Some doubt has been cast on whether there will be a particularly observable effect: such a range of unknown variables are involved that an assessment must be highly speculative.

What may be fairly certainly envisaged, however, is that the social consequences of AIDS will be high, and that these will carry in their wake renewed political mobilisation which may involve very considerable direct costs. These costs are likely to be incurred at the expense of more developmentally oriented spending. An understanding of these issues, well before the actuality suggested by the statistical projections comes into being, may help to develop planning and communication in the formation of preventative policies.

References

1. Much of the analysis of the economic impact of AIDS in South Africa to date has been based on comparative reference to the literature on developing countries, notably those in Africa, or to industrial societies. While methodologically useful, this is of generally limited direct applica-

bility. Cf. D. Nabarro and C. McConnell, 'The impact of AIDS on socioeconomic development', *AIDS*, III (1989), pp. 265–72, and A. Whiteside, 'AIDS in Southern Africa', May 1990, position paper for the Development Bank of Southern Africa.
2. M. Byerley, 'AIDS and small town South Africa', *AIDS Analysis Africa*, I, 6 (1990), p. 3.
3. Cf., for example, J. Simon, *The Ultimate Resource* (Princeton University Press, 1982).
4. For an interesting discussion of one aspect of the economic costs of the massive prospective growth in the number of unemployed in South Africa cf. J.L. Sadie, 'The avoidable costs of population', *South African Journal of Demography*, I, 1 (1987), pp. 20–5.
5. Cf., for example, I. Livingstone, 'Structural adjustment and long-term interactions between demographic and economic variables in Africa', School of Development Studies, *Discussion Paper No. 201* (University of East Anglia, 1987).
6. Cf. *Aids Analysis Africa*, I, 1 (1991), p. 12.
7. World Bank, *Population Change and Economic Development* (Washington, DC: International Bank for Reconstruction and Development, 1984).
8. A.J. Coale, *Lectures on Population and Development* (Islamabad: Pakistan Institute for Development, 1990).
9. For example, Coale, the leading international demographer, feels unable to derive any standard set of indicators from a 25-year study of fertility patterns for the whole of Europe undertaken by the Princeton European Fertility Project.
10. R. Lesthaege, 'Social organisation, economic crises, and the future of fertility control in Africa', in R. Lesthaege (ed.), *Reproduction and Social Organisation in Africa* (Berkeley: 1989).
11. World Development Report, *Poverty* (Oxford University Press World Bank, 1990), p. 231, Table 27.
12. J.L. Sadie, 'A reconstruction and projection of demographic movements in the RSA and TBVC countries', Bureau of Market Research, University of South Africa, Research Report No. 148, 1988.
13. Cf. H.L. Zietsman, 'Regional patterns of migration in the Republic of South Africa 1975–1980', *South African Geographical Journal*, 5, 3 (1988); also P.S. Hattingh, 'A model of adaptive population migration in South Africa', *Journal of Population Studies* (Taiwan, 12 June 1989).
14. J. May, 'The migrant labour system: changing dynamics in rural survival', in N. Nattrass and E. Ardington (eds), *The Political Economy of South Africa* (Oxford University Press, 1990).
15. S.S. Brand, 'Demografie, skuld en ekonomiese ontwikkeling', *South African Journal of Economics*, 57, 4 (1989).
16. S. Van den Berg, 'On interracial income distribution in South Africa to the end of the century', *South African Journal of Economics*, 57, 1 (1989).
17. Cf. for example, 'Changing gear in the South African economy', scenario plan prepared by the PERM/Nedkor team, January 1991, manuscript.
18. T. Thormeyer, and G.F. Ortmann, 'A macro- and micro-level perspec-

tive of a "Traditional" rural area in Southern Africa', *Quarterly Journal of International Agriculture*, XXIX, 3 (1990).
19. A. Spiegel, 'Dispersing dependants: a response to the exigencies of labour migration in the rural Transkei', in J. Eades (ed.), *Migrants, Workers, and Social Order* (Anthropology Society of Africa, 1987).
20. Cf. J. Sharp, 'Relocation, labour migration and the domestic predicament: Qwaqwa in the 1980s', in Eades, *Migrants*, for an account of the typical implications of unemployment for rural households.
21. J. Seekings, J. Graaff and P. Joubert, 'A survey of residential and migration histories of residents of the shack area of Khayelitsha', Department of Sociology, Occasional Paper No. 15, April (University of Stellenbosch, 1990).
22. Cf. May, 'Migrant Labour System'; also T.J. Bembridge, 'The role of women in agriculture and rural development in the Transkei', *Journal of Contemporary African Studies*, VII (1988). For an interesting analysis of constraints on local income-earning activities by rural women, cf. J.S. Sharp and A.D. Spiegel, 'Women and wages: gender and control of income in farm and Bantustan households', *Journal of Southern African Studies*, XVI, 3 (1990), pp. 527–49.
23. J.S. Sharp, and A.D. Spiegel, 'Vulnerability to impoverishment in South African rural areas: the erosion of kinship and neighbourhood as a social resource', *Africa*, LV, 2 (1985).
24. M. de Klerk, 'Seasons that will never return: the impact of farm mechanisation on employment, incomes and population distribution in the Western Transvaal', *Journal of Southern African Studies*, XI, 1 (1984).
25. For a wide-ranging elaboration of this hypothesis cf. W.H. McNeill, *Plagues and People* (Harmondsworth: Penguin, 1979).
26. J. Nattrass, 'The dynamics of black rural poverty in South Africa', Working Paper No. 1, Development Studies Unit (University of Natal, 1983).
27. Centre for Policy Studies, *South Africa at the End of the Eighties: Policy Perspectives*, (Witwatersrand: Centre for Policy Studies, 1989), pp. 201–2.
28. Cf. J.L. Sadie, 'Address to the Social Issues Task Group', Witwatersrand, 1986. Cited in Centre for Policy Studies, *South Africa*.
29. Cf. G. Frame, P. de L.G.M. Ferrinho and G. Phakathi, 'Patients with sexually transmitted diseases at the Alexandra Health Centre and University Clinic', *South African Medical Journal*, 80 (19 October 1991), Table II.

8 The Economic Impact of the AIDS Epidemic in South Africa
Jonathan Broomberg,
Malcolm Steinberg, Patrick Masobe
and Graeme Behr

INTRODUCTION

Despite growing understanding of the dynamics of HIV/AIDS in South Africa, and the emergence of increasingly reliable models of the likely spread of the disease in the country, analysis of the economic and social impact of the epidemic has remained limited and superficial. What research does exist has, in most cases, come from highly specific and often parochial sources, such as insurance companies or industrial consultants with limited areas of interest.

More thorough work on these issues is urgently needed in South Africa. It is crucial that we understand the extent to which this disease will have an impact on specific economic sectors and on the economy as a whole. It is also vital that we understand the effect of AIDS on the health sector, and the consequences of this for allocation of resources, both to that sector and within it.

These are obvious reasons for undertaking this kind of investigation in all countries affected by AIDS. In South Africa, however, there are some specific and pressing reasons that give this task added urgency. One of these is the fact that the HIV/AIDS epidemic in South Africa is at an early stage compared to the rest of Africa. Present data suggests that the South African epidemic is lagging approximately 4–9 years behind the epidemics in most other African countries.[1]

This presents important opportunities for significant preventative measures. It also allows a unique opportunity to predict, and plan for, the impact of the epidemic at all levels of society. Such planning and the implementation of effective policies are, however, crucially dependent on a clear and detailed understanding of the impact of

HIV/AIDS throughout the society. Closing the present gap in such research must therefore be regarded as an urgent priority.

This chapter presents the initial results of one attempt to remedy this gap. Our approach has been to develop a spreadsheet-based economic impact model that takes as inputs projections of the numbers of HIV positives, people with AIDS, and deaths from AIDS, and attaches costs to these projections. The costs included in the model are: the costs of medical care, prevention and research (direct costs), and the cost of lost production due to illness and premature death from AIDS (indirect costs).

The projections of the spread of the HIV/AIDS epidemic are derived from the actuarial projection model developed by Peter Doyle, which is described in detail in Chapter 5. We regard this model as one of the most sophisticated and reliable yet developed in South Africa.

Modelling any epidemic is a hazardous process, and faulty assumptions may generate spurious results. One implication of this is that all results should be treated with caution, and should be judged on the strength of the data and assumptions that underpin the models. Another is that results should not be projected too far into the future. The model we use here does project to the year 2010, but we regard only the projections to the year 2000 as sufficiently reliable bases for modelling the economic implications of the epidemic. Although we have included some estimates for the year 2005, we do not regard these with as much confidence as the estimates for earlier years.

The overall structure of the chapter is as follows: we begin with a brief description of the methodological approach adopted in developing the economic impact model, and then present the results of the first run of the model. These are located in the context of international and local research, before discussing their implications for South Africa. Full details of the methodological approach and the results are available elsewhere.[2]

The authors share certain views relating to the AIDS epidemic in South Africa which we do not make explicit or expand upon in the text for reasons of brevity. These include the perception that the socio-economic realities of the lives of most South Africans, including migrant labour, the disruption of family life and other legacies of apartheid play a fundamental role in the ongoing and rapid spread of the disease in South Africa. Second, we believe that both the state and the private sector have been negligent in failing to devote adequate resources early enough to the prevention of the spread of

AIDS. We also believe that it is not too late to remedy this. One of the major aims of work of this kind should be to generate the evidence that prompts the allocation of substantial resources to efforts to slow the spread of HIV in South Africa, and to attempts to mitigate the impact of the already inevitable epidemic.

ASSESSING THE ECONOMIC IMPACT OF HIV/AIDS IN SOUTH AFRICA: METHODOLOGICAL APPROACH

General Approach

We have adopted a stepwise approach to assessing the overall economic impact of HIV/AIDS in South Africa. The predictions generated by Doyle's model (see Chapter 5) are taken as inputs for an economic impact model. This allows us to estimate the total direct and indirect costs of the disease, and the costs per affected individual, for each year under study, as well as cumulative costs over a particular period. The implications of the cost estimates for the health sector and for the economy as a whole are then analysed.

The estimation of direct and indirect costs was done by the construction of a spreadsheet-based model. This model is designed to generate estimates of the direct and indirect costs of the disease for each year from 1991 to 2000, using a prevalence-based approach: that is, the costs of all cases of HIV/AIDS existing in that year are calculated. Indirect costs and direct costs are calculated separately for each year, and then summed to give total costs per case per year.

Since there is inadequate data on which to base a retrospective analysis of utilisation of resources, or of morbidity and disability patterns in HIV/AIDS, a hypothetical model must be constructed. The model used here assumes that new HIV-infected individuals will live a further 9 years, and that aside from those who contract active TB, all HIV-positive individuals remain asymptomatic in the first five years. In years 6–8, it is assumed that some individuals will experience some symptoms that will cause them to seek health care, and to lose work time. It is further assumed that all individuals will have clinical AIDS at the beginning of the ninth year, and will die at some time during the following 2 years.

The Indirect Cost Model

This component of the model generates estimates of the costs of morbidity, disability and premature mortality associated with HIV/AIDS for each year. We use the human capital approach, which takes lost earnings as a proxy for lost production attributable to the disease. The value of lost production is given by the sum of lost earnings due to morbidity, disability and premature mortality. The approach used in the model is to attach average earnings data, by age, gender and race group, to the number of HIV/AIDS-induced lost work years in each of these groups. The values of lost earnings due to morbidity and disability are calculated for the year under study, while that for premature mortality is given by the total value of the future stream of earnings of all those dying from HIV/AIDS-related illness in that year, discounted (at an assumed social discount rate) back to the year under study.

The impact on those active in the informal sector and those formally employed are calculated separately for each year, and then summed to give the total indirect costs for that year. In the presence of large-scale unemployment, it is likely that a significant proportion of those disabled by, or dying from, HIV/AIDS will be replaced. The model thus adjusts estimates of total production losses in both the formal and informal sectors downwards to account for replacement of a proportion of lost workers in these sectors. Note that non-marketed production (such as household work) has *not* been included in the calculation of lost production costs.

The Direct Cost Model

The direct cost model estimates the personal and non-personal costs of dealing with HIV/AIDS for each year. These are summed to give total direct costs for the country as a whole for that year. The figures for each year can then be summed to give an estimate of the cumulative costs of HIV/AIDS over the period under study.

Direct personal costs
Since no retrospective data on utilisation of health services by those with HIV/AIDS is available, we estimate direct personal costs through the construction of a hypothetical model of the utilisation of all health care resources. This model uses the simplified model of the

disease described earlier, and then makes assumptions about the numbers of those at each stage of the disease (such as active TB, asymptomatic HIV, and AIDS) who will require health care, the numbers who will actually gain access to health services, and the likely utilisation of resources by each of these groups.

Assumptions are not based on a best-care hypothesis, but rather on what we regard as a realistic assessment of the care that people are likely to receive. Thus we assume that no cases receiving care from the public sector will receive AZT (since this is currently the policy), while a proportion of those with access to the private sector are assumed to receive the drug. The major component of direct costs is hospitalisation. It is possible that, as the epidemic increases in size, large numbers of those who would normally require hospitalisation will be treated either in hospital or in their homes. The model allows for this adjustment, but we have assumed that those requiring hospitalisation, and who gain access to a hospital, will be admitted and treated.

Since race and access to private-sector health care are likely to affect access to, utilisation and cost of health services fundamentally, these factors are built into the model. The model thus generates estimates – by race, and for the public and private sectors, and for the country as a whole – of the costs per case treated (since not all HIV positives will receive treatment), and the costs per HIV-positive individual.

Direct non-personal costs
We calculate the cost of HIV testing based on an analysis of the numbers of tests being performed in the public and private sectors at present, and making certain assumptions about how this will change over the next few years. The cost of research and education are based on an analysis of how much has been spent thus far, and on conservative assumptions about how such spending might change in the future (rather than on a normative approach of what should be spent). Direct non-personal costs should ideally include the costs of informal care in the home of people with AIDS. These have been omitted from our calculations due to the difficulty of attaching costs to this kind of care.

Methodological Problems

The approach adopted here suffers many of the important flaws characterising current international research on these issues, as well as certain problems unique to South Africa.

The estimate of indirect costs suffers the general defects of the human capital approach in imperfectly valuing economic losses by measuring lost earnings, and by making implicit distributional assumptions in doing so. This is especially important in a country like South Africa, where the vast majority of those with HIV/AIDS will be in lower-income groups, where large numbers will be unemployed, and where large numbers of sick workers may be replaceable from the pool of the unemployed. Indirect costs measured on the basis of lost earnings as a proxy for lost production are thus likely to be much lower than would be the case if HIV/AIDS affected wealthier, more highly employed sections of society more profoundly. The omission of household work from the calculations of total lost production is also an important weakness. These estimates also suffer from the generally very poor data on employment, earnings and skill level profiles for the South African population.

Direct cost estimates are fundamentally hampered by the lack of reliable data on utilisation of resources by those with HIV/AIDS. This is in part a function of the early stage of the disease in South Africa; but the virtual data vacuum is also typical of the health services in South Africa. Of course, the problem with the hypothetical modelling approach we have adopted is that all the assumptions are only best guesses, based on currently available data, and may have serious flaws.

RESULTS OF THE ECONOMIC IMPACT MODEL FOR TOTAL DIRECT COSTS

Table 8.1 summarises the direct costs of HIV/AIDS for the years 1991, 1995, 2000 as well as cumulative costs for the whole period. These figures are in 1991 Rands. As the table indicates, the model predicts that total direct costs will increase from approximately R94 million in 1991 (the average of the low and high figures) to R7.4 billion in the year 2000. This amounts to a 79-fold increase. Most of the increase in total costs is attributable to the substantial increase in the total projected case load. The costs of treatment and average non-personal expenditure per patient increase by only 3.8-fold over this period. If the treatment patterns we have projected are maintained, our estimates suggest that, by the year 2005, total direct costs will have risen to R18.9 billion.

Table 8.1 The direct costs of HIV/AIDS (1991 R rounded millions)

	1991	1995	2000	Cumulative costs 1991–2000
Personal costs				
TB	25	207	677	
Asymptomatic HIV+	0.3	32	421	
AIDS				
low	27	371	3 395	
high	65	944	8 689	
Total				
low	52	610	4 493	
high	90	1 183	9 787	
Non-personal costs				
HIV testing	16	65	196	
Research	0.6	0.9	1	
Prevention	6	11	23	
Total	23	77	220	
Grand total				
low	75	687	4 713	14 846
high	113	1 260	10 007	30 079

Table 8.2 and Figure 8.1 show the proportion of total health expenditure accounted for by the total direct expenditure on AIDS in the years under study. The table assumes that public-sector health expenditure will grow at the same rate as the economy as a whole – 2.5 per cent per year in real terms – and that private-sector expenditure will grow at the same real growth rate as it has over the last decade. The additional expenditures on AIDS are excluded from the projections of total health expenditures. As noted in the table, the proportion of total health expenditures accounted for by HIV/AIDS begins to increase rapidly after 1994, reaching a peak of between 18 per cent and 40 per cent of all health expenditures by the year 2000. Figure 8.1 also shows that, by the year 2005, health expenditure on HIV/AIDS could reach 34–75 per cent of total health expenditures.

Figures 8.2 and 8.3 show the proportions of total health expenditure spent on AIDS in the public and private sectors respectively. As

Table 8.2 Direct costs of HIV/AIDS as a proportion of total health expenditure

Year	Percentage	
	Low*	High[†]
1991	0.50	0.76
1992	0.85	1.37
1993	1.42	2.41
1994	2.33	4.13
1995	3.68	6.75
1996	5.52	10.42
1997	8.02	15.60
1998	10.69	21.88
1999	14.58	30.33
2000	18.76	39.83
2005	33.64	75.12
Cumulative (1991–2000)	07.60	15.40

* Low = total direct cost of AIDS on the assumption of low hospital costs.
[†] High = total direct cost of AIDS on the assumption of high hospital costs.

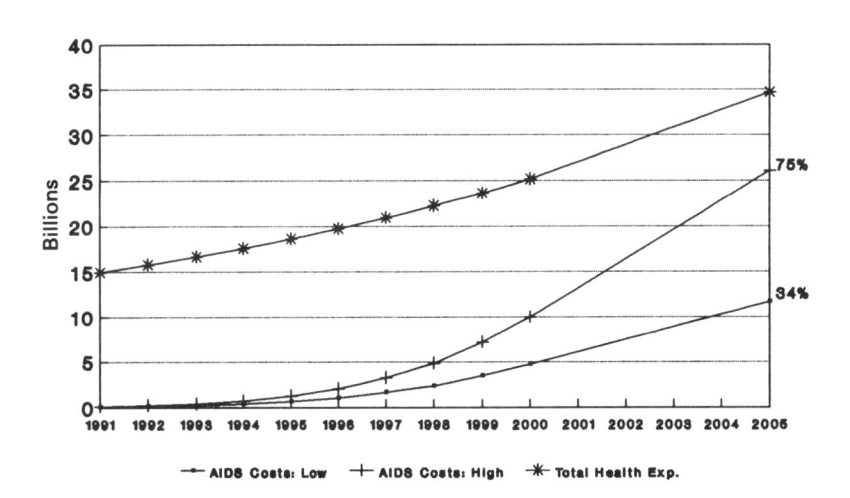

Figure 8.1 Total direct costs of HIV/AIDS versus total health expenditure

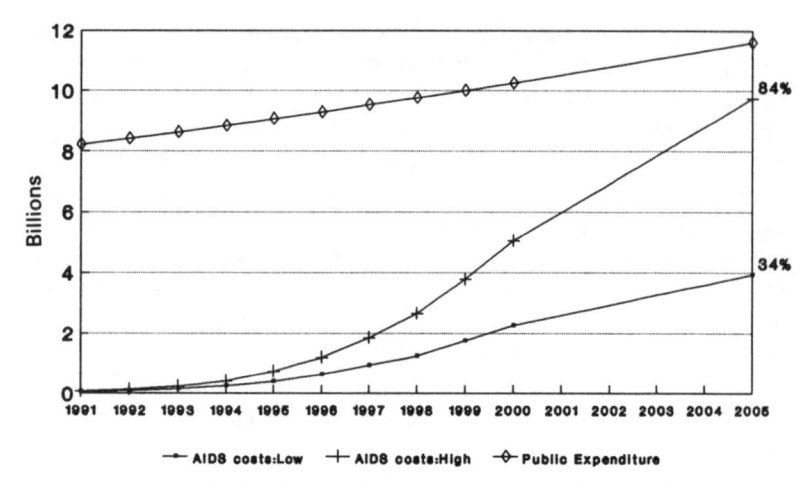

Figure 8.2 Direct public sector costs of HIV/AIDS versus total public health expenditure

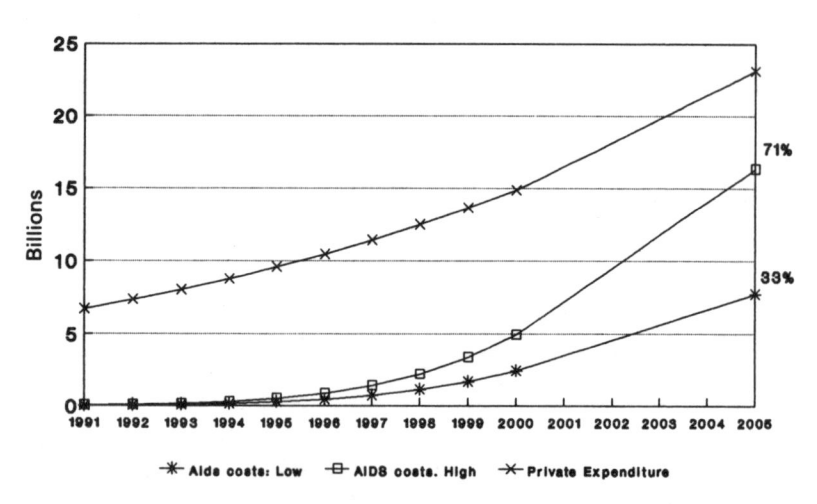

Figure 8.3 Direct private sector costs of HIV/AIDS versus total private health expenditure

demonstrated in the figures, the trends in both sectors are very similar to that for the health sector as a whole, although the proportions are slightly higher in the private sector than in the public sector. In the case of the public sector, the figures are 16 per cent in 1991 and 36 per cent in 2000 while, for the private sector, the equivalent figures are 20 per cent and 42 per cent.

Our model suggests that in the initial stages of the epidemic, public-sector health care costs will predominate, accounting for 64 per cent of total direct costs in 1991. However, this trend changes as the epidemic progresses, so that public-sector costs account for just over 50 per cent of total costs in the year 2000. By the year 2005, the model estimates that private-sector costs will predominate, accounting for 63 per cent of total costs. These trends are explained by the model's assumptions that the proportion of those with HIV/AIDS receiving care in the private sector remains constant, and that private-sector costs escalate more rapidly than inflation, while most public-sector costs do not show real increases.

Table 8.2 also shows that the cumulative total costs of HIV/AIDS between the years 1991 and 2000 amounts to between 7.6 and 15.4 per cent of cumulative health expenditures over this period.

The Components of Direct Costs

Personal versus non-personal costs
Table 8.1 shows that the predominant component of direct costs are the personal costs of treating patients at various stages of HIV/AIDS. This component accounted for 69 per cent of total direct costs in 1991, and for 95 per cent of the total in 2000. This arises from the rapidly increasing case load as the epidemic progresses.

Within total personal costs, the dominant component is the cost of treating AIDS patients, as opposed to those with TB or those at the asymptomatic stages of HIV infection. This is confirmed in Table 8.1, which shows that the estimates of total costs for AIDS care range from 52 to 72 per cent of total personal costs in 1991, and from 76 to 83 per cent in 2000. The reason for this is the high cost of hospitalisation, which is not a feature in the other categories of personal costs. The increase in AIDS costs over the years is once again a function of the increasing case load, while the increasing relative contribution of AIDS costs is due to the greater number of AIDS sick as the epidemic matures.

INDIRECT COST MODEL

Total Lost Work Years

Table 8.3 shows the total work years lost as a result of HIV/AIDS in the years 1991, 1995, 2000 and cumulatively. Adjustment 1 assumes that 100 per cent of those in the unskilled category are replaceable when

Table 8.3 Total work years lost

	1991	1995	2000
Unadjusted	22 175	156 804	2 568 732
Adjustment 1	17 764	108 463	1 996 150
Adjustment 2	14 322	60 702	1 622 494

they become disabled. Adjustment 2 further assumes that 50 per cent of those in the semi-skilled category are replaceable when they become disabled.

The Total Value of Lost Production

Table 8.4 summarises the first-run projections for the total value of lost production. Lost production in both the formal and informal sectors is projected to increase from approximately R296 million in 1991 to R9.3 billion in the year 2000, using unadjusted figures. The table also shows the projection for adjustment 2, and cumulative losses in production (on adjustment 2) over the whole period. Our calculations for 2005 indicate that the value of lost production at that stage will be approximately R22.8 billion.

Adjustment for Replacement of Workers

Adjustment 1 generates a 20 per cent reduction in total lost work years, but only a 2.3 per cent reduction in the value of lost production in 1991. Similarly, adjustment 2 produces a 35 per cent reduction in total work years lost, but only a 3.5 per cent reduction in the value of lost production. The obvious explanation in both of these cases is the extremely low level of earnings (relative to the average) of workers in both the semi-skilled and skilled categories. Thus, eliminating all the losses due to unskilled workers and 50 per cent of skilled workers results in a substantial decrease in lost work years, but a much less significant decrease in the value of lost production. A similar pattern in maintained throughout the years under study.

The Components of Lost Production

The values of the different components of lost production for 1991, 1995 and 2000 are shown in Table 8.4. Using figures for adjustment 2,

Table 8.4 Indirect costs of HIV/AIDS
(1991 R, rounded millions)

	1991 Unadjusted	1991 Adjusted	Cumulative costs 1991–2000 1995 Unadjusted	1995 Adjusted	2000 Unadjusted	2000 Adjusted	1991–5 Unadjusted	1991–5 Adjusted
Morbidity								
TB	3		28		90			
Other	1		18		256			
Total	4		46		346			
Disability	15	13	142	114	879	639		
Premature mortality	277	268	1 826	1 727	8 121	7 198		
Grand total	296	285	2 014	1 887	9 346	8 183	34 111	30 598

Adjusted = adjustment 2.

the table indicates that in 1991 lost production as a result of morbidity accounted for 1.4 per cent of total indirect costs, disability accounted for 4.5 per cent and premature mortality for 94 per cent. In the year 2000, morbidity accounts for 4.2 per cent of the total, disability losses for 7.8 per cent and premature mortality for 88 per cent of the total.

Formal and Informal Sector Contributions to Indirect Costs

Using current employment data, the models predict that the informal sector makes an extremely small contribution to total indirect costs of the HIV/AIDS epidemic. In 1991 the informal sector contribution amounted to only 0.8 per cent. This increases to 5 per cent by the year 2000. The extremely low level of contribution from this sector is a result both of lesser numbers of cases in this sector, and of the extremely low average earnings in this sector relative to average earnings in the formal sector.

TOTAL COSTS OF HIV/AIDS

The total costs of the HIV/AIDS epidemic are given by the sum of the direct and indirect costs for each year, given in 1991 Rands. Table 8.5 shows unadjusted total costs for the years 1991, 1995 and 2000, and cumulative costs over the period. Table 8.6 shows these costs for the same year, adjusted according to adjustment 2.

Table 8.5 Total costs of HIV/AIDS, unadjusted (1991 R, rounded billions)

	1991	%	1995	%	2000	%	Cumulative costs 1991–2000
Indirect	0.30	72	2.01	62	9.35	48	34.11
Direct							
Low	0.08		0.69		4.71		14.85
High	0.11	28	1.26	38	10.01	52	30.08
Total							
Low	0.37		2.70		14.06		48.96
High	0.41		3.27		19.35		64.19

Table 8.6 Total costs of HIV/AIDS, adjusted* (1991 R, rounded billions)

	1991	%	1995	%	2000	%	Cumulative costs 1991–2000
Indirect	0.30	72	1.89	61	8.18	46	30.60
Direct							
Low	0.08		0.69		4.71		14.85
High	0.11	28	1.26	39	10.01	54	30.08
Total							
Low	0.36		2.57		12.90		45.44
High	0.40		3.14		18.19		60.68

* Adjustment 2.

As the tables show, the total costs, unadjusted, are predicted to rise from approximately R390 million (average of the high and low estimates) in 1991, to approximately 16.7 billion in the year 2000. Using adjustment 2, the equivalent values are R380 million in 1991 and R15.5 billion in 2000. In the year 2005, total costs are estimated to reach R41.6 billion.

It is also critical to assess the size of these costs relative to the economy as a whole. We have adopted two different methods of calculating the proportion of GNP accounted for by the costs of AIDS. The first, Method 1, involves a calculation of the *current costs* of AIDS in a particular year as a proportion of GNP in that year. The costs used in this calculation are the morbidity and disability costs of the current year only, to which are added the earnings, in that year, of all people dying in that year, as well as the potential earnings, in that year, of all those who have died of AIDS prior to that year. This is divided by the projected GNP for that year, corrected for AIDS-induced losses of all previous years.

The second approach, Method 2, gives the relationship between the *total costs* of HIV/AIDS and net present value of the GNP for each year under study. In this instance, total costs are the direct costs in each year, to which are added the total value of all potential future earnings of those who died in the year under study. These future potential earnings are then discounted back to the year in question (at a rate of 4 per cent on this run). The GNP is projected over 30 years from the year in question, and is then discounted back to the year under study at 4 per cent per year.

The calculation of the precise period over which to project GNP is extremely complex and, since the majority of people dying from AIDS would have been expected to work for between 20 and 35 years, we have projected GNP for 20, 30 and 40 years to test the effects of these different projections on the overall proportion of GNP accounted for by AIDS costs. Although the impact is significant in percentage terms, it makes very little difference to the overall conclusions with respect to the proportion of GNP. Ideally, this calculation should include an adjustment to the GNP denominator for the losses due to AIDS in each year. This would reduce the total net present value of GNP in each year, and would thus push up the proportion of GNP accounted for by losses due to AIDS. We have been unable to do this adjustment since we cannot calculate the losses due to AIDS for the years required (up to 2030). However, we do not believe that this adjustment would change the overall trend of our observations.

In addition to distinguishing between absolute and relative costs, it is also necessary to distinguish between the *financial costs* and the *economic costs* of the epidemic. Financial costs are represented by the sum of all costs, direct and indirect. The bulk of these total costs are not necessarily a direct loss to the economy since they are represented by expenditure on health-related services, much of which occurs in the form of wages and the consumption of other goods in the economy. Health expenditure cannot therefore be taken as a direct measure of the loss in potential consumption. It does, however, represent a shift towards a less productive form of consumption than might otherwise have been the case. Such a shift may well have important multiplier effects on the economy.

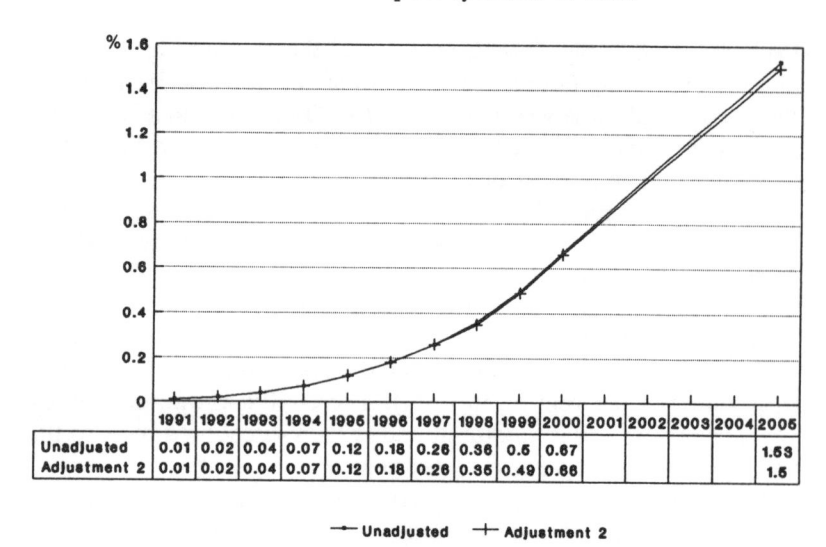

Figure 8.4 Current lost earnings as percentage of current GNP

Year	1991	1992	1993	1994	1995	1996	1997	1998	1999	2000	2001	2002	2003	2004	2005
Unadjusted	0.01	0.02	0.04	0.07	0.12	0.18	0.26	0.36	0.5	0.67					1.53
Adjustment 2	0.01	0.02	0.04	0.07	0.12	0.18	0.26	0.35	0.49	0.66					1.5

Using Method 1, we estimate that the total current cost of AIDS will reach 2.3–4 per cent of current GNP by 2000, and may reach levels as high as 5.1–9 per cent by 2005. However, only a small proportion of these current costs are due to lost earnings, and thus can be considered a directly measurable economic cost to the economy. For example, we estimate that the current lost earnings will reach 0.67 per cent of current GNP by the year 2000, and that by the year 2005 this proportion is likely to reach 1.53 per cent. The equivalent adjusted figures are 0.36 per cent and 1.28 per cent. These results are shown in Figure 8.4. This suggests that the directly measurable economic impact of AIDS is likely to be sustainable, at least over the period mentioned here.

The remainder of the costs are due to direct health expenditures. The very large proportion of current GNP accounted for by these direct costs is shown in Figure 8.5, in which direct costs rise to 3.6 per cent of corrected current GNP in 2000, and to 8 per cent in 2005. This observation has two important implications. Health expenditures are discretionary, and may well be reduced by policy measures or by overburdening of the health care system. Second, expenditures in the health care system are not direct losses to the economy as noted

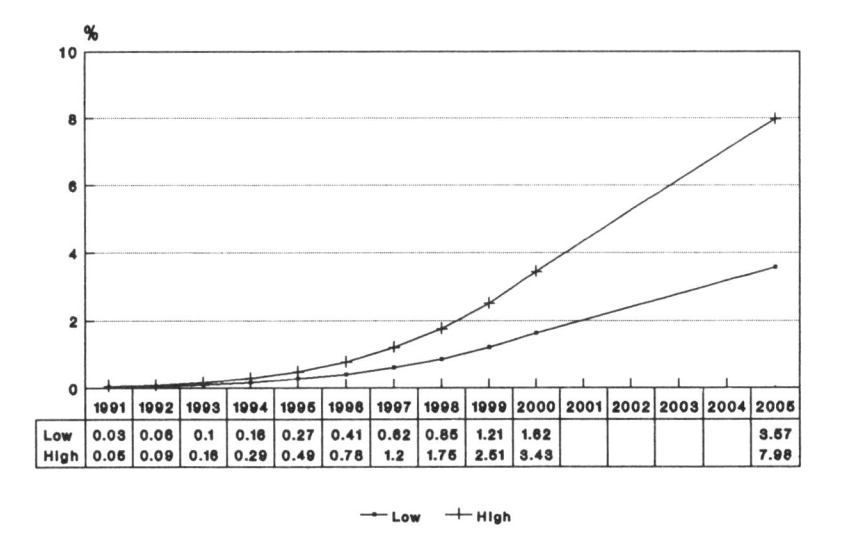

Figure 8.5 Total direct costs of HIV/AIDS as percentage of current GNP (unadjusted)

above. We have omitted to model the actual economic impact of these health expenditures because of the difficulty of predicting the effect of the shift of resources towards health services, and because these expenditures are discretionary, and may be reduced. The omission of the multiplier effects of additional expenditures on health services probably leads us to underestimate, to some extent, the total economic impact of AIDS.

We have attempted to estimate the effects of the epidemic on per capitum GNP, which would give an indication of the economic impact of AIDS on those who survive the epidemic. For the reasons cited here we have to conclude that the impact on per capitum GNP is ambiguous. If we deduct only lost earnings from GNP, then the economic effects of AIDS are less serious than the demographic impact, so that survivors appear to be better off. For example, we estimate that, by 2005, per capitum GNP would be 5.6 per cent less, in real terms, than it is in 1991, while in the presence of AIDS, per capitum GNP is likely to be only 1.8 per cent less than it is in 1991. However, the deduction of all (or even a part of) the health expenditures on AIDS would reverse this observation. In this instance, the economic effects become more severe than the demographic effects. Note that these calculations are dependent on underlying assumptions

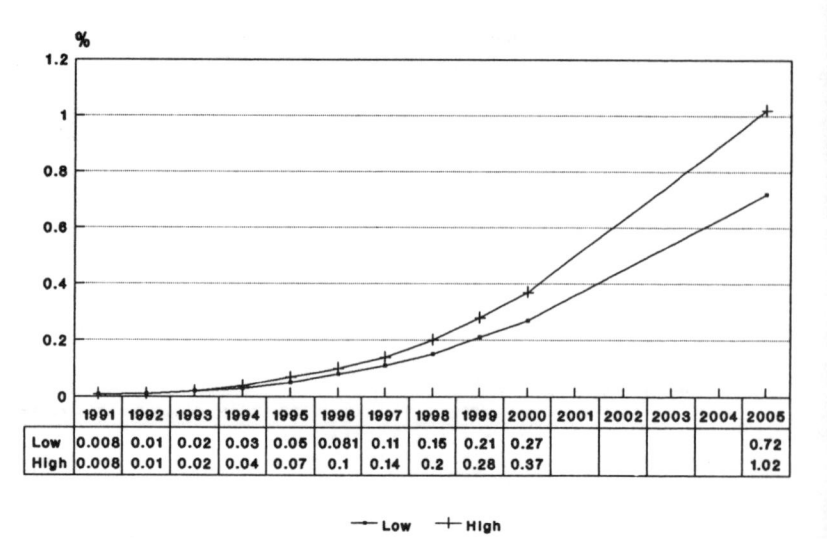

	1991	1992	1993	1994	1995	1996	1997	1998	1999	2000	2001	2002	2003	2004	2005
Low	0.008	0.01	0.02	0.03	0.05	0.081	0.11	0.15	0.21	0.27					0.72
High	0.008	0.01	0.02	0.04	0.07	0.1	0.14	0.2	0.28	0.37					1.02

— Low —+— High

Figure 8.6 Total costs of HIV/AIDS as percentage of GNP projected over 30 years (unadjusted)

as to the growth rate of the economy and of the population. We have maintained an assumption of 2.5 per cent growth in GNP per year, and have used the same population growth rates as used in the actuarial model of the AIDS epidemic.

Using Method 2, we estimate that when GNP is projected over 30 years, AIDS costs will account for 0.27 per cent to 0.37 per cent of GNP in 2000, and 0.72 per cent to 1.02 per cent in 2005. This is shown in Figures 8.6 and 8.7. The results here suggest that, despite the large absolute size of the total cost estimates, these will constitute a relatively small fraction of the total present value of the economy in the years in question.

The Contribution of Direct and Indirect Costs to Total Costs of HIV/AIDS

Tables 8.5 and 8.6 also show the relative contribution of direct and indirect costs to total costs. In the unadjusted calculations, the indirect costs account for 72 per cent of total costs in 1991, and 48 per cent in 2000. Note that these calculations are performed using the low estimate of total costs. If we use the average of the low and high total cost figures, then indirect costs account for 76 per cent of all costs in

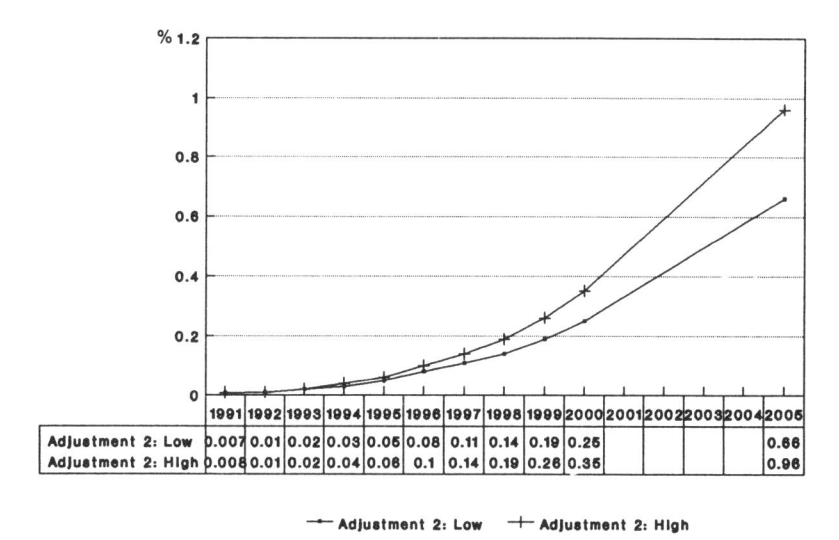

Figure 8.7 Total costs of HIV/AIDS as percentage
of GNP projected over 30 Years (Adjustment 2)

1991, and for 56 per cent in 2000. The decreasing contribution of indirect cost over the years results from the assumptions, built into the model, that direct costs of care and non-personal costs per case will escalate more rapidly, in real terms, than the indirect losses per AIDS case.

SIMULATING THE EFFECTS OF AIDS POLICY MEASURES

The model permits simulation of the effects of different health policy measures, as well as of other interventions, on the total costs of the AIDS epidemic. Extensive exploration of these issues is beyond the scope of this study, but it is worthwhile demonstrating the major impact that certain measures may have, and some of these are briefly presented here.

Changing Roles of the Public and Private Sectors

We noted above that the private sector contributes disproportionately to total costs of the epidemic, especially in the later years we have modelled. Figure 8.8 demonstrates the effects on total health

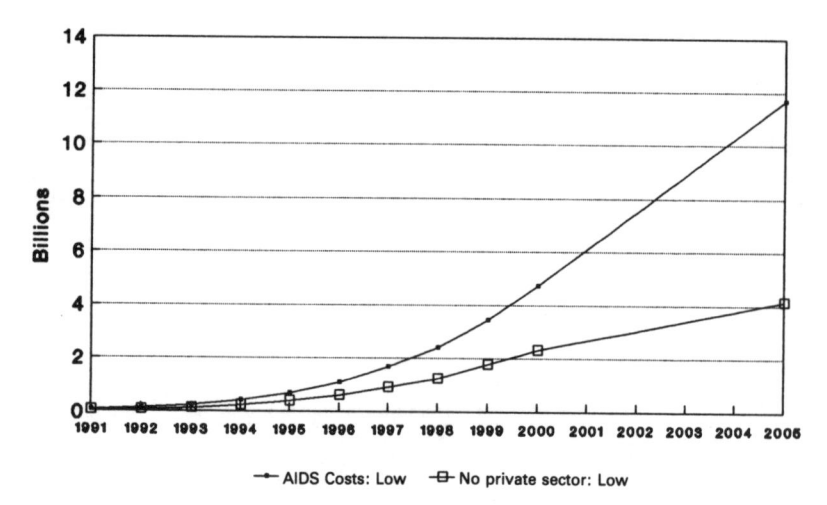

Figure 8.8 Effects of transfer of all patients to public sector

expenditures of a complete shift away from private-sector care, with all health care for HIV/AIDS-related conditions being provided by the public sector. As shown there, this would dramatically reduce total health costs (by approximately 46 per cent in 2000, and 60 per cent in 2005).

This observation should not be taken as an argument for the shifting of the responsibility of the private sector for AIDS care. It is our belief that the private sector must bear full responsibility for the care of those people with AIDS who have access to the private sector. However, it does demonstrate how costly health care in the private sector is, and will be in the future.

What is required instead are cheaper care settings in both the public and private sectors. Figure 8.9 shows the potential impact of a reduction in hospital costs to the current low estimate of public-sector hospital costs (R138 per day in 1991), in both the public and private sectors (note that the no real cost escalation is assumed for subsequent years). As shown in the figure, this would reduce total costs by 22.5 per cent in 2000, and by 33 per cent in 2005.

We have shown that hospitalisation of AIDS patients is the major contributor to health care costs. In Figure 8.10, we show the potential impact of a policy that reduced hospital admissions in both the public and private sectors by 50 per cent. This would generate a 24 per cent reduction in total costs in 2000, and a 43 per cent reduction in 2005.

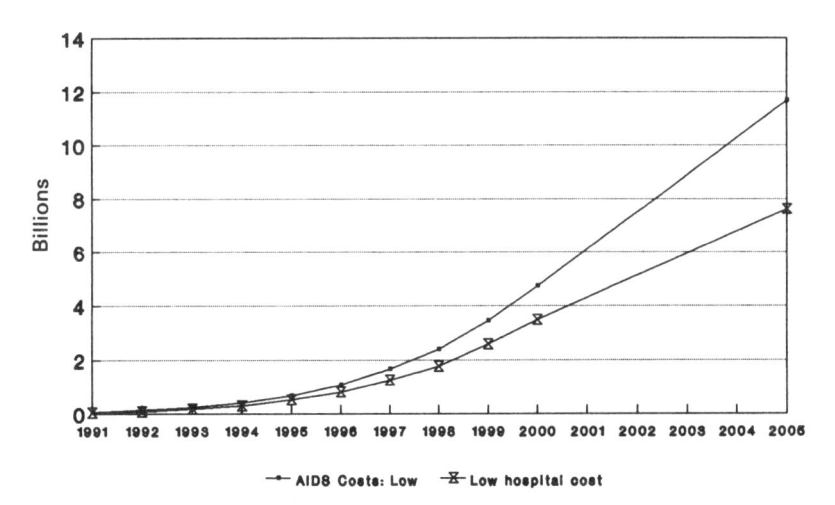

Figure 8.9 Effects of low-cost hospital accommodation (R138 per day)

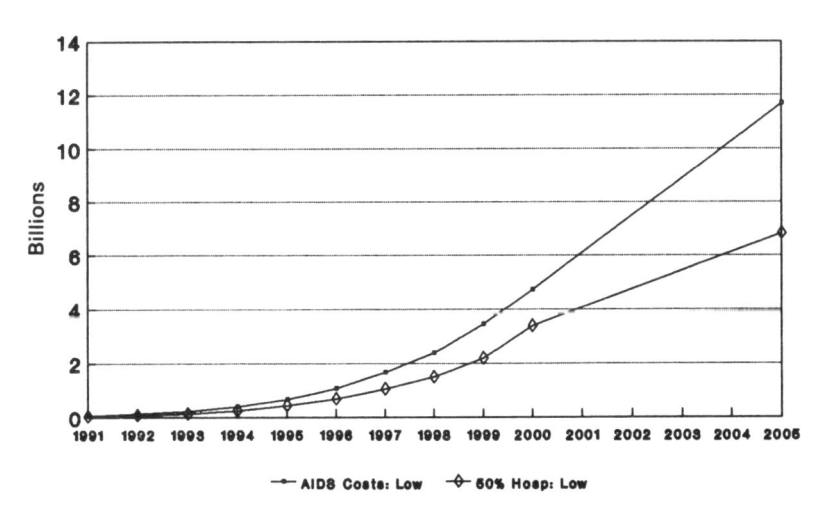

Figure 8.10 Effects of 50% reduction in hospital admissions

The combined effects of some or all of these measures, and additional ones not mentioned here, would clearly have a dramatic impact on the total health care costs of AIDS.

IMPLICATIONS OF THE ECONOMIC IMPACT MODEL: DIRECT COSTS

We have presented the results of a hypothetical model of the costs of a package of care likely to be received by those people with HIV or AIDS who gain access to health services. This excludes the very significant proportion of people both at the asymptomatic stage and even at the symptomatic stage of AIDS whom we believe will not gain access to health services at all. We have also assumed that all those who present themselves for care will receive it. It is possible that future policy decisions – for example, on whom to treat and where and how to treat them – will reduce these costs by reducing the level or cost of care, but this seems unlikely for the next few years at least.

Cost per Person Treated

Our estimates for the 1991 costs per person treated are in a similar range to some of the crudely derived estimates for the years 1988 and 1990 generated by other South African models.[4] It is important to note, however, that the total cost projections in these other models differ from ours in two crucial respects; first, they assume that *all* AIDS patients will receive care. This explains why total cost projections in our model are so much lower than most of the other predictions. Second, the other models hold the costs of medical care constant over time, while our model builds in cost escalations for various components of medical care. As a result, our projection for the cost per case treated in the year 2000 is approximately double that of the 1991 cost.

The costs per person treated projected by our model are significantly lower than equivalent costs for most of the developed countries, and are far higher than the equivalent costs in the poor developing countries for which there is data available. Interestingly they are quite similar to the estimates cited for Brazil.[5] The fact that our cost projections are in a similar range to those of a middle-income country like Brazil confirms the observation that expenditure on AIDS increases in direct proportion to total health expenditure per capitum, which is in turn a direct function of per capitum GNP.

Our projections of costs per case treated include all stages of HIV-related illness, whereas most other studies only focus on the AIDS stage. If we exclude the other stages from our cost analysis, a similar pattern emerges: cost projections for South Africa are still much higher than equivalent costs for the developing countries, and substantially lower than for the developed countries.

In terms of the components of direct costs, our model projects very similar patterns to those projected from studies in all other countries. As in those studies, by far the most dominant component of direct costs is the cost of hospitalisation in the AIDS stage. Our estimates of non-personal costs, such as those of research, prevention and HIV testing, suggest that these occupy a very similar proportion of the direct costs to the estimates from other countries (approximately one-third). As noted earlier, we are concerned that we have underestimated present expenditure on prevention, particularly through lack of information about current activity in the private sector.

Total Direct Costs of HIV/AIDS

Our total direct cost projections are comparable to some of the currently available South African projections, and substantially lower than some others (for the reasons described above, and because of lower total case load projections). Existing estimates for 1995 range between 197 million and 2.97 billion.[6] Our figures are R686 million to 1.26 billion for 1995. For 2000, the range of other South African projections is from 6 to 90 billion, while ours is 4–10 billion.

One useful way to judge the impact of the epidemic on the health services is to project the proportion of total health expenditure that will go on care for those with HIV/AIDS. Our model predicts that the consumption of health care resources on the care of people with HIV/AIDS will initially be small in relation to total health expenditures, but will become an increasingly important feature after 1995, reaching extremely high levels by the year 2000 (with even more disturbing figures in 2005). This will obviously be a far greater burden than that imposed by any other disease on either sector at that time.

These figures are far higher than the equivalent for developed countries, since health expenditure in these countries is much higher and the size of the epidemic is projected to be much smaller than the one predicted here. Our projections are much closer to the situation in developing countries, where AIDS is already consuming a vast share of total resources for health care. As noted earlier, we are lagging some years behind most African countries, and our projections of the proportion of the total health expenditure by the year 2000 are in a similar range to those for Zaire (19 per cent) and

Tanzania (31 per cent) which were calculated for 1988.[6] A more recent figure for Zaire suggests that, at present, 57 per cent of total health resources go on AIDS-related care (Dr A.J. van der Merwe, personal communication). Personal communications with AIDS Control Programme officials from a range of African countries confirm that expenditure on HIV/AIDS is already consuming, or is expected to consume, a substantial proportion of total health expenditure in all these countries.

Even in a well-endowed health care system, the order of expenditure we are projecting from 1998 onwards would have a drastic impact on the health services. In the light of the current shortage of resources for health care in South Africa, and the likelihood that this shortage will become worse through population growth and competing social spending demands, this expenditure will be unsustainable.

This observation has several further possible implications. One possible scenario is that substantially more resources will be devoted to health care than is presently the case. For obvious reasons we believe that this will not occur. One clear danger is that there is likely to be substantial reallocation within the health services away from the treatment of other diseases and towards the treatment of people sick with AIDS. This will result in 'crowding out' of non-AIDS patients from the health care system, and in deterioration of all non-essential health services (especially preventive services, and others that are not strongly demanded by individuals). It is also likely that large numbers of AIDS patients will simply be refused care as the health services are overburdened. All of these phenomena are already commonplace in several African countries.

Some of these devastating effects for the health services can be avoided in South Africa if urgent policy decisions are made soon, and rational planning is undertaken. Debating these options is beyond the scope of this chapter, but areas of attention should be primarily focused on attempting to cut down on hospitalisation costs through the development of hospital admissions policies, and possible alternative treatment settings, such as low-cost hospices and community-based care systems.

The potential impact of such policies on costs is well illustrated by the major differences between the high and low estimates of AIDS health costs. The explanation for the differences is found in different assumptions as to the number of hospital days per AIDS case per year, and in the cost per hospital day. In the absence of rational policy decisions, the majority of patients who present for care will be admitted, and will probably spend long periods in hospital, so that the high figures are likely to be realistic. However, an effective and rational hospitalisation policy might mean that the costs could be kept to the low estimates or even lower. This was demonstrated by the simulations presented earlier.

Another area of policy which requires urgent attention concerns the respective responsibilities of the public and private health sectors. Our estimates of health care costs assume that the current functioning of the public and private sectors with respect to AIDS care will remain constant. However, several possible factors could alter this; the private sector could attempt to rid itself of all responsibility for the care of AIDS patients (our model assumes that the private sector provides comprehensive AIDS care for 30 per cent of medical aid members). This would place a greater burden on the public sector, but it would also reduce total costs substantially as the simulation showed. On the other hand, the development of cheaper treatment settings by the private sector could both reduce total costs substantially, and reduce the burden on the public sector.

There is also an urgent need for investigation of how to minimise the potential impact of HIV-related TB, and of treatment protocols for all aspects of HIV-related illness.

We are at an early enough stage in the epidemic that such policies, if implemented effectively, could mean that all those with AIDS who require care could be given some form of decent care at an affordable cost, without devastating effects on the rest of the health care system. In the absence of such planning, however, care for AIDS patients will continue on an *ad hoc* basis. The epidemic will inevitably overwhelm the health services, with drastic consequences for those with AIDS and for all those who depend on the public health system.

INDIRECT COSTS

We have attempted to measure the value of lost production due to HIV/AIDS on the basis of lost earnings caused by morbidity, disability and premature mortality resulting from the disease. Measured in this way, total production losses are relatively low in 1991, but increase dramatically by 2000, and can be expected to escalate even more rapidly as greater numbers of people become ill and die in subsequent years.

No other assessments of indirect costs have yet been performed for

South Africa, and the very different employment and earnings profiles in other countries render comparisons with our results inappropriate. One common pattern, also demonstrated in our results, is the fact that the costs of premature mortality constitute the bulk of indirect costs. This is explained by the fact that death from AIDS occurs when people are in their most productive years. In this respect the average indirect costs per person of AIDS are likely to be very similar to other causes of mortality at a young age, such as motor vehicle accidents and violence. In the present context in South Africa, then, these factors are far more important causes of lost production than is AIDS. By the year 2000 and thereafter, though, AIDS will exceed all other factors as a cause of mortality at these ages.

One interesting difference as regards the international data is found in the relationship between direct and indirect costs in our model. Most other studies have found that indirect costs exceed direct costs by a factor of 5 or 6. The ratio in the earlier years of our study is 3.2:1 (using the average of the low and high total cost estimates), and decreases over time so that the final ratio for 2000 is 1.3:1. One explanation for this significant difference with international findings may be that high unemployment and low average earnings have a negative impact on indirect costs in South Africa compared to other countries, while the relatively sophisticated health care infrastructure means that direct costs per case are much higher than would be expected in a country with similar employment and earnings profiles.

We should stress once again here the very important limitations inherent in using this method to measure the economic impact of a disease. The first limitation concerns the inadequacy of data; the data on employment and earnings, in both the formal and informal sectors in South Africa, are inaccurate, and changes to these data inputs will have a substantial impact on the model results. There are also no data as to the differential impact of AIDS on different economic sectors, such as the employed versus the unemployed, or different skill categories; significant differences here would also have an important impact on these measures.

The second limitation concerns the question of whether lost earnings can really be taken as a proxy for lost production. As we noted earlier, the presence of large-scale unemployment means that a sizeable proportion of potential lost work years are likely to be saved through replacement of lost workers. Our calculations suggest that replacement of unskilled workers and half of the dying semi-skilled workers would save a substantial fraction of projected lost work years (although their lower levels of earnings means that this adjustment has much less impact on total lost earnings). It is possible that, in reality, all but the most highly skilled employees (and perhaps even these) could ultimately be replaced in the presence of high unemployment. This would obviously have important frictional costs, but these would only be a fraction of the total costs of lost earnings over the lifetime of a worker who could not be replaced. In this case, the major costs to the economy would be the frictional costs of recruiting and training, and perhaps some temporary labour supply bottlenecks, rather than the permanent lifetime losses that would result from labour shortages in a fully employed economy.

We also recognise that the impact of AIDS on the labour market could cause increases in average wages, as well as in labour participation rates, which would themselves affect the predictions of this model. These effects have not been adjusted for due to the complexity of the modelling involved.

We conclude that, in an economy like South Africa's, the use of potential lost earnings as a proxy for overall economic impact should be viewed with extreme caution. This does not mean, however, that there is no value to this measure. If the total costs of AIDS measured in this way are calculated to constitute a substantial proportion of total potential production, then even replacement of a large number of earners is unlikely to completely mitigate the effect of the disease on the economy. We thus believe that the value of these calculations lies in their ability to give some indication of the size of potential losses relative to the potential size of the economy as a whole. We take this issue further in the discussion of total costs below.

On the other hand, a different problem is that production losses are undervalued because a large proportion of labour in the economy earns no income at all (for example, domestic work by housewives). A fuller estimation would have to attach a shadow wage to these sorts of economic activity.

A final problem with this method of measuring total costs of a disease, as mentioned earlier, is its implicit distributional assumptions. High unemployment and low average earnings among many of those affected will generate much lower estimates of total costs than in a more fully employed economy with higher average earnings.

TOTAL COSTS OF HIV/AIDS AND OVERALL ECONOMIC IMPACT OF THE DISEASE

Although the predictions of the total costs of HIV/AIDS generated by the model for the next few years are relatively low, they are predicted to rise rapidly over the decade. Looked at in isolation, the numbers become disturbingly large by the end of the decade, and can be expected to reach even more alarming levels as the epidemic progresses further. The calculation of total costs is useful since it provides the basis of cost-benefit analyses of present expenditure on prevention of further spread of HIV/AIDS. In the context of our estimates of total costs for 1991, for example, the state's present allocation of R5 million is obviously grossly insufficient.

However, we have argued that is it crucial to view these costs in relation to the total size of the economy if we are to develop an accurate assessment of the total economic impact of the epidemic, and that it is also necessary to distinguish between the financial costs and the economic costs of the epidemic.

The current cost calculations (Method 1) suggest that the directly measurable economic impact of AIDS (namely, current lost earnings) is likely to be sustainable over the next 10–15 years. It is important to note, however, that this method of calculating the impact of AIDS omits the direct costs of the epidemic. We have omitted to model the impact of these because of the difficulty of predicting the effect of the shift of resources towards health services, and because these expenditures are discretionary and might be substantially reduced either by policy decisions (as shown in the simulations discussed above), or through the inability of the health services to cope with the burden of caring for AIDS cases.

We have also calculated the proportion of GNP accounted for by the AIDS epidemic with all future costs (direct and indirect) included, and with the GNP projected into the future as well (Method 2). The results here suggest that, despite the large absolute size of the total cost estimates, these will constitute a relatively small fraction of the total present value of the economy in the years in question. This remains the case even if we assume that none of those dying from AIDS will be replaced. If we assume, as argued in the previous section, that an even greater proportion of the workforce than we have adjusted for might be replaceable, then the total impact would be a smaller proportion of total GNP than our estimates suggest. Of course, the frictional costs involved in such replacement should be included in the calculation, but these are likely to be insignificant relative to total lost earnings over a lifetime.

The critical implication of this analysis is that the total costs generated by the AIDS epidemic, although large, will not have a devastating effect in macro-economic terms, at least to 2005. Our estimate of directly measurable losses in potential consumption suggests that these will be a small proportion of GNP in 2005. We have argued that health expenditures may be reduced well below the levels we have estimated here. If this does not occur, the resulting shift towards unproductive expenditure will certainly have a detrimental impact on the economy. Whether or not health costs are reduced, however, we believe that the overall macro-economic effects will be sustainable, and that other macro-economic variables (including cyclical phenomena) are likely to be as important as AIDS in the next decade. Even after that, we believe that indirect costs, while large, will be sustainable. However, by 2005, the potentially negative effects of massive health expenditures will become more important, and overall economic consequences will be more serious if these are not contained.

It is, of course, crucial to note that these comments are limited to the time frame to 2005. Since deaths from AIDS are likely to peak in around 2010, the peak economic impact will only be felt during the 20 or 30 years after this, when those who died at the peak of the epidemic would otherwise have been contributing to the economy. It is thus possible that, in the years after 2010, the epidemic could pose a major threat to continued economic growth.

Observations by the WHO Global Programme on AIDS suggests that for most developing countries, the overall economic impact of even massive epidemics is likely to be sustainable. In the case of African countries, one major explanation for the relatively low total costs of the epidemic is the very low expenditures on health care (Dr J. Chin, personal communication).

These estimates and observations should not be taken as an argument for complacency in the face of this epidemic in South Africa. Instead, we regard these conclusions as vital in overcoming the paralysis induced by many of the previous 'doomsday' analyses of the impact of HIV/AIDS in South Africa, and thereby strengthening the arguments for urgent interventions so as to minimise the effects of the epidemic.

The doomsday economic predictions of the impact of AIDS in South Africa suggested that the major mechanisms by which AIDS would affect the economy would be through labour supply shortages, and through significant reductions in aggregate demand (via reductions in total consumption). It is our view that the impact of AIDS by means of these mechanisms has been exaggerated in both cases. As we argued earlier, in the presence of high unemployment, even the large numbers of deaths from AIDS that our model projects are more likely to result in temporary labour supply bottlenecks and frictional replacement costs, rather than substantial and lasting labour supply shortages. The fact that population growth will remain positive throughout all phases of the epidemic for the period under review strengthens this view. It is possible, however, that certain industries or sectors will experience transient labour shortages more seriously than others.

Our projections also suggest that the overall effect on consumption will be less than that predicted by others. High unemployment means that only a proportion of deaths due to AIDS actually have consequences for total consumption in the economy. We have also suggested that a substantial proportion of those who are employed will be replaced when they become ill or die, so that they will not represent a permanent loss in consumption potential. In addition, continued population growth – albeit at a lower level than in the absence of AIDS – is likely to maintain consumption growth.

Another postulated mechanism for decreased demand is via reduced demand for our exports from neighbouring countries whose economies are predicted to be affected in an equally serious way. We have not researched this issue at all, and prefer not to make detailed comments. However, it is our suspicion that similar trends to those predicted for South Africa would apply in most of these countries. Even though several of them already have an extremely high prevalence of HIV in the labour force, this has not appeared to affect their formal economies drastically, and the formal economies are responsible for the bulk of imports for South Africa. Once again, then, AIDS will have some negative impact here, but is unlikely to be a devastating one.

We are also not able to give any predictions about the effects of AIDS on specific sectors of the economy. It is very likely that the epidemic will differentially affect certain industries and sectors, both in terms of labour supply and demand for goods. It is also likely that some industries, or economic sub-sectors, will be very seriously affected. However, projections of these effects require extremely detailed analysis, and data (for example, the differential distribution of HIV in the labour force) which is simply unavailable. We thus regard all current sectoral analyses as speculative at best. The only exception here is the work emanating from the insurance sector and from the mining industry, both of which have made a careful analysis of the impact of AIDS in their own areas. Further detailed sectoral analyses are thus an urgent priority in South Africa.

CONCLUSION

We have attempted to develop a model that will generate estimates of the total cost of the AIDS epidemic to the country, given certain projections about the dynamics of the disease over the next decade.

Although it is at an early stage in development, we believe that the results generated by the model are useful for gaining an overall understanding of the impact of the epidemic on the South African economy and society. There are several fundamental messages that emerge at this stage which should inform both further research and present policy decisions at all levels.

The first observation is that the impact of AIDS on the health services will be profound, and may well be devastating. These effects will only be mitigated if major policy decisions that will protect the health services and ensure adequate care for those with AIDS are taken soon, and if action based on these decisions is undertaken as a priority.

Our second conclusion is that the total costs of the epidemic have the potential to grow to enormous proportions, with a noticeable impact on consumption, but that the overall economic impact is likely to be sustainable to the end of this decade. Thereafter our estimates suggest that, if significant prevention efforts and health services policies are not in place, the epidemic may begin to pose a serious threat to ongoing economic growth. It is also possible that, in the next decade, some sectors of the economy will be seriously affected. Which these are, and the extent of the impact, is an urgent priority for further research.

It is also important to note that a model measuring potential GNP losses at a point in time omits several other factors that may have a significant effect on the economy. These include the potentially negative impact of AIDS on the country's ability to attract foreign investment, skilled immigrants and tourism, all of which are crucial for ongoing economic development. This static model also excludes the potentially important multiplier effects of the GNP losses caused by the epidemic.

We have also omitted analysis or discussion of some of what may be regarded as potential 'benefits' of the epidemic. These might include potentially positive, longer-term economic effects of reduced population growth rates and size. These latter issues have been omitted because we believe that the negative effects of the epidemic in human terms (and almost certainly in economic terms) far outweigh these 'benefits', and also because of the extreme complexity of modelling such effects.

Our general conclusion, that the overall effect of the AIDS epidemic will be a sustainable one for the South African economy in the next 15 years, should be seen in the correct context. We believe that this problem is still a *desperately serious* one for our society, in both economic and human terms. Although the economic costs are likely to be sustainable over the next 10–15 years, they are substantial and will expand rapidly with the epidemic. We have also argued that a static model, such as this one, may underestimate the total economic impact of this epidemic on our society.

Third, a macro-economic view also hides the devastating economic consequences of this disease for affected individuals and their families. If the experience of other countries and current trends in South Africa are any indication, there is likely to be increasing discrimination in the work place, resulting in large numbers of those who are HIV positive losing their jobs. The burden on families who have to care for (and bury) people dying of AIDS, and those who lose breadwinners, will be enormous. This will be aggravated by unemployment, by inadequate social support services and transfer payments, by discrimination in access to insurance and housing, and by the predicted inability of the health services to offer adequate care to affected individuals and support to their families.

Finally, and most importantly, the AIDS epidemic in South Africa will be an awful and enormous human tragedy, through the potentially avoidable loss of hundreds of thousands, and ultimately millions, of lives.

Taken together, these observations constitute powerful arguments for current expenditure on interventions that will diminish the projected size, and hence the cost, of the epidemic. We have not calculated the potential savings to be made from even small reductions in the spread of the HIV, or the cost-effectiveness of expenditure on prevention. Such calculations should be undertaken as a priority.

Even without calculations, however, it is obvious that both the state and the private sector have been grossly negligent in providing resources and the attention they have paid to this problem so far.

Perhaps the most important message of this research is the urgent policy and research agenda which it defines. We have touched on several issues requiring action in terms of policy decisions and/or further research. The responsibility for such action lies with all the relevant state agencies, as well as with a range of private-sector organisations including the trade unions and employers. It is already too late to stop the hundreds of thousands of deaths of those who are now carrying the HIV virus. It is not too late, however, to prevent further millions from dying, and to mitigate the impact that this epidemic will have on our health services and on our society as a whole. Whether or not we can succeed will depend on actions taken now and in the immediate future.

Acknowledgements

We gratefully acknowledge the Economic Trends Research Group for commissioning the research on which this publication is based, and Francie Lund for much initial encouragement. We also acknowledge the extensive help of our colleague, Dr Max Price. Thanks also to Professors Charles Simkins, John Sender and Rob Dorrington, Debbie Budlender, Dr D. Sifris, Dr N. Padayachee, Dr S. Miller, Dr D. Martin, Gary Taylor, Dr A. Roukens de Lange and several others who generously offered extensive advice and information. We are especially grateful to Peter Doyle and his colleagues at Metropolitan Life for allowing us access to the actuarial model, and for much time spent in discussion. Thanks also to Jennifer Harris for assistance in production.

References

1. P. Doyle, 'The impact of AIDS on South Africa's population', in *AIDS in South Africa: Demographic and Economic Implications* (Johannesburg: Centre for Health Policy, September 1991).
2. J. Broomberg, M. Steinberg and P. Masobe, 'The economic impact of AIDS in South Africa', Report to the Economic Trends Group, Centre for Health Policy, Johannesburg, July 1991.
3. Estimates are given by the following authors: J.A. van der Merwe, 'AIDS', unpublished paper, SANLAM, 1988; A. Spier, 'Medical Aid',

Aids Analysis Africa, 1, 1 (June/July 1990), p. 5; W.A. van Niekerk, Minister of National Health and Population Development, November 1988, cited in Retrovir slide presentation, undated; G. Taylor, personal communication, calculation of 'best care' hypothetical model for a patient in the private sector, 1991; E. Osborne, 'Aids – what if?', in *Nedbank Guide to the Economy*, (Johannesburg, August 1990); A. Whiteside, 'AIDS in Southern Africa', a position paper for the Development Bank of Southern Africa, Economic Research Unit, University of Natal, Durban, 1990.

4. H. Cordeiro, 'Medical costs of HIV and AIDS in Brazil', in A.F. Fleming, M. Carballo, D.W. FitzSimons, M.R. Bailey and J. Mann, *The Global Impact of AIDS* (New York: Alan R. Liss, 1988), pp. 119–22.
5. These are derived from van de Merwe's low figure and Whiteside's high figure: see p. 3.
6. M. Over, S. Bertozzi, J. Chin, B.N. Galy and K. Nyamuryekung'e, 'The direct and indirect costs of HIV infection in developing countries: the cases of Zaire and Tanzania', in Fleming *et al.*, *The Global Impact of AIDS*.

9 Some Reflections on a Human Capital Approach to the Analysis of the Impact of AIDS on the South African Economy
George Trotter

The first section of this chapter contains an explanation of the 'human capital approach', and then briefly outlines the relevance of the concept to health economics in general and to an analysis of the impact of AIDS in particular. Some indication of the educational investment lost through AIDS deaths will be given in the second section. The third section will consider the implications for mortality cost estimates of different assumptions about: (i) the skills distribution of AIDS deaths; (ii) the length of working life lost as a result of these deaths; and (iii) the annual rates of discount and of increases in earnings.

The fourth section presents some estimates of recruitment, adjustment and retraining costs, at different skill levels. The conclusion addresses the spread of AIDS, rather than attempting to present firm estimates of the indirect or human capital costs of any aspect of the AIDS epidemic in South Africa (see Chapter 8). The emphasis throughout is on highlighting the sensitivity of any estimates and projections to changes in some of the underlying parameters.

THE HUMAN CAPITAL APPROACH

The basic idea behind the theory of human capital is that the economic capabilities of people are a produced means of production, so that the embodiment of skills through education and training is as much a form of investment as is the purchase of a machine.[1] The origins of human capital theory can be traced back to Adam Smith, as indicated by the following quotation from *The Wealth of Nations*:

> A man educated at the expense of much labour and time . . . may be compared to [an] expensive machine. The work which he learns to perform, it must be expected, over and above the usual wages of common labour, will replace to him the whole expense of his education, with at least the ordinary profits of an equally valuable capital. It must do this too in a reasonable time, regard being had to the very uncertain duration of human life, in the same manner as the more certain duration of the machine.[2]

This quotation is particularly relevant to the human capital aspect of health economics. If the uncertainty surrounding the 'duration of human life' can be reduced (and some improvement in the quality of that life can be secured) the productivity of the individual will be increased.

There are undoubtedly analogies between education economics and health economics.[3] Both health and education expenditures are an 'investment in people', and both contain some element of consumption. Viewed as investments, they may often be regarded as joint investments made in the same person. This could make the measurement of the benefit to be derived from either form of expenditure rather difficult; improving an individual's state of health will increase the return to be derived from further education, while raising someone's productivity through education is likely to increase the return to investment in his or her health.

Taken separately, expenditure on health, like expenditure on education, will raise lifetime earnings. This is most clearly true when mortality is prevented, but it also applies to other forms of health and medical expenditure when periods of illness and disability are shortened. Apart from the benefit derived by the individual, society will also benefit from having a healthier population. So there is no doubt that the expenditure on AIDS – whether it be for AIDS education and awareness campaigns, research, or the prevention or postponement of seroconversion – is an investment which is both privately and socially beneficial.

Improving a person's health has an obvious effect on the quality of labour, in a way which is sometimes difficult to measure. One cannot, for example, easily estimate the effect that the later stages of the HIV infection will have on the productivity of an employee, whether he or she is a weekly-paid factory worker, a piecework labourer, or someone who is self-employed. But health expenditure also increases the more readily measurable quantity of labour, either by reducing the amount of labour time lost through illness or, in the more extreme case, by making available more person-years of labour when the incidence of mortality is cut. The treatment of HIV-positive cases is undertaken in order to lengthen the period between infection and the onset of fully-blown AIDS, as well as to alleviate suffering during the later part of the HIV stage. (For someone who has contracted AIDS, death seems inevitable at this stage of our knowledge.) Expenditure is also incurred for education and awareness programmes which are aimed at decreasing the number of infected people, and for research into more effective treatment regimes and ultimate cures.

An important difference between the economic analysis of education and that of health is the fact that opportunity costs are treated somewhat differently in a cost-benefit analysis. The educational opportunity cost is generally added to the direct costs associated with schooling, and this total cost is then compared to the benefits in the form of earnings differentials. In the case of health economics, the benefits are the reductions in productivity losses, generally measured by the earnings not forgone as a result of the treatment (or other health expenditures); health economists refer to these as indirect costs. The true opportunity cost of the health expenditure (the alternative use to which the equivalent amount of funds could be put) is not generally taken into account at all (see Chapter 8).

In a cost-benefit analysis of education,[4] the direct and indirect costs are added together and set against the productivity benefits; in health economics, the only meaningful way of undertaking a similar form of cost-benefit analysis is to compare the direct costs (both personal and non-personal) with the benefit in the form of reduced indirect costs (or reduced productivity losses). The resulting cost-benefit ratio enables comparisons to be made between competing health programmes, or between health expenditure and other forms of social investment.

Perhaps the most obvious similarity between the economics of education and health is to be found in the technique of analysis known as cost-effectiveness. This is used as an alternative to cost-benefit analysis, particularly in cases where it is impossible, or extremely difficult – or perceived to be undesirable – to measure certain benefits, which are nevertheless clearly identifiable. A frequently-used example concerns defence: while it may be impossible to put a monetary value on 'national security', which simply does not have a market price, it may nevertheless be feasible to compare different weapons systems capable of achieving a certain level of security.

Instead of asking, 'What productivity losses can be averted by spending a certain amount of money on different ways of treating AIDS?' one might ask, 'If there are two (or more) ways of treating AIDS patients, and these different methods have the same overall result, which one uses fewer resources?' There may be a very strong argument for this approach on humanitarian grounds: the 'overall result' referred to above may be the saving of a life, whether it be the life of a city-dweller or a rural worker, an unskilled labourer or of a highly-paid professional.

Unfortunately, as Blaug points out,[5] cost-effectiveness is seldom so simple that we can rely exclusively on one (unquantifiable) objective. For one thing, decisions on alternative expenditure packages almost invariably involve multiple objectives, with no one objective dominating the others; for another, except in the most artificial of circumstances, some comparison of outcomes is inevitably necessary, and such comparison presupposes an ability to rank these outcomes.

In Chapter 8, Broomberg and his colleagues, while discussing the 'limited policy applicability' of existing South African research, refer to the 'initial concentration on computing the total costs of the disease, rather than on more detailed cost-effectiveness or cost-benefit studies'. There is at least one study undertaken elsewhere in Africa which is concerned with these aspects.[6] The authors first calculate the discounted total number of future years of healthy life lost by an average person infected by 14 different diseases, and this provides a basis for the allocation of health care expenditures within the health budget. Next, a monetary value is attached to each productive healthy life year. The authors point out that these calculations could guide resource allocation in general if the expenditure of a certain magnitude could result either in a measurable benefit in (say) the transport sector, or in a certain number of cases of HIV infection prevented. Either one of these approaches would require knowledge of the cost of various health programmes per case prevented.

To what extent could the empirical work undertaken by Broomberg and his colleagues be used to provide the basis for further cost-benefit studies? It would be necessary to gather information on alternative possible uses to which funds could be put, either within the health sector (to compare alternative medical programmes) or outside health (to compare other possible social investment programmes). This would make it possible to compare the cost-effectiveness of expenditure on HIV and AIDS patients with alternative expenditures. But the benefit:cost ratio could be calculated only if it was possible to estimate the reduction in indirect costs which would result from an additional amount spent on AIDS. From a purely economic point of view, if the benefit:cost ratio of additional AIDS expenditure exceeded that of additional expenditure on some other disease, the AIDS expenditure would have been chosen. If the ratio exceeded that of some other form of social investment, the medical outlay would once again have been 'justified'.

LOST EDUCATIONAL INVESTMENT

The eventual demise of an individual AIDS sufferer effectively implies that the past investment in education and training is 'wasted'. This should not be added to an estimate of costs since it is not an amount that would be avoided if the illness was more effectively treated so that morbidity and mortality were averted, and neither is it in the proper sense of the word a 'cost', direct or indirect, associated with contracting the HIV infection; but it does add to the concept of 'waste' which is incurred by AIDS.

In 1987, a report was compiled which identified and aggregated the social costs of all formal and specified types of non-formal education in South Africa.[7] The total of all educational costs for 1985 was R10 292 million, and this was disaggregated by race group as well as by level of education as shown in Table 9.1. Table 9.2 shows the average cost attributable to, or 'investment in', each pupil or scholar, calculated from these totals.[8]

The educational qualifications of the economically active population are changing rapidly: for example, the proportions with no

Table 9.1 Disaggregation of total social costs, 1985 (R millions)

	Primary	Secondary	Tertiary	Total
Blacks	1 250	1 263	1 110	3 623
Coloureds	369	373	328	1 070
Indians	178	179	158	515
Whites	1 755	1 772	1 557	5 084
Total	3 552	3 587	3 153	10 292

Source G.J. Trotter and A.J. Shave, *The Total Social Costs of South African Education* (Durban: Economic Research Unit, University of Natal, 1988).

Table 9.2 Average 'educational investment' per capitum (1985 Rand)

	Primary	Secondary	Tertiary
Blacks	259	1 059	17 666
Coloureds	615	1 950	14 849
Indians	1 226	2 050	7 018
Whites	3 071	4 452	7 647

Sources G.J. Trotter and A.J. Shave, *The Total Social Costs of South African Education* (Durban: Economic Research Unit, University of Natal, 1988); and *South African Labour Statistics 1990* (Pretoria: Central Statistical Services, 1990), pp. 2.62 and 2.63, Table 2.1.9.

Table 9.3 Distribution of economically active population by race group and educational level (%)

Educational level	Whites	Coloureds	Indians	Blacks
None	0.5	10.5	2.7	22.0
Up to std 3	0.5	17.0	4.8	21.4
Stds 4–5	0.6	22.4	11.0	22.0
Stds 6–8	28.4	37.2	44.0	26.0
Stds 9–10	37.0	7.8	26.3	7.0
Post-secondary	32.1	4.7	11.1	1.7

Source *South African Labour Statistics 1990* (Pretoria: Central Statistical Services, 1990), Table 2.1.9.

education and with bachelor's degrees changed between 1980 and 1985 from 24 to 17 per cent and from 1.3 to 1.7 per cent respectively. For blacks, the proportion with 'no education' fell from 34 to 25 per cent. It would thus be inappropriate to use the proportions as indicated for 1985 and apply these to the 1991 AIDS death figures. In the absence of more recent data, the 1985 percentages have been modified slightly to reduce the percentages in the lowest levels of education. The data are aggregated into six educational groups, and the percentages used are shown in Table 9.3.

In the absence of more specific data, Whiteside's suggested ratio of deaths among blacks to total deaths (66.67 per cent)[9] will be used to distribute the 1273 AIDS deaths, predicted for 1991,[10] between blacks and the other population groups; the balance will be distributed equally among coloureds, Indians and whites. Table 9.4 shows the resulting cross-tabulation of these deaths by race group and educational level, using the percentages from Table 9.3.

Table 9.4 Distribution of estimated 1991 AIDS deaths by educational level, using the proportions for the economically active population

Educational level	Whites	Coloureds	Indians	Blacks
None	1	15	4	187
Up to std 3	1	24	7	182
Stds 4–5	1	31	16	187
Stds 6–8	40	52	62	221
Stds 9–10	52	11	37	60
Post-secondary	45	7	16	15
Total	140	140	142	852

Table 9.5 Cumulative cost per capitum within each educational group (1985 Rand)

Educational level	Whites	Coloureds	Indians	Blacks
Up to std 3	11 114	2 500	5 130	1 036
Stds 4–5	20 356	4 051	8 141	1 694
Stds 6–8	32 813	7 851	12 604	3 722
Stds 9–10	43 048	13 332	18 220	6 717
Post-secondary	56 064	31 173	30 279	27 953

Source Calculated from Table 9.2.

Table 9.5 shows the amount 'invested' in each person with the specified level of education expressed in 1985 values.[11] This obviously varies according to the number of years of schooling received; for example, someone with a bachelor's degree will have spent seven years in primary school, five in secondary school and three in a tertiary institution. These values are then multiplied by the appropriate figures in Table 9.4 to calculate, in 1985 Rands, the human capital 'lost' or 'wasted' within each educational group when someone dies of AIDS, as shown in Table 9.6. The final figure in this table (just under R27 million) is extrapolated from the sum total using the inflation rate over the period 1985–91. It represents an estimate of the total investment of educational human capital (in 1991 Rands) for those who are likely to die of AIDS during 1991.

A major limitation of this method of calculating the costs per person educated is that 1985 figures are used, despite the fact that the people concerned were obviously educated at different times in the past: cohort analysis, rather than cross-sectional data, should ideally

Table 9.6 Total investment of human capital for the estimated number of AIDS deaths in 1991 (assuming the proportions for the economically active population are used) 1985 (Rand)

Educational level	Whites	Coloureds	Indians	Blacks
None	0	0	0	0
Up to std 3	11 114	60 005	35 913	188 519
Stds 4–5	20 356	125 580	130 253	316 784
Stds 6–8	1 312 524	408 248	781 458	822 619
Stds 9–10	2 238 472	146 654	674 151	403 007
Post-secondary	2 522 864	218 212	484 469	419 298
Total	6 105 329	958 699	2 106 243	2 150 227
Grand total	11 320 498			

Adjusted for inflation over the period 1985–91:
R26 875 554

Source Calculated from Tables 9.4 and 9.5.

Table 9.7 Distribution of 1991 AIDS deaths by educational level, skewed towards the lower educational levels

Educational level	Whites	Coloureds	Indians	Blacks
None	6	35	25	300
Up to std 3	25	60	55	300
Stds 4–5	25	33	40	191
Stds 6–8	75	9	11	50
Stds 9–10	10	2	6	5
Post-secondary	0	1	4	5
Total	141	140	141	851

Source Arbitrary modification of Table 9.4.

have been used. Moreover, the upward adjustment of the 1985 figures to take account of inflation obscures the fact that the racial educational spending pattern is changing rapidly. What is of greater interest than the absolute total of R26.9 million, which is only a crude approximation, is the extent of the variation in this amount if the hypothetical educational distribution of the AIDS deaths was modified.

Two alternative possible extreme distributions of the AIDS deaths are now considered. Assume first that the distribution of AIDS deaths was skewed towards the uneducated, as indicated in Table 9.7. The average 'investment' values for each group, as given in Table 9.5,

Table 9.8 Total investment of human capital for the estimated number of AIDS deaths in 1991 (assuming these are skewed towards the lower educational levels) 1985 (Rand)

Educational level	Whites	Coloureds	Indians	Blacks
None	0	0	0	0
Up to std 3	277 848	150 013	282 171	310 746
Stds 4–5	508 896	133 682	325 632	323 560
Stds 6–8	2 460 982	70 658	138 646	186 113
Stds 9–10	430 475	26 664	109 322	33 584
Post-secondary	0	31 173	121 117	139 766
Total	3 678 201	412 191	976 887	993 768
Grand total	6 061 048			

Adjusted for inflation over the period 1985–91: R14 389 298

Source Calculated from Tables 9.5 and 9.7.

Table 9.9 Distribution of 1991 AIDS deaths by educational level, skewed towards the higher educational levels

Educational level	Whites	Coloureds	Indians	Blacks
None	0	0	0	20
Up to std 3	0	10	0	50
Stds 4–5	0	20	5	200
Stds 6–8	10	60	55	260
Stds 9–10	80	30	55	170
Post-secondary	51	19	26	150
Totals	141	139	141	850

Source Arbitrary modification of Table 9.4.

can be applied to these numbers of AIDS deaths to give new aggregate amounts, as shown in Table 9.8; the final inflation-adjusted figure for the overall 'investment' lost if there were to be 1273 AIDS deaths during 1991 now falls to just over R14 million, or 53.5 per cent of the former total. On the other hand, if the distribution of AIDS deaths was skewed towards the more highly educated (as indicated in Table 9.9) the grand total of the human capital invested in these people would be R41 million, as shown in Table 9.10: this is nearly 54 per cent higher than the first total amount. The three results are summarised in Table 9.11.

Table 9.10 Total investment of human capital for the estimated number of AIDS deaths in 1991 (assuming these are skewed towards the higher educational levels) 1985 (Rand)

Educational level	Whites	Coloureds	Indians	Blacks
None	0	0	0	0
Up to std 3	0	25 002	0	51 791
Stds 4–5	0	81 020	40 704	338 806
Stds 6–8	328 131	471 056	693 229	967 787
Stds 9–10	3 443 803	399 965	1 002 116	1 141 853
Post-secondary	2 859 246	592 289	787 261	4 192 985
Totals	6 631 180	1 569 331	2 523 310	6 693 221
Grand total	17 417 041			
Adjusted for inflation:	R41 349 122			

Source Calculated from Tables 9.5 and 9.9.

Table 9.11 Total educational human capital invested in 1273 estimated 1991 AIDS victims, with three assumed educational distributions

	Amount (R millions)	Index
Distribution as for economically active	26.9	100.0
Biased towards uneducated	14.4	53.5
Biased towards educated	41.3	153.9

Sources Tables 9.6, 9.8 and 9.10.

MORTALITY COST ESTIMATES

Detailed data on the skills distribution of the incidence of AIDS are not yet available in South Africa.[12] This section will test the sensitivity of the mortality component of indirect human capital cost estimates to different assumptions about the skills distribution of AIDS deaths, and also about the number of years of productive activity lost on average as a result of an AIDS death.

Four categories of skill level are identified:

(a) professionally qualified and experienced specialists, and middle management (hereafter referred to as 'management');

Table 9.12 Median annual salaries by race and skill level: estimates for 1991 (Rand)

Grade	All groups	Whites	Indians	Blacks	Coloureds
Management	95 566	95 162	71 701	57 071	53 727
Skilled	57 369	58 435	52 754	42 394	42 045
Semi-skilled	32 540	34 823	30 463	23 804	26 768
Unskilled	17 118	23 030	19 527	16 445	17 086
Informal*	8 559		9 763	8 223	8 543

* The earnings of informal sector workers are arbitrarily assumed to be equivalent to one-half of the wages of unskilled workers.

Source See n. 16.

(b) skilled, technical and academically qualified employees, and junior management ('skilled');
(c) semi-skilled;
(d) unskilled.

To these four categories must be added the informal sector, for the demise of members of this sector will also reduce the output of the economy. The size of the informal sector was estimated at 3 000 000. This was derived by subtracting the total formal sector personnel strength of 6.06 million plus the probable number of unemployed – about 1.8 million[13] – from the total economically active mid-year estimate for 1989 of 10.86 million.[14]

Table 9.12 indicates the median annual salaries of the various skill levels, derived from a salary survey for September 1989, and escalated at a rate of 10 per cent per annum.[15] The earnings of informal sector workers are arbitrarily assumed to be equivalent to one-half of the wages of unskilled workers. Table 9.13 shows the distribution of the 1273 AIDS deaths anticipated for 1991, based on the skills distribution of the economically active population: Assumption (A).[16] Two further assumptions are examined: for Assumption (B) the distribution of deaths is skewed towards the lower skill levels, while the converse is the case for Assumption (C). These two cases are illustrated in Tables 9.14 and 9.15 respectively.

The calculation of the indirect costs of AIDS mortality in terms of lost production requires four further assumptions, the first being that the average number of future 'healthy life years' lost when someone dies of AIDS must be estimated. Over *et al.* calculated this figure at 8.8 years for Tanzania and Zaire,[17] and Broomberg and his

Table 9.13 Assumption (A): distribution of 1273 deaths in 1991 according to the distribution of skill levels in the economically active population

	Totals	Whites	Indians	Blacks	Coloureds
Management	102	46	17	29	10
Skilled	135	48	39	31	17
Semi-skilled	444	47	50	290	57
Unskilled	146		4	128	14
Informal	445		31	371	43
Total	1272	141	141	849	141

Source See n. 17 and 18.

Table 9.14 Assumption (B): distribution of 1273 deaths in 1991 skewed towards the lower skill levels

	Totals	Whites	Indians	Blacks	Coloureds
Management	0	0	0	0	0
Skilled	0	0	0	0	0
Semi-skilled	166	81	25	50	10
Unskilled	540	60	40	380	60
Informal	567		76	420	71
Total	1273	141	141	850	141

Source Arbitrary modification of Table 9.13.

Table 9.15 Assumption (C): distribution of 1273 deaths in 1991 skewed towards the higher skill levels

	Totals	Whites	Indians	Blacks	Coloureds
Management	431	78	52	240	61
Skilled	433	48	45	300	40
Semi-skilled	320	15	35	240	30
Unskilled	59		4	50	5
Informal	30		5	20	5
Total	1273	141	141	850	141

Source Arbitrary modification of Table 9.13.

colleagues have obtained detailed figures for the number of AIDS deaths occurring in each age, race and sex group.[18] Those figures are not actually published in Doyle and Millar's article.[19] In the sensitivity analysis that follows, estimates will be derived for 5, 10, 15 and 20 years of life lost on average: the lost earnings (as a proxy for production) were subsequently discounted to obtain present values.

Second, an assumption must be made about the levels of skill for which vacancies can be filled from the ranks of the unemployed. Following Broomberg and his colleagues, two sets of estimates, referred to as 'unadjusted' and 'adjusted' respectively, have been considered.[20] In the first, full mortality costs are estimated, while the second possibility assumes that all the unskilled labour force and one-half of the semi-skilled can be replaced so quickly from the ranks of the unemployed that no productivity losses are suffered from the demise of members of this group.

Third, the rate of discount is usually related to the prevailing structure of interest rates, although there may be reasons why some different social discount rate might be preferred. Mortality cost estimates were derived for real rates ranging from 0 per cent to 8 per cent.

Finally, the rate of increase of salaries and earnings over the next 10–20 years is clearly a matter of debate at present, and much will depend on the progress of the economy in a post-apartheid South Africa. There seem to be as many economists who believe that earnings will increase in real terms as those who hold the opposite view.[21] The sensitivity of estimates to a range of real rates from −2.5 per cent to 5 per cent is examined below.

The indirect costs of mortality are calculated by summing, for each individual, the discounted flow of earnings for the years assumed to be lost as a result of each individual AIDS death. This is then multiplied by the expected number of deaths in the group in question, and aggregated over all groups.

Given the vast number of possibilities if the three parameters were varied simultaneously,[22] the sensitivity analysis was undertaken in two steps.

Step 1

Using a real discount rate of 4 per cent and a real rate of increase in earnings increase of 2.5 per cent, the effect of the three different 'skill distribution' assumptions for each of the 'adjusted' and 'unadjusted'

Table 9.16 Total productivity losses, 1991 (R million)

	5 years	10 years	15 years	20 years
Unadjusted				
Assumption A	113	218	316	407
Assumption B	67	130	188	242
Assumption C	199	384	557	717
Adjusted				
Assumption A	71	138	200	257
Assumption B	9	17	24	32
Assumption C	181	349	505	651

Source Calculated from Tables 9.12–9.15.

cases was tabulated for the four alternative assumptions in respect of the number of years of life lost on average. The results are shown in Table 9.16, where it can be seen that the mortality cost estimates vary from R67 million (Assumption (B), 5 working years remaining) to R717 million (Assumption (C), 20 years remaining) in the case of the 'unadjusted' figures, and from R9 million to R651 million after the unemployment adjustment. The difference caused by the adjustment for unemployment is of little significance if deaths are skewed towards the highly skilled members of the labour force, but very marked if the opposite assumption is held.

Using the numbers of AIDS deaths (231 343) projected by Broomberg and his colleagues for the year 2000, an identical exercise was undertaken and the outcome is shown in Table 9.17. The mortality cost figures (in current Rands) range from R9 billion to R114 billion in the 'unadjusted' case, and from R1 billion to R104 billion in the case of the 'adjusted' totals.[23]

While this type of 'alternative scenario model' is useful for providing some indication of the possible orders of magnitude involved, care must be exercised in the choice of values considered to be appropriate. The critical parameters can change over time. For example, it may be that the number of working years lost from an average AIDS death in 1991 is five, but the average age at death may fall so that by 2000, 20 years may on average be lost. At present the deaths are probably skewed towards the higher skill levels; this may change, and by 2000 the bias may be in the other direction. In that case, indirect mortality costs may not rise from R407 million to R61 billion, as would be suggested by comparing the 1991 and 2000 figures for

Table 9.17 Total productivity losses, 2000 (R million)

	5 years	10 years	15 years	20 years
Unadjusted				
Assumption A	16 830	32 481	47 036	60 570
Assumption B	9 128	17 617	25 510	32 851
Assumption C	31 711	61 200	88 623	114 124
Adjusted				
Assumption A	11 423	22 047	31 925	41 112
Assumption B	1 400	2 702	3 912	5 038
Assumption C	28 849	55 677	80 625	103 825

Note The distribution of the projected deaths was calculated in precisely the same manner as that for 1991, as in Tables 9.13–9.15.

Source Calculated from Tables 9.12–9.15 and n. 20.

Assumption (A) in the 20-year column; rather, the costs today might total R181 million (1991, Assumption (C), 5 years, 'adjusted' figures), and these might rise to R5 billion by the year 2000 (Assumption (B), 20 years, assuming continued unemployment). Although the deaths are expected to increase by a multiple of 182, the costs would increase by an estimated multiple of only 28.

Step 2

Assuming that the average AIDS death will reduce an individual's working life by 20 years, the impact of different rates of discount and of increases in salaries and earnings has been computed in the case of only one of the skill distributions of the AIDS deaths: Assumption (A). The results of this analysis (using both 1991 and 2000 figures, but expressed in 1991 Rands) are indicated in Table 9.18, for both the 'unadjusted' and the 'adjusted' cases. In the former, the costs obviously increase with the rate of increase applied to the salaries and earnings, and decrease as the discount rate increases. The discount rates range from 0 per cent to 8 per cent, and the real rates of increase of nominal earnings range from −2.5 per cent to 5 per cent. The mortality costs vary from R208 million to R769 million in the 'unadjusted' case, and from R132 million to R486 million when the adjustment is made. The differences are even more startling when the projections for the year 2000 are examined; the corresponding ranges

Table 9.18 Total mortality costs for three discount rates and three earnings' increase rates (20 working years lost)

Rate of increase of earnings	Discount rate		
	0%	4%	8%
1991	1991 R millions		
Unadjusted			
−2.5%	370	270	208
0.0%	465	329	247
2.5%	594	407	296
5.0%	769	510	361
Adjusted			
−2.5%	234	170	132
0.0%	294	208	156
2.5%	375	257	187
5.0%	486	322	228
2000	1991 R billions		
Unadjusted			
−2.5%	50	26	14
0.0%	79	39	21
2.5%	126	61	31
5.0%	203	94	48
Adjusted			
−2.5%	34	17	10
0.0%	54	27	14
2.5%	85	41	21
5.0%	137	64	32

Source As for Table 9.17.

are R14 billion to R203 billion in the 'unadjusted' case, and R10 billion to R137 billion in the 'adjusted' case. The choices of discount rate and rate of increase in earnings' are clearly critical to the order of magnitude of the estimated mortality costs of AIDS, both for the current year and particularly for projections into the future.

RECRUITMENT, ADJUSTMENT AND RETRAINING COSTS

The level of unemployment is critical to the estimation of AIDS mortality costs caused by lost production. The costs estimated so far are almost meaningless if high levels of unemployment continue.

Even if the number of unemployed stabilises at the present figure, or falls to as low as 1 000 000 by the end of the decade, there are not likely to be that many vacancies caused by AIDS deaths. So if in future all cases of disability and all deaths caused by AIDS occur at the relatively unskilled level, these cases will merely absorb the continuing large number of unemployed; there will be no productivity lost, and no significant recruitment costs, particularly when unskilled labourers are being replaced. However, there will be training costs, which will differ between skill levels.

It would be totally incorrect to include both productivity losses and replacement costs in the calculation of the indirect costs of AIDS deaths. Two extreme cases may be contrasted. In the first, it is assumed that the level of unemployment is extremely high and that all the vacancies caused by the deaths can be filled within a reasonable period of time. While the impact upon individual families and upon firms would be serious, there would be no long-run production losses for the economy as a whole. The costs would be limited to recruitment, training and the immediate loss of production as new employees settled into the vacancies. Apart from the obvious difficulty of the availability of appropriate skills, this is likely to approximate to the position in South Africa at present.

In the second case, it is assumed that there is virtually full employment, and that all vacancies remain unfilled. The costs of the AIDS deaths would be the full extent of the production losses as calculated above in the 'unadjusted' case. There would be no training costs, and the only recruitment costs would be advertising positions for which there would be no applicants. This is clearly a theoretical extreme since there is always some level of frictional unemployment, and people are in any case upwardly mobile. The situation in the years to come will probably fall between these two extreme cases. The overall costs of mortality will include some productivity losses and some recruitment and training expenses.

Any attempt to establish the average recruitment, adjustment or retraining costs of AIDS-related vacancies for individual firms is fraught with difficulty. Much will depend on the nature of the activity, the level of skills involved, and the particular skill level and employment record of the individual in question. The policy of the company is also relevant; some firms will only promote from within, while others will hire directly from the market whenever possible. In the latter case, recruitment costs would be easier to establish and, provided the person with the correct skills could be found, the training costs may be very low or zero. It is probable that each firm will have its own approach to budgeting for replacements, based on its historical turnover record as well as its perception and experience of the labour market.

It is easier to estimate these costs in respect of the AIDS deaths for the country as a whole. In the absence of more detailed information one might assume that recruitment costs could be represented by the levels of fees charged by employment agencies. It is customary for such fees to be about 15 per cent of the gross annual salary in the case of higher-level employees;[24] this proportion will usually drop to about 10 per cent in the case of employees with basic skills, such as chemical analysts, and will be 5 per cent or less at the lowest skill levels. The recruitment costs below were calculated by using 15 per cent for the two top levels ('management' and 'skilled'), 10 per cent for 'semi-skilled', and 5 per cent for 'unskilled'. No distinction needs to be made between the different population groups.

The two other elements to be included in replacement costs are the loss of productive time during training, and the direct initial on-the-job training costs. Discussions with senior personnel officers indicate that, on recruitment, the number of months of unproductive time is approximately 6, 3, 2 and 1 respectively for the management, skilled, semi-skilled and unskilled levels. The cost of formal training will obviously vary enormously between firms, so the figures used for this component must also be regarded as extremely approximate estimates. Table 9.19 gives the estimated average replacement costs per individual in each skill category for 1991, undifferentiated by population group.

One possible model which might describe the way in which replacement at the various levels takes place is illustrated in Figure 9.1. If there are 102 deaths in the middle management category, these would probably be filled from the 'skilled' level below, implying that the number of vacancies at that level would be 102 places vacated by those moving upwards *plus* 135 vacancies as a result of deaths at this level. The number of vacancies at the semi-skilled level would then be the number of deaths (444) *plus* the vacancies caused by the 237 who moved up, totalling 681, and so on. This model is used in Table 9.20, which shows what the total recruitment costs for 1991 and 2000 would be, assuming that there are 1273 AIDS deaths during 1991 and 231 343 in 2000. Once again, three different possible totals are given for each year, corresponding to Assumptions (A), (B) and (C). The figures in Table 9.20 are calculated by multiplying the average costs in

Table 9.19 Average replacement costs in 1991 per individual (Rand)

	Recruitment	Unproductive time	Formal training	Total
Management	14 335	47 783	2 000	64 118
Skilled	8 605	14 342	1 500	24 447
Semi-skilled	3 254	5 423	300	8 977
Unskilled	856	1 426	200	2 482

Source Table 9.12, and impressionistic data suggested to researcher by discussions with senior personnel officers.

Figure 9.1 Model illustrating the number of vacancies caused at each level if vacancies caused at higher level are filled from beneath: distribution of 1991 AIDS deaths according to Assumption (A).

Unemployed	Unskilled	Semi-skilled	Skilled	Management
Deaths	146 die	444 die	135 die	102 die
Movement 827 →	*681* move up	*237* move up	*102* move up	
Vacancies	827	681	237	

Table 9.20 Total replacement costs assuming all personnel can be replaced (1991 R million)

	1991	*2000**
Assumption (A)	21	4 901
Assumption (B)	3	776
Assumption (C)	62	14 956

* Average replacement costs projected from totals in Table 9.19.

Table 9.19 by the cumulative numbers of AIDS deaths, starting with the highest skill level.

The major limitation of this model is that there is likely to be a barrier between the semi-skilled and the skilled level. This would reduce the training component and greatly increase the lost productivity component at the skilled level simply because there would be very few people qualified to move into the vacancies. While it is possible to calculate the totals for a variety of alternatives, this would be a complex exercise which would require assumptions about the length of time positions remained vacant; the levels of skill, experience and education needed for different positions; and the levels of these characteristics embodied in those who are seeking positions. The figures in Table 9.20 do no more than provide an approximate indication of the order of magnitude of the amounts involved. The replacement costs of all 1991 AIDS death vacancies could be as low as R3 million if these deaths occurred mainly at the lower skill levels, or as high as R62 million if the distribution of the deaths was skewed towards the highest skill levels. The range estimated in this way for the year 2000 is from R0.8 billion to R15 billion.

If there had been full employment in 1991, and no upward mobility at all, then productivity losses somewhere between R67 million and R717 million would have been sustained.[25] With extensive unemployment in the economy, if all the vacancies at all levels could be filled from the ranks of the unemployed, the only costs to be considered would be the replacement costs which, according to Table 9.20, are somewhere between R3 million and R62 million, depending on the skill distribution of the AIDS deaths. Neither of these theoretical extremes will be found in practice. Even when unemployment levels are very low, there will be some possibility of replacing employees either from other skill levels (which will create vacancies there, of course) or, at the lowest levels, from the small number of unemployed. And even when unemployment levels are as high as are presently experienced in this country, it will clearly not be possible to fill all vacancies in the manner suggested in Figure 9.1, for reasons already mentioned. The important point here is that it would be inappropriate to include *both* the life-long productivity losses *and* the replacement costs (which include an element of lost production for the period during which a post remains vacant) for any particular instance of a vacancy caused by an AIDS death.

There is an interesting intermediate possibility. Indirect cost estimates may be formed by adding recruitment costs in respect of the deaths which occur in the unskilled and one-half of the semi-skilled categories to the 'adjusted' mortality cost estimates of the previous section. Assuming that, on average, 20 years of life are lost by each AIDS death, then the mortality costs for 1991 as calculated in Table 9.16 are R257 million for Assumption (A), R32 million for (B) and R651 million for (C). Accepting these costs implies, of course, that the vacancies at the management and skilled levels, and half of those at the semi-skilled levels, will not be filled. It is now necessary to add to these totals the appropriate replacement costs for the unskilled and one-half of the semi-skilled vacancies which, it is assumed, will be

Table 9.21 Total replacement and lost production costs if only the unskilled and one-half of the semi-skilled personnel can be replaced ('Adjusted') assuming 10 working years lost (1991 R million)

	Replacement	Lost production	Total
1991			
Assumption (A)	5.1	257	262.1
Assumption (B)	2.5	32	34.5
Assumption (C)	8.4	651	659.4
2000			
Assumption (A)	2 049	41 112	43 161
Assumption (B)	325	5 038	5 363
Assumption (C)	6 254	103 825	110 079

Source As for Table 9.20, suitably modified.

filled. These are shown in Table 9.21, which repeats the relevant 'lost production' costs and gives the totals of both for each assumption: R262, R35 and R659 million respectively. The inclusion of replacement costs increases the totals by 7.8 per cent in the case of Assumption (B), and by less than 2 per cent in the other two cases. The equivalent projected overall replacement and lost production cost totals for 2000 are R43 billion, R5 billion and R110 billion for Assumptions (A), (B) and (C) respectively.

CONCLUSION

The empirical aspects covered in the three previous sections – the amount of educational investment 'wasted' as a result of AIDS deaths; the sensitivity of mortality costs to various parameters such as the skills distribution of these deaths; and the costs of replacement – are human capital considerations of relevance to the broad macroeconomic implications of the premature mortality which will be caused by AIDS. These implications are of paramount importance to all concerned with the vital issue of resource allocation, both within the health sector and between health and other forms of social investment in South Africa.

There is another set of vitally important decisions which will have to be taken on a continuing basis. Individual firms throughout the country will have to face the possibility – indeed, in years to come, the likelihood – that some proportion of their workforce at all levels will be infected by the HIV virus, which will be converted to AIDS, and they will die. At the moment the probability of this eventuality in any one firm is extremely low, and the proportion of affected workers may remain small for some years to come. But the numbers are expected to grow; in the year 2010, over 750 000 people may die from AIDS.[26] Several questions arise for chief executive officers and personnel managers, particularly of large corporations. How should they plan to modify their training and recruitment programmes in the face of likely labour losses? Which categories of labour would be most likely to succumb, and which most difficult to replace? What would be the implications of ascertaining this information? Could satisfactory steps be taken to avert any large-scale catastrophes for these firms?

Recent research suggests that the macro-economic impact of AIDS in South Africa, while severe, is likely to be sustainable over the next 15 years at least. But the inevitable spread of the disease, particularly in the urban industrial areas, is certain to constitute a vexing and broadly indeterminate parameter in the decision matrix facing individual firms. AIDS will affect their turnover rate in a largely random manner. Each personnel manager could set up different possible scenarios, and evaluate each on a cost-benefit basis; but, as one personnel manager stated in conversation with the author, 'In the absence of sufficient information, would cost-effectiveness analysis of alternative measures itself be cost-effective?'

Discussions held with several senior executives suggest that many firms, while formulating clear (but not always publicly stated) 'AIDS policies' in terms of their approach to the employees who contract the disease, simply feel that they are not in any position to start making contingency plans to counteract the reduction in the labour force: they tend to take a 'wait-and-see' attitude, well knowing that this impending depletion of their employee numbers is going to place a strain on their recruitment budget. In a labour situation such as we have in South Africa, with simultaneous unemployment at the low skill levels, and shortages at higher skill levels, the problems take on a peculiarly worrying dimension. Until more is known about the epidemiology of the infection, and until firms can form a reasonable estimate of the occupations and skill levels most likely to suffer, very little detailed advance planning can be undertaken.

Acknowledgements

The author is grateful to the co-editor, Alan Whiteside, Senior Research Fellow, University of Natal, for his encouragement and assistance; and to his colleagues, Julian Hofmeyr and Charles Meth, for their help and advice. Stephen Hosking, from the East London campus of Rhodes University, also made some helpful comments. The author remains responsible for the views expressed, and for any remaining errors.

References

1. For a brief discussion of the concept, see G.J. Trotter, 'The economic rationale for educational planning', *The South African Journal of Economics*, 44, 4 (1976), p. 344. Recent interest in human capital formation dates from 1961, when Theodore Schultz delivered his Presidential Address to the American Economic Association on 'Investment in Human Capital'.
2. A. Smith, *An Enquiry into the Nature and Causes of the Wealth of Nations* (1776), Book 1, Chapter 10, pt 1.
3. See, for example, M. Blaug, *An Introduction to the Economics of Education* (Harmondsworth: Penguin 1980), pp. 317–24.
4. Blaug defines cost-benefit analysis as 'a technique for evaluating public investment projects that compete actually or potentially with similar projects in the private sector': Blaug, *Introduction*, p. 120.
5. Blaug, *Introduction*, p. 124.
6. M. Over, S. Bertozzi, J. Chin, B. N'Galy and K. Nyamuryekung'e, 'The direct and indirect cost of HIV infection in developing countries: the cases of Zaire and Tanzania', in A.F. Fleming, M. Carballo, D.W. FitzSimons, M.R. Balley and J. Mann (eds), *The Global Impact of Aids* New York: Alan R. Liss, 1988, pp. 123–35.
7. G.J. Trotter and A.J. Shave, *The Total Social Costs of South African Education* (Durban: Economic Research Unit, University of Natal, 1988). South Africa was taken to include the independent homelands, but Namibia was excluded. Costs of training were excluded from the study.
8. The source of the student or pupil numbers was *South African Labour Statistics 1990* (Pretoria: Central Statistical Services, 1990), p. 2.62–3, Table 2.1.9.
9. A. Whiteside, *AIDS in Southern Africa* (Durban: Economic Research Unit, University of Natal, and Development Bank of Southern Africa, 1990), pp. 32–3, Appendix.
10. See Chapter 8.
11. This is calculated from more detailed information on the educational distribution of the economically active population given in *South African Labour Statistics 1990*. The average figure in each cell of the aggregated

tabulation is the weighted average of the appropriated individual group figures.
12. Broomberg, Steinberg and Masobe use the distribution that applies to the economically active population: Chapter 8, Table 8.3.
13. *South African Labour Statistics 1990*, p. 2.228, Table 2.5.1.1 and p. 2.230, Table 2.5.2.1. The estimates of black, Indian and Coloured unemployment for 1989, according to the Current Population Survey, were around one million. The true figure is probably closer to two million than to one.
14. *South African Statistics 1990* (Pretoria: Central Statistical Services) p. 7.5, and the tabulation of the Personnel Strength by Industrial Sector, Occupational Category and Race Group: 1987–1989 (Department of Labour Manpower Survey 1988). This information, which was the most recent available on these aspects, was kindly supplied on disc by J. Hofmeyr, Senior Research Fellow in the Economic Research Unit, University of Natal.
15. P.E. Consultants, *The South African Salary Survey*, September 1989, Volume 1, Part 1: Median Monthly Salaries.
16. For source see n. 10.
17. Over *et al.* 'The direct and indirect cost', p. 130.
18. See, Appendix I, p. v.
19. P.R. Doyle and D.B. Millar, 'A general description of an actuarial model applicable to the HIV epidemic in South Africa', unpublished paper, 16 October 1990. The assumed average would appear to be about 14 years.
20. p. 34.
21. The author discussed this matter informally with three colleagues, each of whom had a different opinion. One believed there would be an increase in real terms, the second a decrease, and the third felt the most reasonable assumption was constancy. Broomberg and his colleagues assume a real growth rate of 1.25 per cent per annum, without specifying the assumed inflation rate.
22. With unadjusted and adjusted calculations, four possible lengths of working life lost, five discount rates, four alternative rates of earnings increase and three assumptions about the skill distributions, there would be a bewildering 480 figures to compare. This would apply if cost estimates were made for one year (1991) only; the number would double when estimating costs for one other year.
23. See Chapter 8.
24. It is not unknown for some agencies to charge a rate equivalent to 25 per cent of the entire pay package. Subsequent to completing this analysis, the author was shown an anonymous paper entitled 'AIDS and human resource accounting', which suggests that, in Zimbabwe, an executive earning $Z50 000 could cost half that much to replace; a skilled employee, $Z20 000, and a semi-skilled person, $Z8000. These figures are remarkably close to the estimates used in Table 9.19.
25. See Table 9.16 above.
26. Broomberg and his colleagues cite a projection of 794 309 deaths in that year: see Chapter 8.

Part IV

The African Experience

10 The Impact of AIDS on Industry in Zimbabwe
Alan Whiteside

INTRODUCTION

That HIV infection and AIDS present a serious threat to sub-Saharan African economies and society is no longer in doubt. The data available from across the continent points to a burgeoning problem and it is clear that the epidemic will leave no country or aspect of society untouched.

This chapter looks at HIV infection, AIDS and industry in Zimbabwe. It examines and evaluates the available data and all the projections made to date. AIDS will have a particularly significant impact in Zimbabwe. It is the first industrialised African economy to experience the disease, and therefore has many lessons to teach South Africa.

The development of the epidemic in Zimbabwe has been fairly typical of Africa. The first case was seen in the mid-1980s and by 1990 a cumulative total of 5994 cases had been reported. Unfortunately, there was initial disbelief in government circles that the disease represented a serious threat, and for several years the problem was ignored and, in some instances, actively concealed. The appointment of a new Minister of Health helped to change this and there is a growing awareness and openness. The government has begun to address the problem, and there are a large number of private, business and aid agency initiatives.

HIV AND AIDS DATA

One of the basic problems facing planners is the availability and quality of data. This also affects industrialists. Indeed the position may be worse for the latter group since information received here is often secondhand and sources and biases will not be clear. In general, two types of data are available:

(a) AIDS cases: all countries record the actual number of AIDS cases (this comprises the people who have progressed through the various stages of the infection and who are actually ill;
(b) HIV infection: this reflects the number of people who have been infected with the virus and who have been tested. The data will not show how long ago people were infected and almost all HIV data will be biased in some way, either over-representing or underrepresenting HIV positives.

AIDS Data

The number of AIDS cases in a country has been (frequently) likened to the tip of an iceberg as far as the actual AIDS epidemic is concerned. This is because reported AIDS cases only reflect a few of the actual AIDS cases and a small proportion of HIV positivity. AIDS case data in Zimbabwe are shown in Table 10.1.

Zimbabwe currently has the third highest total of reported AIDS cases in the region after Malawi and Tanzania (refer for comparative data to Table 11, Chapter 1). This may be because the coverage is comparatively good and, in recent years at least, the reports have been regularly updated. Even so it is still likely that there is a considerable amount of underreporting and this is hardly surprising. WHO notes:

> where stark differences in the level of health infrastructure development exist between countries, it is not surprising that global data are biased by a wide inter-country and inter-regional variations in completeness of AIDS case detection and reporting. Completeness of reporting is thought to vary from 80 per cent in some industrialised countries to less than 10 per cent in African nations.[1]

There is no doubt that many AIDS victims die without having been seen by the Western medical system. A percentage of those actually seen by government health services will not be recognised or recorded as AIDS cases. Bureaucracy at all levels may hamper reporting: records may not be collected or forwarded to the central point, and medical staff and administrative staff may suffer from weariness with regard to reporting AIDS cases. All this may further reduce the statistical reliability.

Zimbabwe has unfortunately suffered from an initial cover-up. In 1987 the number of reported cases was reduced on the instructions of

Table 10.1 Confirmed AIDS cases in Zimbabwe, 1985–90

Year	Cases
1985–7	119*
1988	202
1989	1311
1990	4362
Total	5994

* The first case was seen in 1985. In 1987 the Ministry of Health revised the number down from 300 to 119.

Source Government of Zimbabwe, Ministry of Health, *HIV and AIDS Surveillance Annual Report* (1990).

the Ministry of Health. In 1988 the Permanent Secretary of Health announced government policy was that the blood transfusion service could only inform doctors and not donors of their HIV status; hospitals were not permitted to inform patients or employers; and doctors were told to report AIDS cases only to the AIDS Control Programme. People with AIDS were officially discouraged from announcing their illness and at one point a ministry spokesman actually accused the medical profession of misdiagnosing cases and thus overreporting.

In 1990 the policy changed, partly because of the appointment of a new minister, Dr Timothy Stamps. Dr Stamps regarded it as essential that the citizens of the country be aware of the true position. More realistic and accurate reports are forthcoming.

Data on actual AIDS cases in Zimbabwe are available from three sources. The first and most comprehensive is the government reporting of AIDS cases; second is the insurance industry; and third, the medical aid societies. The latter two sources will only be accurate if doctors or medical attendants put the cause of death on death certificates so as to reveal that the deceased died of HIV-related illness.

Government data are collected and released by the Ministry of Health in Harare. Cases are reported by the provinces, the central hospitals and the cities as well as private practitioners. Until recently, virtually all testing was done in the Public Health Laboratory, and this facility was also responsible for confirmatory testing. The data are correlated and analysed in the Department of Epidemiology of the Ministry of Health, which then releases the reports on an annual and quarterly basis. The reports provide a reasonably comprehensive look at AIDS data on the basis of cases by sex, age group and province, and also include some information on HIV data. This is shown below in Table 10.2 and Figure 10.1.

The second source of information on AIDS cases is the insurance industry. Most of the insurance companies operating in Zimbabwe have analysed their mortality data to try to identify the number of claims arising from HIV infection. It is, of course, only representative of the people who are insured.

There were an estimated 1 042 000 people in paid employment in Zimbabwe in 1985,[2] and a substantial proportion of these people will have some form of insurance cover. One insurance company estimates that 70 per cent of those in formal employment have group life cover. Old Mutual, the biggest insurance group, has 770 000 policies, of which 450 000 are group life.

The insurance companies have seen a steady increase in the number of deaths due to HIV infection, as shown in Table 10.3 below. Medical aid society data is less complete. Nonetheless, the schemes note that the number of claims that they are receiving for care of patients with HIV-infected disease is increasing. The medical aid societies are not representative of the population, although they have approximately half a million people registered.

Table 10.2 Cumulative AIDS cases by sex and year

Year	Female	Male	Unknown	Total	Cumulative total
1987				119	119
1988				202	321
1989	630	674	7	1311	1632
1990					
1st quarter	357	363	5	725	2357
2nd quarter	350	422	7	779	3136
3rd quarter	944	1150	21	2115	5251
4th quarter	310	420	3	733	5984
1991					
1st quarter	301	419	4	724	6708

Source Government of Zimbabwe, Ministry of Health, *HIV and AIDS Surveillance Annual Report* (1990), and *HIV and AIDS Surveillance Quarterly Report* (April–June 1991).

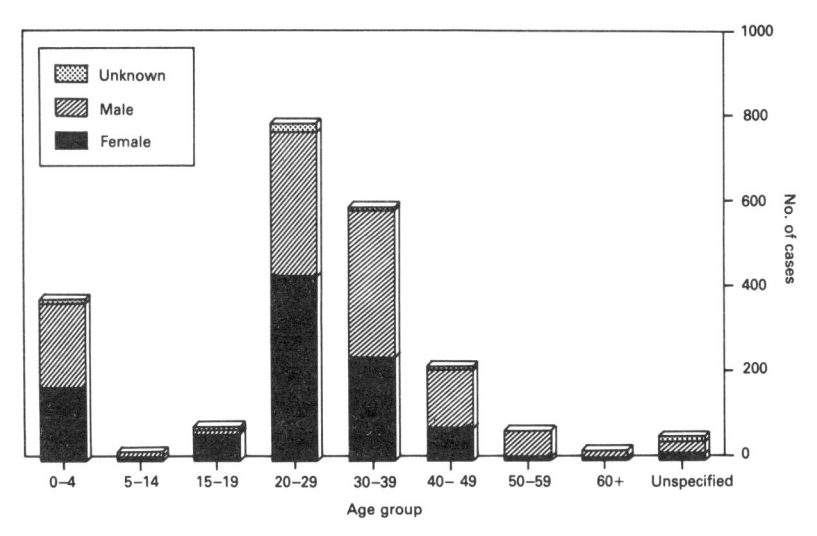

Figure 10.1 Distribution of AIDS cases
by age group and sex

Source Government of Zimbabwe, Ministry of Health, *HIV and AIDS Surveillance Annual Report* (1990), and *HIV and AIDS Surveillance Quarterly Report* (April–June 1991).

Table 10.3 Mortality experience in individual life cover

Year	Policies exposed to risk	Deaths from all causes	AIDS deaths	Overall mortality rate per thousand	AIDS and suspected AIDS mortality rate
1987	275 808	779	9	282	3
1988	323 604	1 067	17	330	5
1989	376 738	1 346	36	357	10
Total	976 150	3 192	62; Average	323	6

Sources Personal communication: unpublished data.

HIV Data

Data on HIV infection are important because of the long incubation period of the disease. These data indicate what will happen in the epidemic in the years ahead.

Sources of HIV data can be divided into three broad groups. The first is incidental testing where a test is carried out as part of a process. Examples are the blood transfusion service, which tests in order to ensure that safe blood is provided to clients; insurance, where testing for HIV infection is intended to protect the industry and policy holders; and clinical testing, where a doctor has a patient tested in order to confirm a suspected HIV-related illness.

The second type of HIV data comes from surveys. These may be done on high-risk groups such as people attending STD clinics or TB patients. Particular categories of workers may be surveyed by employers. The third and most useful type of data are drawn from sentinel surveys, designed to obtain information on the degree of HIV infection across the population.

Blood transfusion data
Zimbabwe was the third country in the world to seek to ensure that blood supplies were safe through testing of donated blood. All blood is tested for HIV I and II. The National Blood Transfusion Service (NBTS) tries to screen out potential HIV-positive donors through a pre-donation questionnaire.

The blood transfusion data will not be representative of the sexually active population for a number of reasons. First, the pre-test counselling should exclude those who are most likely to be carrying the virus. Second, the transfusion service will not take blood in high HIV areas or occupations: for example, it is known that blood is no longer taken from the army or the prisons. This means that the transfusion data may well underrepresent HIV levels in the general population.

Conversely, as there are no free test facilities available in Zimbabwe, individuals may decide to use the transfusion service as a testing centre. If significant numbers do this, it will push up the number of HIV positives recorded. Details on the NBTS HIV antibody results are shown in the Table 10.4.

In the first quarter of 1991 the percentage of HIV-positive blood donors fell from 4.69 to 3.05 per cent, mainly due to a more selective policy towards donors[3]. The bulk of HIV positivity is found in new donors, particularly in the urban areas. At the headquarters, on average 6.84 per cent of new donors are HIV positive, in schools the figure is 1.7 per cent, and in other locations (mainly factories) 14.37 per cent.

The insurance industry
Insurance companies are permitted to test, and do so, for policies of

Table 10.4 HIV positivity in blood donors

Year	Donors tested	Number HIV +	% HIV +
1986	87 376	2 043	2.34
1987	77 759	2 015	2.59
1988	67 002	2 108	3.15
1989	87 666	4 540	5.18
1990	85 161	3 975	4.67

Source Government of Zimbabwe, Ministry of Health, *HIV and AIDS Surveillance Annual Report* (1990).

£100 000 and above. The initial test is an Elisa; if the result is positive or suspicious, a second Elisa and then a Western Blot test will be carried out. Until recently, all tests had to be done through the government health service; however, private pathology laboratories are now being allowed to test.

Precise figures on the number of HIV cases in applicants were not available, the industry indicated that while it was small, it was growing. Certain organisations have been unable to obtain insurance because of high levels of HIV incidence in their members, the example most quoted being the Zimbabwe Owner Drivers' Organisation.

Sentinel surveys
The 1990 HIV and AIDS Annual Report noted:

> In order to get a clear picture of the prevalence of HIV infection in the population, a protocol on sentinel sero-surveillance was developed and sent to all provinces for implementation. Five provinces . . . have already started such studies in six sites . . . The objective of the survey is to get the degree of HIV infection in various groups of the population. The groups were divided into the high risk group and low risk group. The high risk groups includes STD patients. The low risk group includes antenatal and general outpatients. HIV screening laboratories on all these sites are functional.[4]

Some of the results were available and published in 1991; these are shown in Table 10.5. It is evident that levels of HIV positivity were very high among STD attenders. As Zimbabwe had 1 078 293 STD cases in 1989, this is a serious source of concern.

Table 10.5 Summary of selected sentinel survey site results

Type of patient	Negative	Positive	Total	% positive
Midlands Province				
STD	148	48	196	24.5
Antenatal	275	23	298	7.7
Total	423	71	494	14.4
Mashonaland West Province				
STD	106	89	195	45.6
Antenatal	236	59	295	20.0
Total	342	148	490	30.2
Matebeleland North				
STD	97	47	144	32.6
Antenatal	257	32	289	11.1
General outpatient	10	2	12	16.7
Total	364	81	445	18.2
Summary result for all sites				
STD	351	184	535	34.4
Antenatal	768	114	882	12.9
General outpatient	10	2	12	16.7
Total	1129	300	1429	21.0

Source Government of Zimbabwe, Ministry of Health, *HIV and AIDS Surveillance Quarterly Report* (April–June 1991).

PROJECTIONS

The key questions industrialists and businessmen are asking are what is going to happen, how many cases can be expected, and how will it affect their operations? There have been a number of attempts at projecting the incidence of HIV and AIDS in the country and its likely impact on the Zimbabwean economy, society and population.

The first published projection was developed by Peter Fraser-Mackenzie of the Commercial Farmers Union (CFU). This was fairly crude but was important as it was the first attempt to put figures on the possible impact of AIDS in Zimbabwe.[5] Father Brian MacGarry of Silveira House prepared a response to Fraser-Mackenzie and proposed to 'give more precise, less overstated, life expectancies for infected persons and estimates of the chance of HIV transmission from sexually contact with references to recent research on the subject'.[6] The author expects the population to peak in the year 1997 and thereafter to decline. There would be 214 461 cases at the peak in 2017 and in 1997 the number of cases would total 206 118.

The banking and insurance industries have both dabbled in estimating the impact of AIDS on Zimbabwe. The work done by one of the banks concluded that:

> AIDS, however, has changed that dramatic picture of human vitality [referring to growth rates in Harare of seven per cent]. With 30 per cent of mothers testing HIV positive, the population in 2001 may have dropped from ten million to eight million. Harare will no longer be under siege from the countryside. Instead of doubling, it and other urban centres might grow slowly, perhaps only 25 per cent over the decade, or less than two per cent per annum. The urban population would then grow from three now to four million by the year 2000. Under this scenario the rural population would then fall from seven to four million or 43 per cent.[7]

Comments on Modelling

All the early attempts to project the AIDS epidemic in Zimbabwe have been overly pessimistic with regard to the demographic impact. The reasons for this are the assumptions made and methods used. This should not be seen as a criticism of the modellers as they were doing essential pioneering work and did not have access to information currently available.

At the simplest level the epidemic can be expected to follow an 'S' curve as is illustrated in Figure 10.2. The curve will be made up of a number of epidemics according to region, occupational and social group, to name but three of the many variables. The HIV infection levels in the population will follow the curve first, and after a lag of some years it will be replicated by actual AIDS cases and deaths. Key assumptions that need to be made include the following.

1. At what point will the epidemic peak in the sexually active population? That is, when will point 'A' in Figure 10.2 be reached? This includes an assessment of what proportion of the sexually active population (the at-risk population) will be infected – point 'A' – and how long it will take before this happens (point 'D'). It must

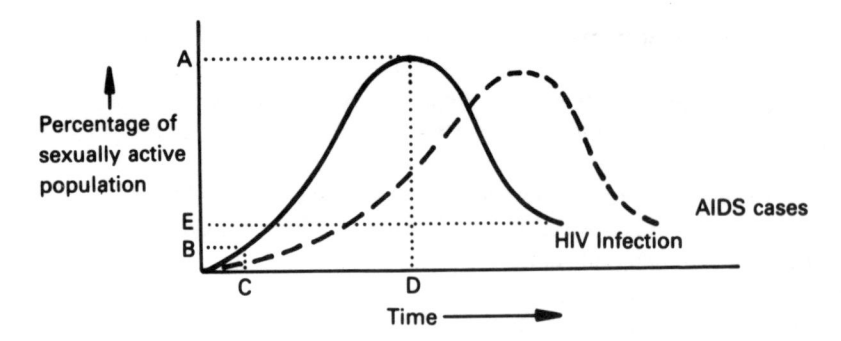

Figure 10.2 The epidemic 'S' curve

be realised that as the virus spreads in an 'at risk population', so the numbers at risk will be reduced. Furthermore, it is possible that the education programmes will reduce the at-risk population.
2. At what point in the epidemic will the rate of growth become exponential? Evidence suggests this may be around 2 per cent (point 'B') and it is therefore academic for Zimbabwe where the level of HIV prevalence is above this.
3. How long will it take for the epidemic to run its course (from point 'C' where it becomes an epidemic to point 'D' where it peaks)? Again, evidence from Africa suggests that this may be a shorter time than generally expected, possibly 6–8 years.
4. Finally, at what level will the epidemic become endemic in a population (point 'E')? There is no firm evidence on this because no country has seen the epidemic run its course yet, but it may be approximately 10 per cent.

It seems that for Zimbabwe the epidemic will probably run its course within a few more years as far as HIV infection is concerned. AIDS cases and deaths will follow the same pattern over the next 5–10 years.

In May 1991, a workshop on modelling the AIDS epidemic was held in Harare. The workshop was sponsored by USAID and run by AIDSTECH, a division of US-based Family Health International (FHI). Participants included epidemiologists and National Aids Control Programme officials from Botswana, Ghana, Malawi, Nigeria, Zimbabwe and South Africa. The Zimbabwean team of four included mainly government officials. Unfortunately, the private sector was not represented.

The conclusions of the workshop were: the level of HIV incidence in a population is unlikely to exceed 35 per cent of sexually active people, and even this may be too high; the progression rate will not exceed 2 per cent per annum; and it is apparent that the virus is not easily transmissible.[8]

Three of the four projections made available in 1991 concluded that the population would actually decline in Zimbabwe over the course of the next decade. This is unrealistic as the percentage of the sexually active population being infected will not reach the levels previously believed. It must be stressed that while the demographic impact will not be as bad as has been predicted, the economic, social and psychological effect can only be surmised.

There is a clear and urgent need for the government to share data and modelling techniques with the private sector. If the ground rules can be agreed then realistic projections can be produced that will allow industrialists to assess the implications of the disease for their operations.

IMPLICATIONS

There can be no doubt that the HIV/AIDS epidemic will have far-reaching consequences for Zimbabwe. It will affect not only the public-sector allocation of provision of services and the demand for health care, but will also influence the business climate.

Demographic

Although the various models still need to be run to determine the precise implications of HIV infection on the population of Zimbabwe, the general conclusion is that there will not be a fall in the number of people. The rate of population growth, currently 3 per cent, is likely to decline, however, and it is possible that by 2010 the population may be stable. Of most demographic significance is the strong probability that the impact of AIDS may not be uniform across the population. Key questions are: will it affect the classes and socio-economic groups differentially; will there be different effects in rural and urban areas; and will it alter the sex and age composition of the population?

The evidence from elsewhere in Africa is contradictory as to the impact on different socio-economic groups. There are data to suggest

Table 10.6 AIDS deaths: one industry experience

Period	AIDS deaths as a percentage of all deaths
1/90–3/90	11.6
4/90–6/90	15.8
7/90–9/90	43.8
10/90–12/90	42.3
1/91–3/91	22.2

Source Personal communication.

that, at least initially, the level of HIV prevalence is highest in the more wealthy and privileged groups. The reasons for such a higher incidence are not hard to find: this group has greater mobility and thus more sexual contacts. The males of the group have greater disposable incomes and some will spend a portion of these incomes on the purchase of beer and sex, with obvious implications for the spread of HIV.

There is currently no published evidence from Zimbabwe to suggest that there are differing levels of infection among the different socio-economic groups. We can speculate that the HIV data from the blood bank showing that new (presumably educated) donors have lower rates than factory workers indicates that higher socio-economic groups are protecting themselves against HIV.

Work done on the socio-economic characteristics of HIV positive and negative male factory workers in Zimbabwe and presented to the sixth International Conference on AIDS provides some pointers. This found that HIV-positive men had fewer years of school (8.07) as opposed to 9.6 for HIV-negative men. In addition, their mean incomes were lower – Z$419.8, as opposed to $494.8 – and they were less likely to have their wives with them or be involved in medical aid and pension plans.[9]

Data from the insurance industry are revealing. Table 10.6 shows how the number of cases rose steadily and in the second half of 1990 approximately 40 per cent of the deaths experienced by one scheme were from HIV-related illness. The experience of this scheme was that people dying from HIV-related illness were younger (40.5 years) than those dying from other causes (44.1 years).

Information provided by one of the other insurance firms allowed analysis of age, occupation and marital status for both individual and group life claims. Before looking at these data, a number of points

Table 10.7 Increasing claims: all group life (by date of death)

Year	Number	Amount	Average claim
1986–7	9	124 312	13 812
1987–8	26	351 991	13 538
1988–9	31	459 842	14 834
1989–90	105	3 058 732	29 131
1990–1*	98	2 553 550	26 057
Total	269	6 548 427	24 344

* Up to 30 April 1991.

Source Personnal communication.

should be made about the nature of the insurance industry. First, the bulk of people with insurance are male: obviously, they are the ones most likely to be working and who have control of the disposable income. Second, the purchasers of individual life cover will be those who either do not have group life cover or who have sufficient income (and vision) to purchase additional cover. Finally, the profile of clients will vary from company to company.

The data from the insurance companies are particularly valuable for industry as they reveal a great deal about the type of employees who are likely to contract the disease – and also, the significant rate of increase in infection (Table 10.7). This in turn can be analysed for the effect on employee benefits, skill availability and shortages and training needs. Tables 10.8 and 10.9 show the experience to date.

Some significant points emerge from these tables. The average age at death was quite high, which means not only will employees have completed their education and/or training, but they will also often be experienced. Nearly all were married, so for every death shown on these tables another three or four may occur; each individual will probably infect his spouse; the youngest children may be infected; and at least one other person must have been involved to introduce the infection into the family unit. Finally, there is a higher incidence among people who are mobile, especially those who move without their spouses.

The question of differential rural urban impact has also been debated in Africa. There is evidence to suggest that the virus may spread more slowly in rural areas depending on the particular circumstances in the country or province. Nonetheless, it will spread

Table 10.8 AIDS deaths: group life policy-holders by occupation, average age and marital status

Occupation	Number	% of total	Average age at date of death	% married at date of death
General worker	76	28.3	36.8	84.2
Clerk	30	11.2	35.9	82.4
Miscellaneous skilled	26	9.7	35.7	80.0
Mineworker	17	6.3	36.9	73.3
Driver	17	6.3	41.2	80.0
Supervisor, etc.	16	5.9	44.1	87.5
Miscellaneous semi-skilled	15	5.6	30.1	88.2
Machine operator, etc.	14	5.2	35.2	66.7
Manager	10	3.7	39.0	85.7
Salesman	10	3.7	36.9	100.0
Welder	7	2.6	37.0	100.0
Miscellaneous unskilled	6	2.2	41.0	100.0
Tailor	6	2.2	39.5	75.0
Electrician	5	1.9	31.4	73.1
Mechanics, etc.	5	1.9	38.8	66.7
Miscellaneous professional	4	1.5	40.5	66.7
Average			37.5	81.8

Notes Professional: Accounts officer, auditor, nurse, teacher.
Skilled: Tailor, receptionist, computer operator, license inspector, customs clearer, sales assistant, fitters (4), builders (2), carpenters (2), bakers (3), weaver, spinner, plumber, printers (2), laboratory technician, cashier.
Semi-skilled: Postman, phone operator, hide handler, skinner, lorry assistant, sprayer, waiters (2), barman, beef operator, depot assistant, spray painter, locomotive driver.
Unskilled: Security guards (4), peasant farmer.

Source Personal communication.

and will probably run its course in these areas as it does in the urban areas, only more slowly.

Zimbabwe, with its long history of labour migration from rural to urban areas, may experience more uniform and more rapid spread than much of Africa. This is borne out by Davies, who astutely observes:

> Although rural urban migration is important through the developing world, in Zimbabwe it has historically been a dominant feature of the labour market. People from all socioeconomic groups retain their links with 'home areas' and travel there relatively frequently.

Table 10.9 AIDS deaths: individual policy holders by occupation, age and marital status

Occupation	Number	% of total	Average age at date of death	% married at date of death
Soldier	44	38.6	31.1	65.9
Miscellaneous skilled	20	17.5	35.6	50.0
Teacher	12	10.5	34.4	66.7
Miscellaneous professional	10	8.8	31.9	57.1
Clerks	7	6.1	31.0	80.0
Police	6	5.3	32.8	80.0
Miscellaneous semi-skilled	6	5.3	38.0	90.0
General hands	5	4.4	40.6	100.0
Unskilled and unemployed	3	2.6	32.0	66.7
Average			34.2	72.9

Notes Professional: Training officer, medical practitioner, lecturers (2), manager, director, businessman, engineer, cost accountant, planner.
Skilled: Nursing aid, electricians (3), plumber, mechanics (2), printer, secretary (2), receptionist, salesmen (4), locomotive inspector, bakers (2), musician.
Semi-skilled: Supervisors (3), powersaw operator, barman.
Unskilled and unemployed: Unemployed (2), peasant farmer.
Source Personal communication.

This would tend to make the virus spread more uniformly throughout the population. In addition, the high number of workers whose wives live in rural areas will tend to increase the number of partners and thus the rate of spread.[10]

The impact of AIDS on the demographic structure will not be as great as is generally expected, and the dependency ratio will not be significantly altered. This is because AIDS deaths will occur in both the working and non-working groups. Two points should be made with regard to this: first, adults and children who die will not necessarily come from the same families, and second, it is likely that there will be a significant increase in the number of orphans requiring care.

Costs

The costs of the AIDS epidemic may be divided into direct and indirect costs. There has been some work done on this in Africa. The bulk of the costs of AIDS to society will be indirect. The greatest part of the indirect cost will be morbidity (time lost because a person is sick) and mortality (years lost because of premature death). It is difficult to produce a valid computation to show the resultant loss to society,[11] especially since various weightings need to be considered.

The direct cost of AIDS is hard to estimate for African countries. Zimbabwe is unusual in that there is a large private medical sector which has been concerned about the likely effect of HIV for some years. The main medical aid society, CIMAS, has established an AIDS Research Unit responsible for establishing the cost of AIDS to the society (see Chapter 11).

The bulk of the Zimbabwean population relies on the state for medical care and so it is here that most AIDS cases will be seen. Since independence in 1980, Zimbabwe has made substantial gains in the areas of education, health, population and small-holder agriculture. The achievements in health during the 1980s have been impressive: the percentage of children fully immunised has more than tripled from 25 to 86 per cent; infant mortality has declined from 86 to 61 per 1000 births; life expectancy has increased from 55 to 59 years; and fertility has declined rapidly and, consequently, the population growth rate fell to an estimated 2.8 per cent per annum in 1989 and is still declining.

The health budget (see Table 10.10) increased in real terms at an annual rate of 4.7 per cent, roughly 50 per cent faster than the rate of economic growth. Over the period up to 1994/95, the health budget is projected to grow annually at approximately the same rate, with the share of GDP remaining constant and the proportion of central government expenditure rising slightly.[12]

The health gains made since independence will inevitably be affected by the AIDS and HIV epidemic. As Zimbabwe moves into the Structural Adjustment Programme, the commitment is to maintain the level of health services in the country. The Ministry will find it difficult to do this in the face of growing demands for health care.

The Ministry of Health currently is not aware of the cost of an AIDS case to the budget. Each case is treated to the best of the ability of the medical services at whatever level it is seen. It is possible that the patient will be referred up through the system until reaching the central or general hospitals.

Apart from the direct cost of the additional patients seen by the health services, there is also the danger of crowding out as HIV-related patients take up beds which would otherwise be available to other patients. It is the intention of the Ministry to institute a system

Table 10.10 Sectoral budget projections: health and education, 1990/91–1994/95

	1990/91	1991/92	1992/93	1993/94	1994/95
Health budget					
Nominal terms (Z$m)	460	552	651	756	872
Real terms (Z$m)	460	484	510	538	565
Proportion of GDP (%)	2.77	2.77	2.77	2.77	2.77
Proportion of government expenditure (%)	5.6	5.9	6.2	6.4	6.5
Education budget					
Nominal terms (Z$m)	1532	1797	2097	2408	2747
Real terms (Z$m)	1532	1576	1642	1714	1778
Proportion of GDP (%)	9.97	9.72	9.47	9.24	9.01
Proportion of government expenditure (%)	18.5	18.0	17.6	17.1	16.7
Memorandum items					
GDP growth rate (%)	4.3	4.4	4.6	4.8	5.0
GDP deflator	0.16	0.14	0.12	0.10	0.10

Source Government of Zimbabwe, *Zimbabwe: A Framework for Economic Reform* (1991–95).

of referring patients to the primary care levels. Nonetheless, treatment will be needed and AIDS will have a negative effect on resources as it does not replace, but rather exists in addition to, other diseases. Furthermore, the bulk of cases will come from a sector of society which does not normally make demands on medical services: the young and middle-aged adults.

INDUSTRY AND AIDS

Extensive fieldwork was carried out in May 1991 to assess the impact of AIDS on industry. Although many companies have experienced the loss of workers from HIV-related infection, numbers have not yet been significant. In general, industry believes that there will be a rapid rise in cases and that they will lose significantly more workers in the years ahead. The year 1995 is regarded as the point at which the effects of the epidemic will really begin to be felt.

The concerns expressed by industry are to protect workers, employee benefits and business activities. The Confederation of Zimbabwe Industries (CZI) has established an AIDS Committee headed by Peter Harding, president of the Matebeleland Chamber in Bulawayo, who regards the epidemic as an immense political, social and economic problem for the country.

Obviously the industrial sector is not homogeneous. The response to, and perception of, HIV infection will vary from company to company depending on the size, location, activity and attitudes of senior management. Nonetheless, there are certain common concerns and responses.

Industrialists expect the impact of the disease to be two-fold. Initially, the concern is with manpower and, in the long run, it will be with the markets.

In the manpower field the effect will be on (i) recruitment procedures; (ii) training and development; and (iii) employee benefits. These issues have been explored extensively in papers presented at seminars by a number of authors. Particular reference can be made to the work done by Tony Devlin of Anglo-American[13] and Helen Jackson of the School of Social Work,[14] both based in Harare. The general consensus is that pre-employment screening of potential recruits is undesirable. It is recognised that the test is not reliable in the early stages of infection; it will not be cost-effective; those infected may remain healthy for long periods; and there are legal constraints on screening. It is further suggested that an individual can be employed for a particular job, but nonetheless excluded from certain benefits because of a medical condition, not just HIV-related illness.

The policy that has emerged is that employees are not tested prior to employment, and so being HIV-free is not a necessary qualification for employment. Where employees are found to be HIV positive, they are employed until such time as they are no longer able to work, at which point their employment is terminated. In general, they are to be treated in exactly the same manner as any other person with a 'dread' disease. Employee benefits for HIV-positive employees are exactly the same as for other employees.

Devlin suggests two areas for consideration by employers: the setting-up of accurate attendance registers, and a review of medical, pension and disability benefits. The completion of attendance registers is necessary in order to pick up absences due to HIV infection, which will register a pattern of absence. Where appropriate, a company should terminate the employee's service with access to appropriate benefits. These benefits may be provided without undue strain on existing schemes or other members.

The issue of testing people offered scholarships and employees prior to training is one that is increasingly debated. It is suggested that testing prior to training may be justified as money is to be invested in a person which will only be paid back in years ahead.

In general, experience shows employees only remain with a company for an average of seven years after they are trained and, as HIV-positive people can remain healthy for lengthy periods, there can be no justification for discriminating against them. If, however, the training period is long and expensive, then this puts a different complexion on the matter and a case could be made for screening. This issue is not just faced by the private sector but is also a source of concern for government and donor agencies. It is worth noting that where overseas training is contemplated, the trainee may be required to be free of HIV by the host country.

Employee benefits are an increasing source of concern. Medical aid schemes face escalating costs as medical intervention becomes more sophisticated, and AIDS is no exception to this. The medical aid societies are aware of the danger that AIDS poses to their costs and to their existing members, and indeed CIMAS recently sought to establish a $21 million reserve fund to cover this eventuality. They requested funding from member companies; however, the response was poor and the decision by the revenue office to disallow contributions as tax benefits had a negative impact on contributions.

Medical aid schemes have a number of options.

1. *Pay All Claims*: this is the popular call which means treating AIDS claims like any other illness. Unfortunately it will be expensive. One scheme in South Africa notes that if only 1 per cent of their members had AIDS this would result in a 31 per cent direct increase in subscriptions. Most medical aid committees believe that this (on top of the usual annual increase of 20–25 per cent) will be totally unacceptable to the low-risk members of that scheme who feel that AIDS is an avoidable illness which they do not wish to subsidise.
2. *Severe Limits*: there is a feeling within schemes that AIDS, like alcohol- and drug-induced illnesses (which generally have limited medical aid benefits) are avoidable. While this strategy protects the interests of the medical aid scheme, the employer will soon be faced by infected employees seeking loans to cover the bills not refunded by the medical aid. Furthermore, since practitioners are not compelled to stipulate diagnosis on their accounts, doctors may well hide an HIV-related treatment as 'pneumonia' or something similar in order to bypass low limits. This ensures that the patient gets covered by medical aid, that the doctor gets paid, and

that even more cross-subsidisation takes place as the subscriptions soar!
3. *Managed Health Care*: early studies in San Francisco showed how the greater use of home-care and hospice facilities substantially reduced the medical costs to AIDS patients without adversely affecting the quality of health care.[15]

In Zimbabwe, CIMAS restricts expenditure on drugs to $1000 per patient per year, but otherwise has no limits. The policies of the other schemes vary. It is generally believed that AIDS will lead to societies reviewing their policies and limits, and obviously as experience accumulates this can be done in an informed manner.

The impact on pension benefits is unlikely to be considerable as the earlier payment of pensions will be probably offset by the shorter period of payment. It is a harsh truth that potential claimants against pensions who are HIV infected are likely to die before they claim, as will their spouses, and very rarely is there a provision for payments to other dependents.

Lump-sum death benefits are likely to see increasing claims. One way around this will be to restrict lump-sum benefits to death in service; therefore, claimants with HIV infection are likely to have service terminated prior to death.

Most companies are seeking to create AIDS awareness among their work force. The CZI is trying to get its members actively involved in creating AIDS awareness and is doing this on a regional basis. Companies are attempting to place counsellors in the workforce and to encourage the use of prophylactic measures. Where possible, a range of activities is being used, including drama groups. Concurrent with this is pressure for better health facilities.

A particularly serious problem is that the economic recovery put forward in the Structural Adjustment Programme will require increasing levels of skilled manpower. If the AIDS epidemic spreads at the rate expected then there will be less manpower available at this level. Clearly, this could have serious implications for the projected economic growth of the country in the years ahead.

Although this chapter focuses on industry in Zimbabwe, the experience of the Commercial Farmers Union (CFU) is instructive. The CFU felt the impact of AIDS before industry, and the farmers were among the first employers to recognise the threat of AIDS to their operations. This appears to have been largely due to the initiatives taken by the CFU AIDS Coordinator, Peter Fraser-Mackenzie. The CFU has established a policy on AIDS and a network of branch AIDS coordinators.

The CFU policies may seen at first sight rather patronising and symbolic of the employer–labour relationship in the rural areas; if they are successful, then they should be widely replicated. Significant losses of labour in both commercial and communal land will have a detrimental effect on the production of both cash and subsistence crops with negative consequences for the Zimbabwean economy.

The consequences of the HIV epidemic for commercial farmers has been further explored by Peter Fraser-MacKenzie. He suggests that the cost of ill health and termination of employment benefits will have to be reviewed. The labour force may become younger and have more female members. Commercial farmers may be badly hit by the loss of skilled labour because of the nature of their operations: skilled workers have considerable autonomy and are required to make important decisions, and thus their loss could be significant. Conversely, the relationship between farmers and their labour force could be such that they can do a great deal in educating and changing behaviour.

Farmers will also face problems with the impact of AIDS beyond the farm. It could affect organisations which supply services, such as the marketing boards, the electricity supply and telecommunications services and so on. The banks may lose staff, and may also try to insure themselves against AIDS hitting their debtors. These problems could equally apply to industry.

Organised labour has responded through the Zimbabwe Congress of Trade Unions (ZCTU). The ZCTU acknowledges that the early response to HIV was slow and, indeed, it was marginal to a number of other issues. In 1989 a policy workshop was held on AIDS and a similar policy to that of the WHO was adopted. This was not widely put into practice. In May of 1991 a workshop on 'AIDS and Workers in Zimbabwe' was held by the ZCTU. This tried to develop ways of turning policy into practice. The ZCTU felt that, until recently, the issue was dominated by the government which was the only voice heard in international fora and the CZI. Unions were excluded and this has only recently been addressed. The involvement of unions is, however, regarded as crucial if the issue is to be realistically addressed.

The workshop noted that broader social and economic factors lead to the spread of AIDS. These include:

poverty and joblessness; female unemployment leading to sexual partners as a means to socio-economic security; social poverty and under-development in communities that lead to alcohol consumption and sex as a form of social relief; lack of accommodation and the break up of family units associated with urbanisation and some forms of employment; traditional and contemporary social attitudes towards male and female roles and status, towards sex, towards multiple partners, towards condom use, and so on.[16]

The government put a short-term programme in place initially and this was followed by a medium-term programme intended to run from July 1988 to June 1993.[17] The short-term plan received financial support from WHO and other donor agencies and began in August 1987. The medium-term plan was expected to cost US$13 million over the five years. It was reported in the press that Zimbabwe's underestimating of the problem of AIDS resulted in donors not providing as much money as was needed at the first donor conference.

Apart from actually dealing with the AIDS problem, the government has reacted by setting out a policy on AIDS. The policy notes that (i) pre-employment screening as part of the assessment of fitness to work is not justifiable and therefore should not be done; (ii) for persons already in employment HIV screening is not justifiable and should not be done; (iii) employees and their families should have access to information and educational programmes on HIV AIDS; (iv) HIV-infected employees should not be discriminated against, including access to, and receipt of any benefits; (v) HIV infection is not a cause for termination of employment: as with any illnesses, persons with HIV-related illness should be able to work as long as they are medically fit for available and appropriate work; (vi) workers, employees and their organisations should create an atmosphere conducive to caring for and promoting the health of all workers. All these policy statements on HIV infection/AIDS and the workplace apply for all forms of employment, including food distribution and the service sector.[18]

There is currently no legislation governing AIDS and HIV infection. The Public Health Act includes provisions aimed at controlling the spread of venereal disease but, presently, AIDS and HIV infection are not encompassed by any of the provisions of the Public Health Act.[19]

CONCLUSION

This chapter has looked at the position of the HIV/AIDS epidemic in Zimbabwe with particular emphasis on its likely implications for industry. It is apparent that there is both good news and bad news for the country.

AIDS will not cause the population to decline. The doomsday predictions as to its economic and demographic impact can be largely discounted. The bad news is that the epidemic means Zimbabwe is going to have to face serious social and economic implications. The need for all parties to get together and address the problem should not be delayed, although the true impact cannot yet be assessed. The level of activity in the country is impressive, but this needs to be coordinated better than is currently the case.

The response of industry to date has been to examine the effect AIDS could have on employee benefits and to put AIDS awareness and education programmes in place. These are intended to reduce the levels of HIV infection among employees. It is clear that industry needs to begin looking at the impact HIV infection will have on their operations as well.

AIDS is not a problem for the government, or the industry, or the unions alone. AIDS is a problem for all and must be addressed by everyone. It is clear from the research that Zimbabwe has the will and has the ability to make a serious attempt to address the AIDS crisis. What is needed is a united approach and an acknowledgement of the seriousness of the problem.

Acknowledgement

I should like to express my gratitude to SAFER who invited me to do the work on which this chapter is based. The work could not have been done without the generous cooperation of a range of Zimbabweans who gave information and answered all my questions to the best of their ability. If a frank acknowledgement of the problem was all that was needed then Zimbabwe would have conquered its AIDS problem. The information in this paper based on interviews was obtained in May 1991.

References

1. P.A. Sato, J. Chin and J.M. Mann, 'Review of AIDS and HIV infection: global epidemiology and statistics', *AIDS*, 3 (1989), suppl. 1, pp. 301–7.
2. Government of Zimbabwe, *Statistical Yearbook* (Harare: Central Statistical Office, 1989).

3. Government of Zimbabwe, Ministry of Health, *HIV and AIDS Surveillance Quarterly Report*, April–June 1991.
4. Government of Zimbabwe, Ministry of Health, *HIV and AIDS Surveillance Annual Report*, 1990.
5. J.P. Fraser-Mackenzie, 'Man in the face of disaster', *Zimbabwe Quarterly*, October 1989.
6. B. MacGarry, 'AIDS and the future', *Zimbabwe Quarterly*, 1990.
7. E.G. Cross, N.E. Reynolds and J. Robertson, 'Zimbabwe: preparing the economy for closer regional co-operation', paper presented at the symposium on Regional Economic Integration and National Development, 14 March 1990, p. 4.
8. I was able to attend some of the sessions of this workshop. The conclusions here are based on my interpretation of material presented there and on informal discussions.
9. M.T. Bassett, J.C. Emmanual and D.A. Katzenstein, 'HIV infection in urban men in Zimbabwe', sixth International Conference on AIDS, San Francisco, 1990, abstract no. Th.D. 581, 1990.
10. R. Davies, 'The political economy of AIDS in Zimbabwe', undated mimeograph.
11. M. Over, S. Bertozzi, J. Chin, B. N'Galy and K. Nyamuryekung'e, 'The direct and indirect cost of HIV infection in developing countries: the cases of Zaire and Tanzania', in A.F. Fleming, M. Carballo, D.W. FitzSimons, M.R. Bailey and J. Mann (eds), *The Global Impact of AIDS* (New York: Alan R. Liss, 1988), pp. 123–35.
12. Government of Zimbabwe, Ministry of Health, *National Sexually Transmitted Diseases Prevention and Control Programme*, 1991.
13. A.C. Devlin, 'Considerations for recruitment, manpower planning and training', paper presented at a seminar on the implications of HIV infection and AIDS for industry, Harare, undated.
14. H. Jackson, 'AIDS and the work place', paper presented at the Symposium on AIDS and its socio-economic implications for Zimbabwe Harare, 14 March 1990; H. Jackson, 'Approaches to the AIDS problem at work', synopsis presented at the Labour Relations and Productivity Conference, 19–20 July 1990.
15. G. Taylor, 'The medical aid response', *AIDS Analysis Africa* (Southern Africa Edition), 2, 2 (August/September 1991).
16. Zimbabwe Congress of Trade Unions, 'Report of the workshop on AIDS and workers', Harare, 1991, mimeo.
17. Government of Zimbabwe, Ministry of Health, *Medium-Term Plan for the Prevention and Control of AIDS*, 1988.
18. Confederation of Zimbabwe Industries, Labour and Legislation Department, *Bulletin No. 490*, Bulawayo, 10 May 1990.
19. G. Feltoe, 'AIDS and the law', *Legal Forum*, 1, 6 (1989).

11 The Medical Costs of AIDS in Zimbabwe
Richard Hore

INTRODUCTION

Zimbabwe, with a population of just over 9 million, is estimated to have over 500 000 people infected with the HIV virus. This study is concerned with the potential impact of the AIDS epidemic on direct health care costs and the continued viability of medical aid societies. Clearly, the main focus is on those in employment, but the broad picture which emerges has major implications for how Zimbabwean society as a whole responds to this crisis.

In Zimbabwe, health care is financed by two parties, the public sector and voluntary health funds, which are known as medical aid societies. Government provides a free health service only for those earning less than Z$150 per month. All those who earn in excess of Z$150 have to meet direct health care costs whether the service is provided by the government or the private health sector.

Zimbabwe has a sophisticated private health sector which is financed almost completely by those in the employment sector. Employers and employees have created medical aid societies to which both parties contribute, in most cases on an equal basis, to meet direct health care costs which are raised on a fee-for-service basis by the providers of health services. Membership of medical aid societies is voluntary, with the employee electing to be a member if he or she is prepared to meet the employee portion of the monthly contribution. The benefit coverage of these societies is extended to the whole family. Contribution rates are graduated in accordance with the monthly salary or wage of the individual, so there is a subsidisation from the higher to the lower paid worker.

Medical aid societies are 'not for profit' organisations and contribution rates are set on historical performance. As medical aid societies have had no past experience of an epidemic of the magnitude of AIDS, they fear that direct health care costs could escalate to the extent that either contribution rates will have to be increased to a level that will make them affordable only to a few, or that such societies will become unviable.

Before addressing the above issues directly, it is first necessary to look at the population of Zimbabwe, its age structure, the known AIDS cases and the projected seroprevalence of HIV infection.

AIDS IN ZIMBABWE

The population of Zimbabwe in 1990 (which is being used as the base year) was estimated at 9 316 332. Table 11.1 indicates that about 43 per cent are under 15, and about the same percentage are in the sexually and economically active bracket (15–44).

Table 11.2 indicates that AIDS deaths are currently sharply concentrated amongst those in the 20–29 bracket, and the under 5s.

The cumulative reported AIDS cases for 1987 to May of 1991 numbered 7230. AIDS cases reported for 1990 were 4362. Of the 26 315 patients tested for HIV infection, 11 788 (or 44.80 per cent) were positive.[1]

Whilst the reported total of cases for 1990 was 4362, it is estimated that the actual figure was 17 992 (four times the actual cases) because of underreporting.

The medical aid society on whose figures this chapter has been based has provisionally identified 1046 AIDS cases. If the figure for the society is proportional to the number of AIDS cases for the whole country, the figure would be 1505. This could well be the true figure for, as will be explained, there are gaps in the society's identification systems which are currently being corrected.

The number of new infections is the most important figure but also

Table 11.1 Age structure of the Zimbabwe population

Age groups	Number of group	% of population
0–4	1 506 451	16.17
5–14	2 677 514	28.74
15–24	1 951 306	20.95
25–34	1 341 086	14.39
35–44	776 982	8.34
45–54	504 945	5.42
55–64	304 644	3.27
>65	253 404	2.72

Table 11.2   AIDS cases by age group and sex in Zimbabwe, 1990

Age group	Female	Male	Unknown	Total	%
0–4	415	460	7	882	21.33
5–14	10	16	0	26	0.63
15–19	88	15	4	107	2.51
20–29	718	562	3	1 283	31.20
30–39	412	759	3	1 174	28.54
40–49	130	284	0	414	10.09
50–59	47	152	0	199	4.85
>60	2	33	0	35	0.85
Unspecified	95	124	23	242	
Total	1 917	2 405	40	4 362	100.00
Total by sex	44.41%	55.59%			

the most elusive. It depends upon accurately identifying *all* AIDS cases and monitoring the increase month by month. This is more difficult than it sounds as the symptoms are many and various. However, it is possible to set estimates derived from these sources against the results which emerged from studies of specific groups in order to help to establish more precisely the scale of the impact.

Risk Groups and HIV Incidence

Of the total population of Zimbabwe, 51 per cent fall in the three high-risk age groups which account for 81 per cent of the total reported AIDS cases: that is, the 0–4, the 20–29 and 30–39 age groups.

Another major risk group, overlapping the high-risk age groups, is that of those with STDs. Reported cases increased from 659 551 in 1988 to over 1 000 000 in 1989.[2] A study conducted by the Ministry of Health at the Genito-Urinary Centre in Harare recorded an HIV-positive rate of 51.9 per cent. This figure does not take into account patients treated by private medical practitioners but, at the same time, it does include cases that were treated for more than one STD incidence in a year.

TB cases increased by 70 per cent from 1986 to 1990. The increase from 1989 to 1990 was 30 per cent. The Ministry of Health's TB Unit estimates that between 55 and 70 per cent of all TB cases are HIV positive. Registered TB cases for 1990 were 8919.

Blood for blood transfusions is collected by the NBTS (a registered

244   *The Medical Costs of AIDS in Zimbabwe*

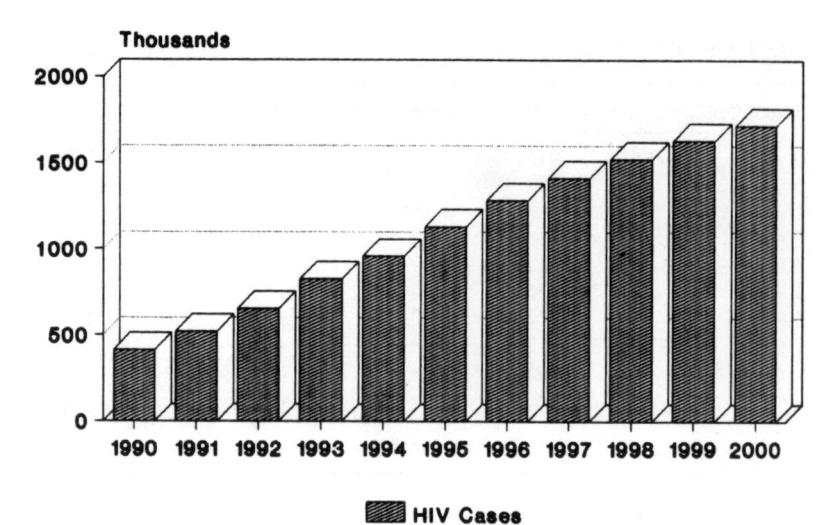

Figure 11.1   Projected HIV cases by year in Zimbabwe: 1990–2000

welfare organisation) from voluntary blood donors. These donors are predominantly in the sexually-active age groups (that is, aged 20–40 years). All blood collected from donors is tested for HIV antibodies.

The NBTS, in addition to its registered donors, has mobile units which visit factories and other work places and (again, on a voluntary basis) collects blood from mainly the same age groups as above. In 1989 the NBTS recorded a 5.18 per cent HIV-positive rate from 87 666 donors. Whilst the percentage positive rate was reduced in 1990 to 65 287, this is probably accounted for by the fact that the mobile units do not return to high-risk sites.[3] In some work forces, the HIV seroprevalence rates are over 28 per cent, and so currently the NBTS is now collecting blood mainly from school children under the age of 16 years, as they are in the lowest age risk category.

The seroprevalence of HIV for 1990 amongst the population as a whole was estimated by the Ministry of Health at 413 043 persons, and is projected to rise to 1 717 391 by the year 2000 (see Figure 11.1).

This projection was based on the following assumptions:

(a) the seroprevalence of HIV was estimated at 7.5 per cent in 1990;
(b) HIV transmission was assumed to have taken off in 1982;
(c) perinatal transmission was assumed to be 30 per cent;
(d) average incubation period for HIV was assumed to be 7.8 years;

(e) average survival time after the onset of AIDS was assumed to be 1.5 years.

The extrapolations of these assumptions agree well enough with the figures from the NBTS of a 5.18 per cent HIV-positive rate in the sexually active groups if applied to the total population. With STDs presenting at a 51.92 per cent HIV rate, as there were over 800 000 STD patients nationwide in 1989 this would suggest a likelihood of over 400 000 HIV cases.

The number of recorded AIDS deaths increased in 1990 over the previous year by 74.53 per cent to 644. Based on the WHO's findings, that only one out of four AIDS cases are reported, this could well also apply to recorded AIDS deaths as it is a known fact that a high percentage of AIDS cases return to their communal homes to die amongst their families. The cause of death is not recorded in these areas.

AIDS and Medical Aid Societies

CIMAS Medical Aid Society is the largest in Zimbabwe, with over 250 000 beneficiaries.[4] Excluded from the statistical data is a scheme for those over 60 years and the scheme for pensioners who reside outside Zimbabwe. This reduces the beneficiary count to 220 340.

The scheme is structured on a three-tiered basis; there is a low-cost primary scheme, and a general scheme with comprehensive benefits (except that private hospitalisation cover is excluded). The third tier is the private hospital scheme which has a full range of benefits and, as its name suggests, covers the full cost of private hospitalisation up to the level of a two-bed ward.

The ethnic group mix is 70.22 per cent blacks, 24.75 per cent whites, 2.61 per cent Asians and 2.42 per cent others. This ethnic group mix applies to all three schemes, with the black members predominant in all schemes. Of the total members of the Society, 69 per cent have elected to join the private hospital scheme.

Table 11.3 shows that the beneficiaries' age groups are very similar to those of the national figures, but the Society has a greater number of beneficiaries in three of the four high-risk age groups. On the other hand, the highest number of beneficiaries are in the lowest-risk age group of 6–15 years.

These figures, provide a typical profile of a medical aid society where the young and healthy subsidise the health costs of the elderly.

Table 11.3 Age groups of beneficiaries (1990)

Age groups	Beneficiaries	Percentage	National %
0–5	33 732	15.31	16.17*
6–15	47 388	21.51	28.74
16–25	41 651	18.90	20.95*
26–35	42 601	19.33	14.39*
36–45	27 250	12.37	8.34*
46–55	14 155	6.42	5.42
56–65	8 294	3.76	3.27
>65	5 271	2.39	2.72

* High-risk age groups.

Table 11.4 Average cost per beneficiary (1990)

Age groups	Cost per beneficiary ($)
0–5	152.82
6–15	111.69
16–25	260.59
26–35	376.56
36–45	412.74
46–55	680.27
56–65	1 006.84
>65	1 586.43

They also clearly illustrate just how vulnerable medical aid societies are to the AIDS epidemic. If the claims expenditure of the high-risk age groups (that is, the 0–5 and the 18–40 year age groups) were to approximate those in the 55–65 age group, total claims expenditure would more than double, and contribution levels would rise so high as to put medical aid cover out of reach of all but the very wealthy.

With the AIDS epidemic beginning to bite in Zimbabwe, and fearing the escalation in claims costs, CIMAS established an AIDS research unit in March 1991. This unit, which is headed by a qualified epidemiologist, has been charged with establishing the actual incidence and cost of AIDS to the Society at present, and to monitor the epidemic's growth on a month by month basis.

To appreciate how difficult this task is, it is necessary to consider the problem of confidentiality. Whilst medical aid societies are billed for the HIV tests carried out on their beneficiaries, the societies are not advised as to whether the tests are positive or negative (to protect the confidentiality of patients), and neither is such a diagnosis given on medical aid claim forms. The Western Blot confirmatory test was stopped two years ago because of its high cost. The cost to the societies of AIDS arises from opportunistic diseases as a result of impaired immune systems, and there is therefore not a single diagnosis to identify but a whole range of diagnoses.

To identify possible AIDS cases, computer programmes have been written to extract all claims of patients who have been referred for HIV tests (Elisa), and these claims are examined for AIDS-related symptoms. Those claims which indicate the possibility of HIV infection are extracted both before and after the HIV test dates, and the patient's claims are followed on a month-to-month basis thereafter. The whole family claiming pattern is also monitored in the same way. This database will take time to produce meaningful figures for the future but historical data has been extracted over the last two years and is providing useful data and guidelines. In addition, all STD cases are being flagged, as are all TB cases.

It is known that a large number of members of the Society are either blood donors or give blood to the mobile unit of the NBTS when their work place is visited. All donors are HIV tested but, as no charge is raised for these tests, there is no way of identifying these members on the computer. This partly explains why, of the known AIDS cases, there is a large percentage of cases where no trace of an HIV test can be found.

In order to try to cover this gap, claims are also being extracted for all persons in the age groups 0–5 years and 20–40 years who have current costs exceeding that for the particular age group for the previous year.

Research Findings

Based only on cases which had been HIV tested, for the period June 1990 to May 1991 no less than 140 definite AIDS cases were identified and 906 probable cases. Of the 140 definite cases, 17 were cases brought forward from the previous year and there were 123 new cases. All the probable cases related to the current year. Fourteen of the definite cases died during the year under review.

Claims expenditure for the two groups came to $1 546 308, with a straight average cost per case of $1478.00. The split of the total expenditure was as shown below.

General practitioners	22.56
Medical consultants	13.32
Hospitalisation	17.29
Drugs	11.15
Others	35.68

Figures were obtained from a different society which had carried out the same extraction with 466 definite cases of AIDS being identified at a total cost of $440 393. The society concerned has just over 47 000 beneficiaries.

The straight average cost per case was $741.00 and the split of expenditure was as shown below:

General practitioners	20.20
Medical consultants	13.16
Hospitalisation	21.58
Drugs	18.16
Others	26.90

The highest costs under 'Others' was for pathology. This society recorded 7 deaths from AIDS in the year under review. All the above figures include a mix of cases, from new cases to full-blown AIDS, and it is therefore wrong to draw the conclusion that the average direct cost of AIDS can be set at the straight averages given above.

To try to arrive at the average direct cost of an AIDS case, the cost of the 14 patients who died of AIDS during the year under review was extracted from the start of treatment until death. This averaged to $3095.00. The equivalent figure in South Africa, with their higher medical fee tariff, would be R9403.00 per patient.

The cost to CIMAS of the $3095.00 per case was $2303.00. The reason for the difference is that the Society has an annual limit of $1000.00 on drugs, and a number of patients not on the Private Hospital Scheme (PHS) were admitted to private hospitals.

Case Histories

Of the 140 definite AIDS cases, the spread over the three schemes was Primary Scheme 33.87 per cent, General Scheme 35.48 per cent and the PHS 30.65 per cent. As the PHS covers 69 per cent of the beneficiaries and the other two schemes share, on almost equal basis, the remainder, the percentage of AIDS cases to beneficiaries covered is very much greater in the two smaller schemes. As these two schemes are mainly made up of the lower-paid workers, this would support the growing belief that it is not the better-off professional classes who are more prone to contract HIV infection as once was the general consensus.

Of the definite cases, 68 per cent were members, 19 per cent spouses and 13 per cent children. The importance of these percentages will be refered to later.

The individual case histories which are examined have been confined to the definite cases, but the indications from the probable cases already examined indicate no serious deviation. Because of the large number in this group, detailed extraction of data is still in the early stages.

The 12 cases detailed below show the large variance in expenditure and in shortfalls (non-medical aid awards) dependent upon which scheme the patient belongs to, the length of hospital stay, personal resources and education.

Case 1
Female, 30 years, 1 dependent child 6 years
Total cost $12 975.00
Medical aid award $5 711.84
Shortfall $7 263.16
Patient first seen 8 January 1990; died 17 March 1991.

Reason for the large shortfall: patient admitted to a private hospital but not on the PHS.

Case 2
Male 32 years, single
Total cost $8534.00
Medical aid award $7366.75
Shortfall $1167.25
Patient first seen 8 January 1991.

Reason for shortfall: exceeded the drug limit of $1000 per annum. Patient was referred to a neurologist in South Africa with chronic neurological problems. Following extensive investigations, including Magnetic Resonance Scans, was tested and found HIV positive. Discharged from hospital and given a prescription for AZT at a cost of $1400.00 per month. The drug AZT is not covered by the Society.

Case 3
Male 38 years, spouse 33 years, 2 children 9 and 7 years
Total costs $4104.00
Medical aid award $821.00
Shortfall $3283.00
Patient first seen 3 November 1990; died January 1990.

Reason for shortfall: private hospitalisation and exceeding drug limit. Patient on Primary Scheme, not entitled to private hospital accommodation.

Case 4
Male 36 years, spouse 23 years, 2 children 9 and 7 years
Total costs $3380.00
Medical aid awards $3139.33
Shortfall $240.67
Patient first seen 10 January 1990; died 5 February 1991.

Member of the PHS, hence low shortfall, applicable only to drugs.

Case 5
Male 45 years, spouse 32 years, 1 child 3 years.
Total costs $3802.91
Medical aid awards $3330.65
Shortfall $472.26
Patient first seen 3 July 1990; last claim 3 May 1991.

A member of the PHS.

Case 6
Female 49 years, no dependants
Total costs $7927.00
Medical aid award $7097.44
Shortfall $829.56
Patient first seen 4 January 1990; died 20 December 1990.

Member of the PHS. Out of the total, hospitalisation came to $5023.57. Shortfall in respect of drugs. Patient admitted 6 times to hospital (February 1990 17 days; March 1990 3 days; March 1990 8 days; April 1990 8 days; November 1990 1 day; and December 1990 6 days).

Case 7
Male 41 years, spouse 36 years, 3 children, 16, 8 and 5 years
Total costs $3829.14
Medical aid awards $2231.48
Shortfall $1597.66
Patient first seen 7 June 1990; died 2 December 1990.

Member of the General Scheme, not entitled to private hospital cover. Admitted to a private hospital for 15 days, shortfall $1531.33.

Case 8
Male 34 years, spouse 39 years, 2 children, 7 and 5 years
Total costs $1974.93
Medical aid awards $1520.95
Shortfall $453.98
Patient first seen 29 January 1990; resigned membership end of December 1990.

Member of the PHS. Shortfall in respect of drugs.

Case 9
Male 31 years, spouse 28 years, 3 Children, 7, 4 and 1 year.
Total costs $845.59
Medical aid awards $753.60
Shortfall $91.99
Patient first seen 2 July 1990, latest claim April 1991. A member of the General Scheme. Hospitalised in a Government Hospital on 5 separate occasions for 1 day each. Shortfall on drugs.

Case 10
Male child 9 months, Father 36 years, spouse 34 years, 1 sibling, 10 years
Total costs $762.70
Medical aid awards $654.08
Shortfall $108.62
Both parents were HIV positive; the spouse first sought treatment on 11 January 1990 and died in September 1990. The father first sought treatment in April 1990 and last claimed on the Society on 14 May 1991. The eldest child shows no sign of being infected.
Patient first seen 1 April 1990; died January 1991.

Father a member of the General Scheme. Shortfall on drugs.

Case 11
Female 27 years, spouse 33 years, 2 children, 12 and 9 years
Total costs $326.90
Medical aid awards $314.50
Shortfall $12.40
Patient first seen 30 April 1990; died April 1991.

Patient on the Primary Scheme. Treatment consisted of General Practitioner visits and injections.

Case 12
Male 32 years, spouse 26 years, 1 child 2 years
Total costs $571.88
Medical aid awards $436.81
Shortfall $135.07
Patient first seen May 1990; died January 1991.

Treatment consisted of General Practitioner visits and injections.

Preliminary Observations

The above data seem to confirm that adult patients becoming symptomatic only live for between 1 year and 15 months, and infected new-born children survive less than a year. It was observed that in the cases where members had died leaving a family, the eldest child in the majority of cases was 7 years of age. As there were no indications that these children were HIV positive, the average incubation period could be less than that estimated for developing countries (7.5–8 years).

In the past, the Society had never bothered to record the date of death of members and their dependants. The examination of individual case histories indicated just how important this information is in further identifying AIDS cases. This has now been programmed into the computer system and there will be monthly extracts of deaths in the high-risk age groups. These cases will be examined for claiming patterns and costs. Any unexplained increase in deaths in other age groups will also be investigated.

As has been stated, STD cases are now flagged on the computer as these cases are 52 per cent more prone to HIV infection in the heterosexual transmission of the AIDS virus, both in becoming infected or in passing the infection on.

Identification of STD cases has only just begun, and the first print-out was for June 1991. This identified 411 cases with a total claims cost of $21 167. Work to establish the seroprevalence level of these cases is still being undertaken.

This Society has always covered the cost of STD claims but there are still a number of societies in Zimbabwe that do not. It has been estimated that a 5 per cent reduction of STDs could result in a 2 per cent reduction in the national seroprevalence level.

The examination of the above data also brings sharply into focus the devastating consequences the AIDS epidemic will wreak on the family. As has been stated, of the identified cases, 68 per cent were the working members rather than spouses. Unless the spouse was in gainful employment, the death of the member will deprive the whole family of medical aid cover. Looking at the age groups infected, mainly 20 and 30 year olds, it is unlikely that the spouse is going to escape infection and, as most of the married couples have young families, they will be orphaned.

Medical aid societies by definition tend to cater for those in employment. With the high level of educated unemployed in Zimbabwe, the member who dies will be replaced, and therefore until the unemployed labour pool is exhausted the membership of the society is unlikely to decrease.

In looking at the drug costs of the cases detailed above, it must be remembered that the drug AZT in not available in Zimbabwe and has to be imported by the individual if prescribed. The current cost of AZT is $1400.00 for a month's prescription and medical aid societies do not include it in the list of prescribed drugs covered by benefits.

Overall Implications

The extraction of all the foregoing data is to establish three major factors: the number of beneficiaries already infected, the number of new infections and the number of AIDS cases. These factors are important in establishing the potential impact of the AIDS epidemic on medical aid societies, both in regard to costs and membership growth. Of the three factors, the most important is the number of new AIDS cases since these persons will be most likely to seek medical attention, the cost of which will have to be born by such societies (either in part or in full).

The projected adult HIV prevalence is estimated by the Ministry of Health to have been 7.5 per cent in 1990, and this will increase to 24.7

254   *The Medical Costs of AIDS in Zimbabwe*

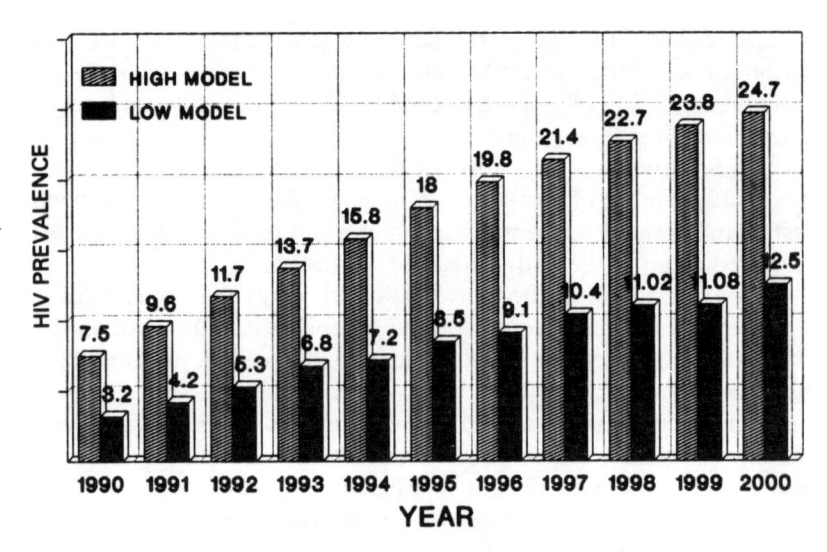

Figure 11.2   Projected adult HIV prevalence

per cent by the year 2000 (see below). The epidemic is not expected to exceed 35 per cent of the sexually active population (see Figure 11.2).

1990	1991	1992	1993	1994	1995	1996	1997	1998	1999	2000
7.5%	9.6%	11.7%	13.7%	15.8%	18.0%	19.8%	21.4%	22.7%	23.8%	24.7%

Based on the figures for Zimbabwe, in 1990 it is estimated that 9769 beneficiaries of the CIMAS were infected with the HIV virus, and this figure will increase to 40 617 by the year 2000 (see Figure 11.3).

The Society has provisionally identified 1046 AIDS cases. (If the figure is based on the number for the whole country, it would be 1505. This could well be the true figure for, as previously explained, there are gaps in the Society's identification systems which are currently being corrected.)

The impact on claims costs
For the first time it has been possible to graph the actual costs of AIDS. Claim costs for the 8 months ending February 1991 were compared with claim costs for the 8 months ending February 1990. The 1990 claims were then adjusted for increases in tariffs since February 1990 and the costs of any new benefits introduced after February 1990 were deducted. The cost per beneficiary was estab-

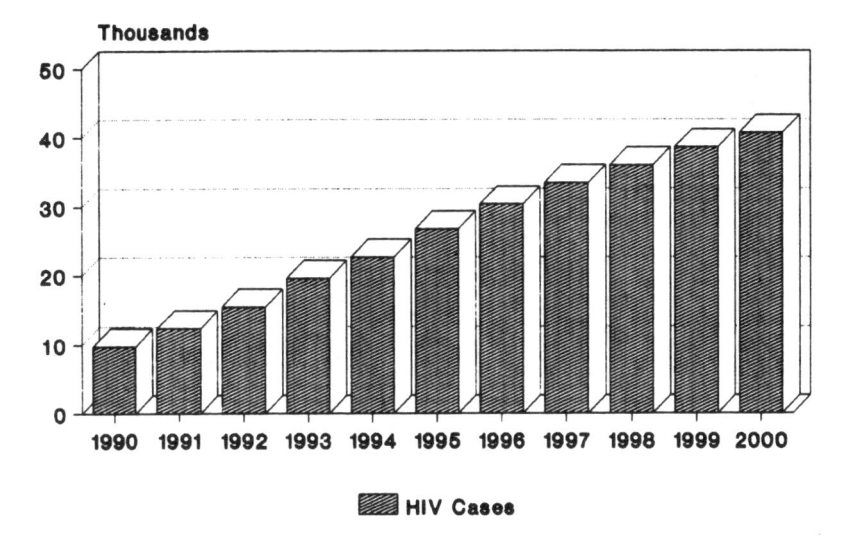

Figure 11.3 Projected HIV cases by year
(medical aid), 1990–2000

lished and the 1990 figures were extended by the increase in beneficiaries since February 1990.

Year after year in the past, when this exercise was undertaken the claim costs per age group reflected a reduction for all but the age groups over 55 years of age. This is accounted for by the fact that the increase in beneficiaries was in the young and healthy. The reduction in claims cost between 1988 and 1989 by age groups may be seen in Figure 11.4. Comparing 1991 with 1990 there was a definite increase in claims costs in the younger age groups (see Figure 11.5).

The direct costs extracted for both the definite and probable AIDS cases came to $1 546 000.00. The increased costs based on the above figures came to $3 245 000.00 and can be seen in Figures 11.6 and 11.7.

From the adjusted figure for current AIDS cases, and taking the current average claim cost per case of $3095.00 (adjusting it for tariff increases that came into effect from 1 July 1991 (30 per cent), and allowing an inflation rate of 15 per cent per annum), the cost of AIDS treatment over the next four years is estimated at $28 million. The Society's liability, based on present benefit levels, is estimated at $21 million.

Potential claims liability against the Society by the year 2000 for the estimated 40 617 HIV-infected beneficiaries would be $500 million,

256   *The Medical Costs of AIDS in Zimbabwe*

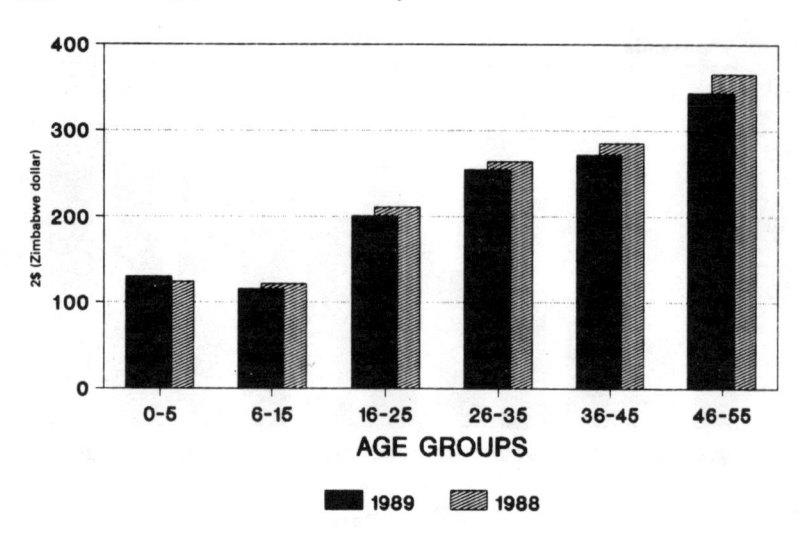

Figure 11.4   Decrease in claims cost: 1989

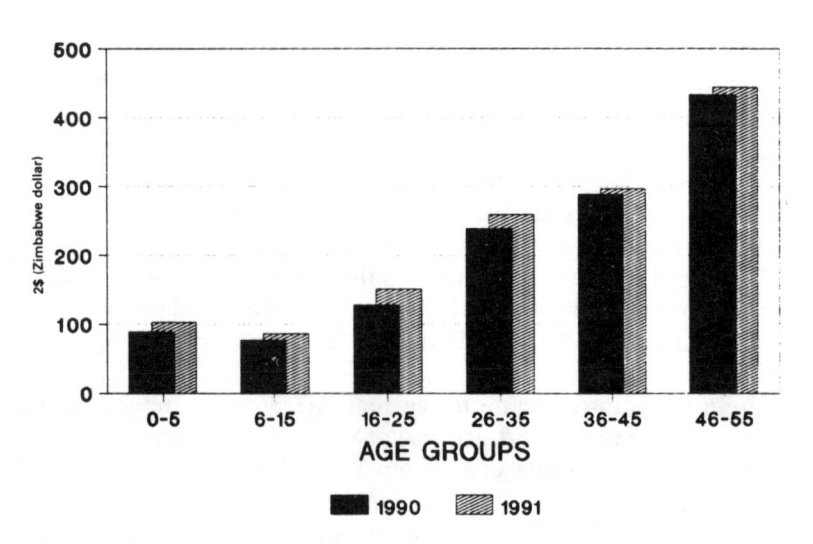

Figure 11.5   Increase in claims costs through AIDS (cost per beneficiary)

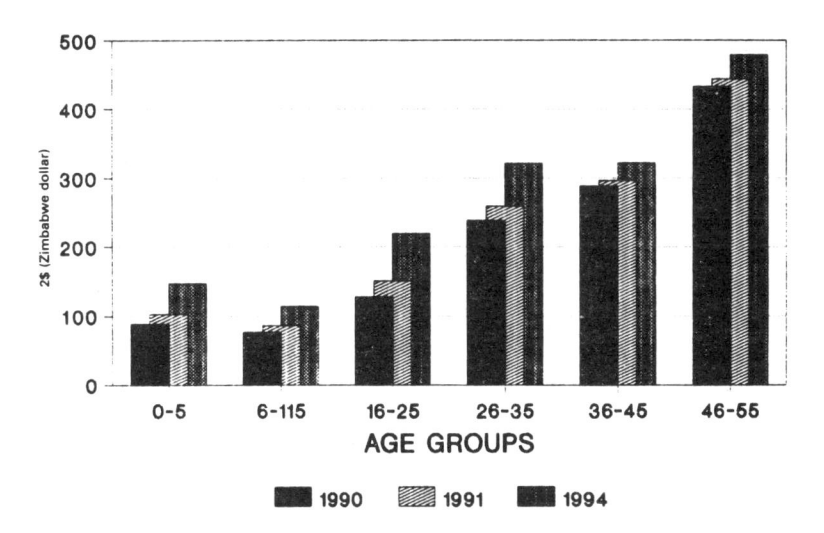

Figure 11.6 Increase in claims costs through AIDS (projected to 1994: cost per beneficiary)

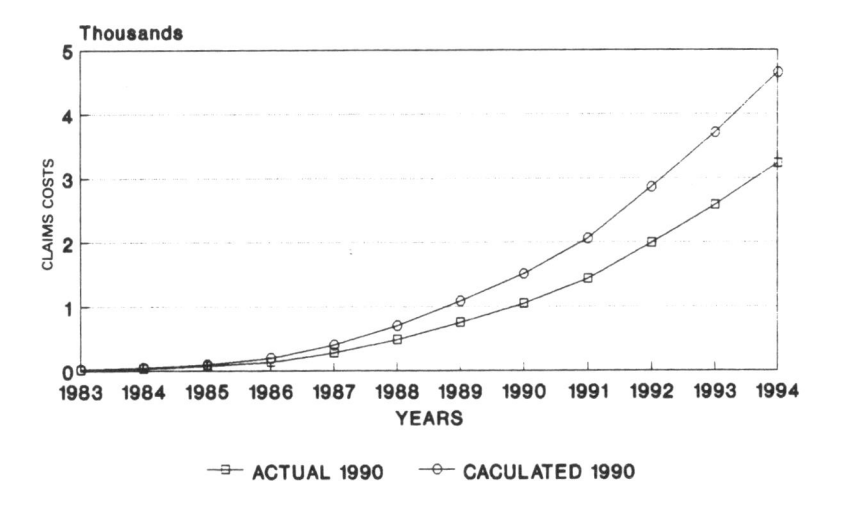

Figure 11.7 Increase in claims costs through AIDS over next four years (Medical Aid Society)

and the Society's liability will be, if current benefit levels are maintained, $372 million. These figures have been based on the current number of beneficiaries and do not take into account membership growth. If membership growth is projected at the current average of 12 per cent per annum, the additional costs, (all things being equal) would increase by a further 177 per cent.

This figure is a straight projection and does not take into account the effects of behaviour change, or the likelihood that over 40 per cent of those reaching the age of 16 will not live to their 50th birthday. At present, by far the most expensive age groups are the 55 plus age group, which have an average claim cost per annum of $1300.00 as compared to $394.00 for the 26–45 age group. Medical aid societies in developed countries are battling to meet the costs of what is referred to as the 'greying of Europe', and this is equally true in America. In industrialised countries it has been estimated that between 1980 and 2040, the average proportion of persons aged over-65 will have increased from 12.2 per cent to 21.9 per cent of the total population. This will not be so in Africa. In Zimbabwe at present the over-65 group represents only 2.72 per cent of the total population. The forced saving in claim costs through the non-'greying of Africa' would have to be taken into account when making any long term projection on costs.

Interventions

All the above figures have been calculated on the current direct costs of the disease and do not take into account a number of interventions that can decrease the cost and spread of HIV infection. Whilst the National AIDS Council has embarked on a massive information and education programme and the nationwide promotion and issue of condoms, there are other more practical interventions which can be introduced.

There are a limited number of beds in private hospitals in Zimbabwe, and all these hospitals are at capacity. In May 1991 it was reported that the largest of these hospitals had 30 per cent of its medical beds occupied by AIDS patients, and the paediatric wards were completely full of AIDS patients. It is understood that a similar situation exists within both government and missionary hospitals.

The answer lies in having these patients removed from hospital, and nursed at home. An investigation has been carried out of the private nursing facilities in the major centres and it was established that they had the capacity to provide this service and were keen to undertake it. This matter was brought before the National Association of Medical Aid Societies, and an acute home nursing benefit was introduced into the national tariff of fees. Previously there was only limited cover for home nursing of chronic cases. The acute care tariff covers in full the cost of providing a 24-hour cover by a Nurse and for daily visits by a State Registered Nurse. The fee for the Nurse Aid for 24 hours is $40.00 and the State Registered Nurse charges on a fee-for-service basis at $24.60 per visit. A two-bed ward in a private hospital cost up to $320.00 per day and this does not include the usual sundry charges. This additional benefit has been well received by the medical profession, and the government is looking at the introduction of a similar benefit. The introduction of this benefit, besides reducing congestion in the hospital, should have a considerable impact on hospital fees.

Another possible intervention is the provision of treatment in pleasant clinic facilities with a pathology laboratory, as well as provision of a counselling service for patients. With the stigma that is presently attached to AIDS victims, the introduction of such clinics may have to wait until the community can accept an AIDS patient as they do any other sick person. The lead in the provision of this type of service has been taken in Puerto Rico, where in 1987 they introduced a comprehensive model that emphasised prevention, education, surveillance, early detection and outpatient care for AIDS victims. It has been reported that in the first year the length of stay was reduced from 22.3 days to 11.3 days, and the annual mean cost of inpatient care was reduced by 74.41 per cent.[5]

CONCLUSIONS

Medical aid societies cannot practically or morally avoid meeting the costs of AIDS patients. From a practical point of view, patients do not die from AIDS but from opportunistic diseases, the signs and symptoms of which are not specific to HIV infection and can be caused by other conditions. Unless medical science can come up with an easily recognisable diagnosis, medical aid administrators will not be in a position to reject claims categorically. From a moral point of view, the whole concept of medical aid is the provision of financial support for the sick and the dying. Cancer kills and is a more expensive disease, yet no medical aid society excludes it from their benefits.

What is frightening about AIDS is that it is a pandemic that is destined to claim millions of lives of young people and infants. Because it is a pandemic it will have far-reaching effects for those who have to meet its costs, whether they are governments, medical aid societies or other institutions. Health care finance planners need to assess accurately their financial liability and then find the resources to meet them. This does not mean that they should be passive; they can be pro-active by coming up with innovative ways of reducing the full impact of the costs. To be successful in this, they must know everything about the effect of AIDS on their society, its effect on claims costs, on membership, on availability of health services and its total effect on all aspects of the economy. This, then, is the challenge, and time is not on our side.

References

1. AIDS Control Programme and Health Information Unit, Zimbabwe (1990/1991).
2. Ibid.
3. Ibid.
4. CIMAS Medical Aid Society, Harare, Zimbabwe.
5. Y.H. Kouri, D.S. Shepard, F. Borras, J. Sotomayor and G.A. Gellert. 'Improving the cost-effectiveness of AIDS health care in San Juan, Puerto Rico'. *Lancet*, 337 (8 June 1991).

12 Simple Methods for Monitoring the Socio-Economic Impact of AIDS: Lessons from Sub-Saharan Africa

Tony Barnett and Piers Blaikie

INTRODUCTION

The WHO estimated in 1991 that as many as 6 000 000 people in the whole of Africa might be HIV positive (the estimate for South Africa is about 100 000).[1] If this estimate is in any way a correct indication of the situation, then the downstream socio-economic effects of AIDS-related illness and death may be very considerable in the next decades.

In Africa AIDS is mainly transmitted heterosexually between adults and, to a lesser extent, from mothers to their unborn and new-born children. Although during the mid-1980s the disease was thought to be predominantly an urban problem, evidence is now accumulating that, in parts of Central and East Africa, HIV I has spread into rural areas.

The AIDS/HIV epidemic has two characteristics which make consideration of, and response to, its social and economic impact of the greatest importance. First, the disease is predominantly sexually transmitted, so it is age-cohort specific in its impact on a population. Second, there is a relatively long time between infection and onset of symptoms. Thus the period of asymptomatic infectiousness makes it a long wave disaster, in contrast to other more familiar disasters such as flood, hurricanes, drought and famine, all of which occur rapidly enough for people to be able to react fairly early.

The first characteristic has considerable long-term implications for social and economic life. Africa is the only continent in which there has been a long-term decline in food production over the past 20 years. It is also a continent where much food production is dependent on the work of farming, fishing and herding households. In these systems of food production, the main productive input is the labour of household members. Unusually high levels of illness and death in young children and in the economically important 15–45 age group will almost certainly reduce agricultural productivity. It will present these already poor societies with huge problems of orphan care as well as care of the terminally ill, in addition to possible declines in food availability.

The second characteristic means that established coping responses are likely to be inadequate to confront the impact of an epidemic which is well established in a population before the first publicly recognisable signs become apparent. Thus the social policy response has to confront a well established epidemic situation rather than one which is easily and early perceived. This means that the costs of dealing with the impact are already huge by the time it is recognised. It is therefore important to have simple monitoring indicators which can provide early warning. We should note, however, that as in the case of famine early warning systems, while indicators are comparatively accessible they have only semiotic status. While they are signs of a developing crisis, they often do not tell us the detail of the processes of the epidemic, which can be expected to differ from one society to another. Thus we should not be seduced by the apparent accessibility of these indicators into disregarding the importance of detailed case studies which focus on the processes which give rise to the signs.[2] Our own work in Uganda has attempted to address some of these issues of process.[3]

OUTLINE

This chapter reviews some of the practical and pragmatic lessons gained from some early AIDS impact research in the rural areas of sub-Saharan Africa.[4] The majority of this work has been done in Uganda, but additional experience has been gained from limited fieldwork in Kenya. The main focus is on the following issues:

(a) the impact on food and cash crop production;
(b) the effect of loss of household members on the community;

(c) the household coping mechanisms developed to cope with the impact of the disease.

The first section outlines the types of study which can be useful in an attempt to establish early understanding of the impact of the disease and to provide some crude (but refinable) instruments for monitoring that impact. The second part describes some of the results of using these techniques. In the third section, some broader implications of the impact are considered in the form of a research agenda. The final section considers some of the broadest equity implications of the impact of the pandemic.

DATA SOURCES AND TECHNIQUES FOR MONITORING AIDS IMPACT

Population Pyramids

This is a very simple technique. Most countries have census data which shows the 'normal' population age and gender distribution. In most African countries this pattern shows a large number of people in the lower age groups and fewer in the older age groups, which approximates to a pyramid. Given the pattern of the disease, one would expect there to be a marked deviation from this expected pattern in a community affected by AIDS. Even in the absence of confirmed diagnoses of the disease, age/gender distributions which deviate markedly from this normal distribution might be interpreted as indications that AIDS is already affecting the population structure. This kind of comparison can be used as a field method in small communities.

Orphan Studies

Another robust but useful indicator of the impact of the disease on the population is the study of the dates of orphaning in a population. If we take a sample or complete enumeration of orphans in a population and graph the year of parental death, then it is possible to compare the actual rate against the assumed 'normal' rate. What this normal rate is will depend upon local circumstances but, in the absence of any known outbreak of disease, famine or other disaster event, it can be expected that the rate might remain constant or exhibit a slow rise consistent with overall population growth. If, however, there is a clear geometric increase in the number of orphanings then, in an area where an AIDS epidemic is suspected, the orphaning curve might be expected to reflect the impact of the epidemic. Studies along these lines have been carried out in Uganda.[5]

Agricultural Impact Simulation Studies

In communities which depend upon subsistence agriculture of whatever kind, from settled cultivation to nomadic herding, the main resource is labour. Loss of labour may be assumed to have serious implications for overall agricultural productivity in an area. However, different farming systems will be differentially sensitive to the loss of labour. One approach to understanding this problem is to simulate the impact of AIDS, given established knowledge of its age-cohort specificity, upon farming systems with a view to arriving at some rough-and-ready ordering of farming systems in terms of their greater or lesser sensitivity to labour loss. This is potentially a powerful policy instrument.

Household Labour Use, Socio-Economic Differentiation and Coping Ability: Parameters for Classification

Disasters, whether earthquakes, floods or famines, do not affect all people in the same way. Differences in wealth and age influence household and individual responses to crisis. This is true of AIDS. Households' and individuals' ability to respond to a crisis depend on a range of resources. Thus some households and individuals are more vulnerable to the socio-economic impact of the disease than are others. Structured analysis of case material can identify the ways in which types of household respond to changes in the labour balance and thus provide an indication of those household situations most likely to face stress.

Household Structure Changes

Research in Uganda suggests that one manifestation of coping strategies adopted by a population is change in the structure of households. This could be a useful indicator, but it is difficult to use as it depends upon the existence of earlier studies or the establishment of sound baseline data from recall interviews, with all the problems that recall data involves. However, if such data are available, they are another useful indicator. Changes in household structure, possibly in response to AIDS, are already apparent in the Rakai district of Uganda.

THE RESULTS WHICH HAVE BEEN OBTAINED FROM THESE STUDIES

Population Pyramids in Buganda

Buganda, in south-western Uganda on the shore of Lake Victoria, is an area where, along with parts of Burundi, Rwanda and parts of Tanzania, rates of rural seropositivity are known to be very high. In February and March 1989, five villages in rural Uganda were surveyed. Four of these settlements were in Buganda and one, used as a control, was in the far west of the country (near the border of Rwanda) where rates of seropositivity and numbers of AIDS deaths were said to be low. Thus we suspected that the village in the west of the country was less likely to be seriously affected by AIDS than those in Buganda.

Of the four Bugandan villages, two villages were known to be likely to have a very high incidence of the disease, and two others were less likely to be so affected. In each village information about the age and gender of those people currently living in a household, and also on those people who were considered as members of the family (this included children and other family members currently living away from the household) has collected. On the basis of this data, and for a small sample, the age and gender structure of these villages can be described in terms both of household and family composition. The distinction is important because in this area men leave for labour migration and women may marry out of the village. It is family data which provides the better account of demographic structure of these communities.

The sample villages were divided into two sets, those assumed to be seriously affected (1 and 2) and those less seriously or not at all (3, 4 and 5). The differences in demographic structure are very marked, as can be seen in Tables 12.1 and 12.2.

There are clear differences between the age structures of the AIDS-affected villages (1 and 2) and the others (3, 4 and 5). There appear to be very few males in the cohort aged 30–34 in villages 1 and

Table 12.1 Comparison of age structure between two sets of villages (males)

Age groups	Villages 1, 2 Number	Villages 1, 2 Percentage	Villages 3, 4, 5 Number	Villages 3, 4, 5 Percentage
0–4	21	16.8	53	12.8
5–9	18	14.4	58	14.0
10–14	16	12.8	52	12.5
15–19	15	12.0	51	12.3
20–24	18	14.4	38	9.2
25–29	11	8.8	38	9.2
30–34	1	0.8	30	7.2
35–39	4	3.2	20	4.8
40–44	7	5.6	18	4.3
45–49	3	2.4	16	3.9
50–54	6	4.8	13	3.1
55–59	0	0.0	4	1.0
>60	5	4.0	24	5.8
Total	125	100.0	415	100.1

Table 12.2 Comparison of age structure between two sets of villages (females)

Age groups	Villages 1, 2 Number	Villages 1, 2 Percentage	Villages 3, 4, 5 Number	Villages 3, 4, 5 Percentage
0–4	21	13.8	47	11.5
5–9	19	12.5	59	14.5
10–14	27	17.8	48	11.8
15–19	27	17.8	53	13.0
20–24	12	7.9	46	11.3
25–29	4	2.6	38	9.3
30–34	10	6.6	25	6.1
35–39	10	6.6	29	7.1
40–44	6	3.9	16	3.9
45–49	7	4.6	13	3.2
50–54	2	1.3	10	2.5
55–59	6	3.9	5	1.2
>60	1	0.7	19	4.7
Total	152	100.0	408	100.1

Table 12.3 Rakai district: seroprevalence by age and gender (%)

Age group	Men	Women
10–14	0.0	5.0
15–19	5.0	30.5
20–24	25.0	42.0
25–29	35.0	31.0
30–34	30.0	22.0
35–39	15.0	22.0
40–44	20.0	20.0
45–49	19.0	15.0
50–54	5.0	14.0
55–59	0.0	9.0
>60	0.0	0.5

Source M. Musagara, S. Musgrave, B. Biryahwaho, S. Serwadda, M. Wawer, J. Konde-Lule, S. Berkley and S. Okware, 'Sero-prevalence of HIV-1 in Rakai district, Uganda', Poster 010 at the Fourth International Conference on AIDS and Associated Cancers in Africa, 18–20 October 1989, Marseilles, France.

2 (0.8 compared with 7.2 per cent in villages 3, 4 and 5). The same is true of females in the 25-29 cohort: 2.6 per cent in villages 1 and 2 compared with 9.3 per cent in villages 3, 4, and 5. These differences could be the result of differences in labour migration and marriage patterns, but it should be recalled that this data describes *families* and *not* households. Thus children of the household who may have migrated or married out of the village are included in these figures. There may have been problems with recall and recording of absent family members, but such errors should be equally distributed between the two sets of villages. For the moment, then, we conclude that these data are an accurate reflection of the age and gender distributions in these villages at the time of the survey. They suggest that something very unusual has occurred in villages 1 and 2. The most likely explanation is AIDS. This hypothesis is strongly supported by the data (from another survey) showing rates of seropositivity in the area. This is shown in Table 12.3, where it can be seen that the highest rates of seropositivity are in the age cohorts five years junior to the age cohorts which are underrepresented in the age pyramid for men and for women. That the assumed rate of progression from initial infection to death is about five years in Uganda lends additional weight to the hypothesis that the observed difference in distribution is AIDS-related.

Orphan Studies in Uganda

Susan Hunter's data are derived from a 100 per cent census of the number of parents dying from all causes since 1971. The aim of the census was to identify the number of orphans in two districts in Uganda. It should be noted that an 'orphan' in Uganda is defined as a child with either one or both parents dead or missing.[6] Figure 12.1 shows the year of death of all parents of 'orphans' in both districts. It is likely that the decline in deaths in Rakai district for 1989 was due to the fact that the survey was carried out before the end of that year. It can be seen that there is a very rapid rise in the percentage of parents' deaths in Rakai district after 1983. Hoima district was severely affected by war in 1978–80, but the rise in mortality during the mid- and late 1980s is also probably due to the AIDS pandemic reaching the district some five years or so after it first appeared in Rakai.

Some more disaggregated data are shown in Figure 12.2 for nine sub-counties from Rakai district. These show the location of the sample sub-counties, and Figure 12.3 shows the cumulative deaths of parents through time for each sub-county. These statistics are uncorrected for population growth. Lack of reliable data on the population as a whole makes correction for this factor impracticable. However, in general the very rapid increase in mortality in some sub-counties is very marked. In the sub-counties of Kakuuto, Kalisizo and Kyebe,

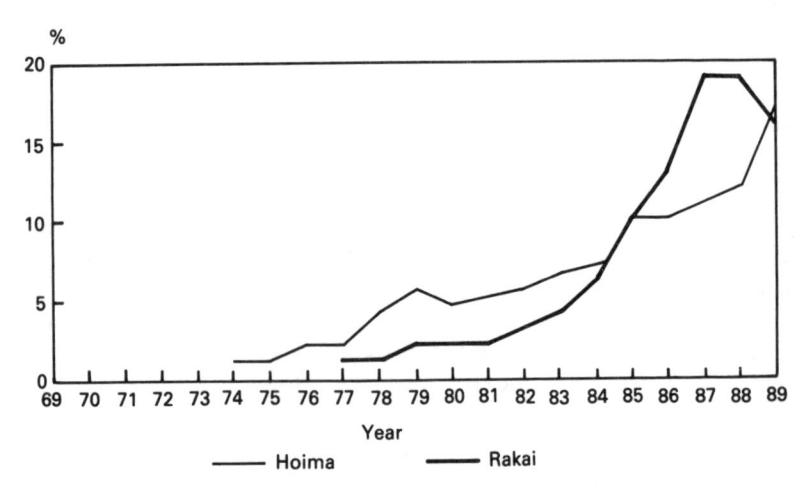

Figure 12.1 Dates of parents' deaths, Hoima and Rakai districts

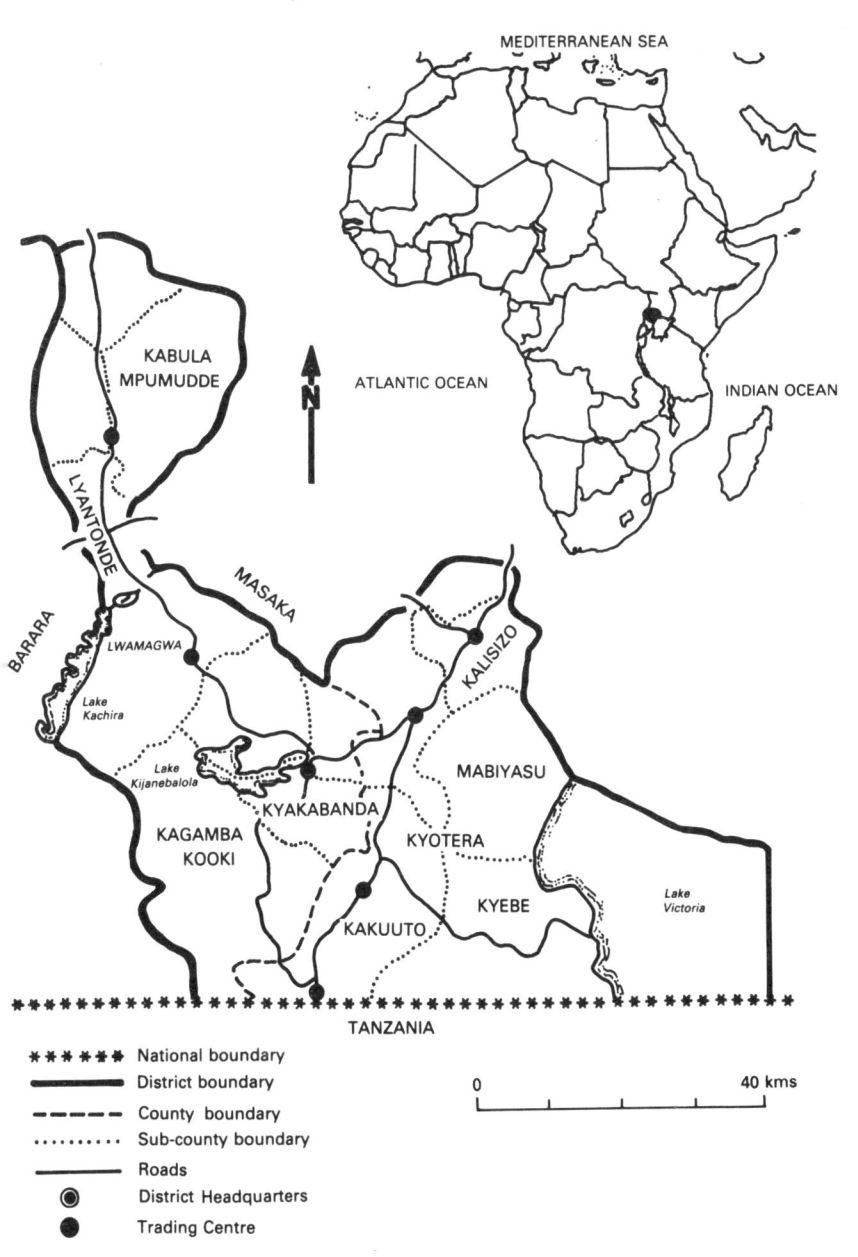

Figure 12.2 The sub-counties of Rakai district
Note Some sub-county boundaries may be inaccurate since their reorganisation

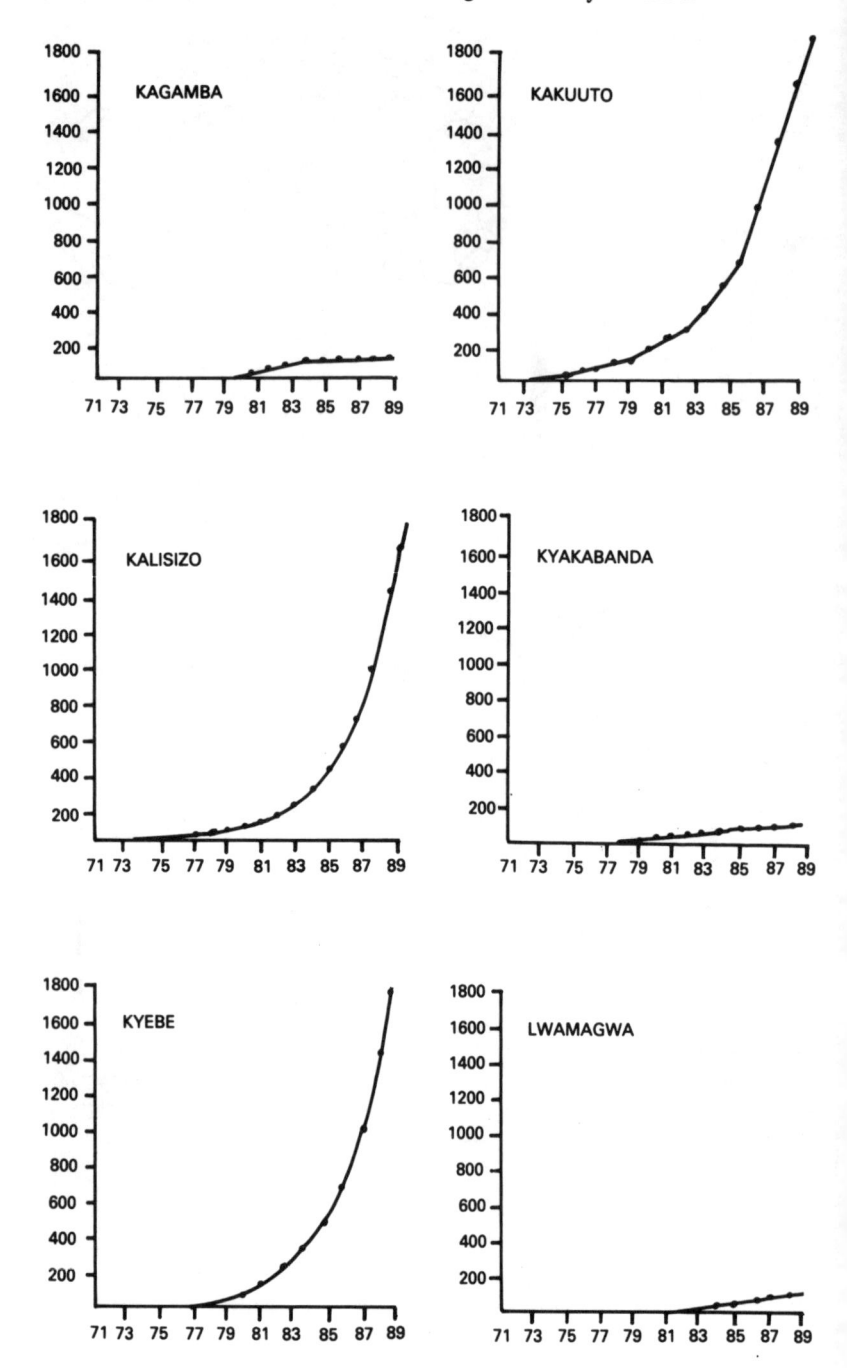

270 *Socio-Economic Monitoring Methods for AIDS*

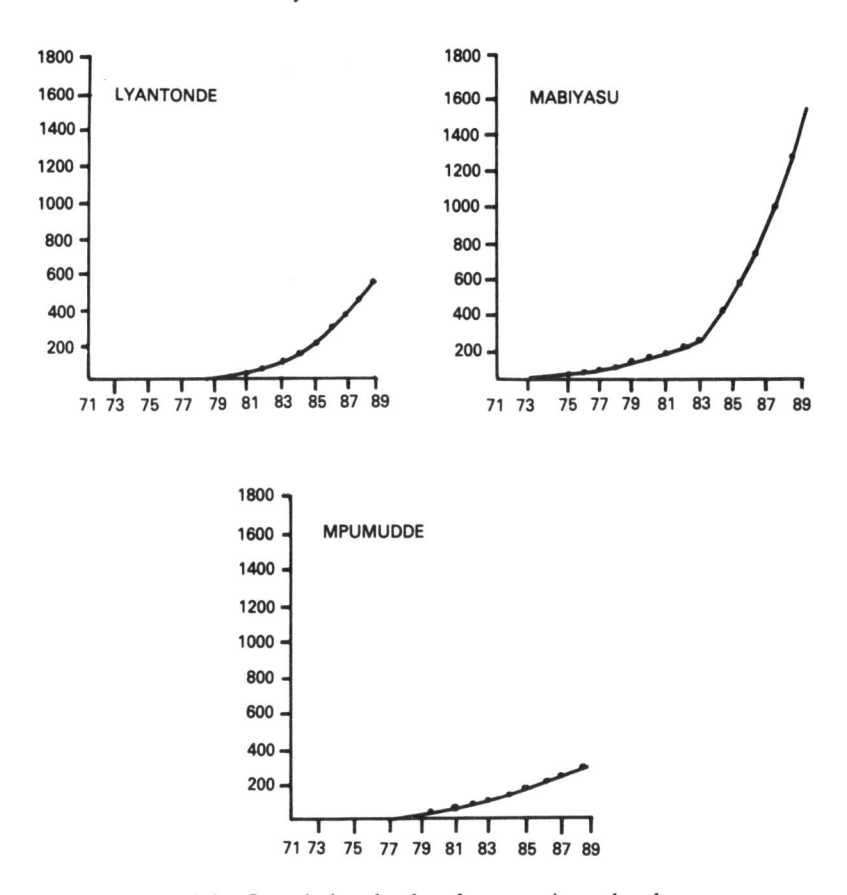

Figure 12.3 Cumulative deaths of parents in each sub-county

mortality increased greatly from about 1982, and Lyantonde is an intermediate case between sub-counties such as Lwamagwa or Kyakabanda and those mentioned earlier. In the worst affected sub-counties, in a population of about 30 000, nearly 2000 parents have already died. Taken together, the age profile of parental fatalities (not reproduced here, but falling in the expected ranges) and the form of the curve both suggest very strongly that AIDS is an increasing contributor to mortality in these sub-counties.

Another important observation from these data is that the spatial pattern of the diffusion of the pandemic as it develops through time means that generalisation at one point in time or space will simply be erroneous. As the pandemic develops, the experience of mortality in any one region will be very patchy. Thus, while the data collected in 1989 indicate that there were 24 524 orphans in Rakai district as a whole (12.6 per cent of all the children under 15 in the district), they were unequally distributed between the sub-counties. It must be emphasised that these data did not indicate the cause of parental death but, given the sudden rise in the rate of orphaning in this area after 1983 and the different pattern of orphaning in, for example, the Luwero area (where there were widespread massacres of civilian populations, and the peak of orphaning occurs during 1982–83),[7] it is safe to assume that many of these cases are the result of the AIDS epidemic.

POLICIES FOR LARGE ORPHAN POPULATIONS

Hunter's techniques can be used as an indicator of the epidemic. Together with other more detailed studies it demonstrates that there is an orphan problem. Case material collected in the course of our own research suggests that certain key policy areas need to be addressed in relation to orphans, and these will be examined next.

Education

Those dealing directly with orphans and their problems see education as a priority. The young children need to start school and the older ones must be kept in school. The associated costs of doing this are considerable for poor households.

Of some importance is the content and quality of the education which these orphans receive. A case could be made that it should be predominantly agricultural or vocational, for all of these children will have to earn their own living from an early age. In Uganda some vocational schools run by the religious orders are accepting a limited number of orphans because they believe that the future of orphans will depend upon their having marketable skills, as all of them will not wish to live by agriculture. However, such a view effectively excludes a very large number of people from other, more academic, types of education, and insofar as Uganda may lose many of its skilled and trained people to AIDS[8] and these will have to be replaced, it can be argued that the orphans created by the epidemic should not be doubly penalised by exclusion from the best education available.

Parenting

In Buganda, parenting responsibilities are usually taken on by a father's sisters and younger paternal grandparents. However, there has to be some doubt whether the full demands of caring for, teaching, socialising and disciplining children can any longer be met by the extended family. The coping capacity of some households and kin networks is already being exceeded. Many influential people in Uganda say that the orphaned children should be absorbed into extended families because it is 'traditional'. This assertion is prompted by an opposition to orphanages which are assumed to take children out of the local community. These arguments ignore the fact that most of the AIDS orphans will probably grow up with non-relatives anyway, and that there is an urgent need to establish institutional care which will be community-based but run by professionals in education, nutritional health and child care. This may also relieve the burden on the grandparents who experience problems in providing adequate care. What is clear is that decisions need to be taken now, and policies developed, to deal with this problem of how best to achieve care within and in relation to the community, without producing a generation of children who are institutionalised and alienated from their society.

Nutrition, Shelter and Clothing

In the great majority of cases these fundamental needs are met. Insofar as rapid appraisal can in any way be a reliable guide, there were few orphans, except at one or two unsatisfactory orphanages, who showed obvious signs of failing to have these needs satisfied. However, there is a noticeable minority of orphans who showed signs of malnutrition, particularly among the under 5s. In addition, some of the older children appeared underfed and ragged. These children were not neglected, but were simply receiving inadequate nutrition, particularly those who were living in poor households. Their condition was a result of being orphans in a poor society, rather than of simply being orphans. In some cases there was not enough food, particularly during the dry season. The special nutritional and care problems of these children need special attention.

Legal Protection of Orphans' Property

Some of the disputes before the local courts in Rakai district involved orphans. These cases concerned the rights of orphans to inherit their deceased parents' tenure of the farm. It would be a worrying precedent if landlords won any of these cases. Clearly these children are vulnerable to pressures from the unscrupulous. Minors are always vulnerable to relatives who may try to cheat them out of their inheritance, or who may divert their wealth to educating their own children; orphans will be no exception. In Rakai a few landlords had started dispossessing the orphans of the rights in land which their parents had enjoyed, and which are widely treated in these communities as heritable. Such widespread insecurity is an additional burden for households already suffering stress through death and illness.

Thus in Uganda there are specific areas of policy to do with orphans which need to be tackled, and tackled soon. However, the underlying policy issue is the choice between targeted and non-targeted assistance. The former may create privileged households and encourage corruption and even orphan-farming; the latter may be seen at best as an inefficient use of scarce resources, and at worst as a threat to the welfare of these children. In general we are talking about very poor people and very poor communities, their poverty made worse by the past traumas they have suffered and the current trauma of AIDS. The choice of how to pass between the Scylla of targeting and the Charybdis of non-targeting must surely be one of the cruellest which this society could have to face, and it is in the care of orphans that it is faced in an acute form.

AGRICULTURAL IMPACT SIMULATION STUDIES

Two studies of the possible future impact of AIDS using secondary data exist. These use data from farm management studies to examine the effects of labour loss upon different farming systems.

Gillespie[9] examined the implications of rising rural seroprevalence rates and resulting morbidity and mortality on the household labour force in Rwanda, and thus on farming systems. He noted the following effects: reduction in labour productivity; reduction of the available labour force; intensified competition between on-farm and domestic work, and reduction in available child labour. The information was collected in 1982–3 from 270 rural households in ten prefectures. The available data contained information on household composition, household members' activities for 15-day periods, and crops and soils. Two projection methods were used to simulate the probability of an average household losing a productive individual over the next ten years. One of the projection methods was the WHO epidemiologically based projection model,[10] and the other was an alternative model derived from current seropositivity data available for Rwanda.

Five different Rwandan farming systems were modelled. These were differentiated by altitude, soil type and population density. An assessment was made of the differential sensitivity of these systems to labour loss. The features of labour organisation and supply considered were: seasonality of labour demand, degree of labour specialisation, degree of interdependence of labour inputs, labour economies of scale, ecological potential for supporting less labour-intensive systems, and possibilities for substituting labour-saving technologies. A labour profile was constructed for each system. The results of this simulation suggest that the five Rwandan farming systems which were considered appear to be differentially sensitive to the loss of household members. The most sensitive systems, based on sorghum and potato cultivation on rich volcanic soils, are found in the highlands. The second most sensitive systems are those found in the Nile–Congo divide, based on fallowing and the cultivation of beans, sweet potatoes and maize. The least sensitive systems are those of the Kagera piedmont type with large landholding and low cropping intensities, and where the main crops are beans, sorghum, cassava, banana and coffee.

The conclusion of this simulation is that AIDS deaths will alter household profiles, reducing seasonal labour balances in all systems, but to different degrees depending on the relative level, type and timing of the labour contribution of the household member or members.

Another attempt at simulation undertook a similar study for Tanzania, using data collected from the Tabora region in 1979–80.[11] This study examined changes in the labour profile of different types of household in different agro-ecological zones. The zones were distinguished as follows: high rainfall, low fertility; low rainfall, medium fertility; and low rainfall, high fertility. They grew crop mixtures as follows: maize, groundnuts, beans and roots, tobacco and marketable food crops; sorghum, maize, groundnuts, roots and marketable food crops; sorghum, maize, groundnuts, roots and cotton, in that order.

The simulation took as its base three different types of household: a couple in their twenties with three children under ten years of age; a man in his fifties with two wives, one in her fifties, the other in her mid-twenties, with six resident children, three under ten and three aged ten to fifteen; a couple in their sixties living in close association with three related couples aged from twenty to forty, and twelve children living with the family, six under ten and six aged from ten to fifteen. Using this as the base, the simulation examined the changing labour profiles of these households as first one and then two members were affected by, and then died of, AIDS. The general conclusion of the simulation was that the effects of AIDS will vary as between households and their initial labour resources and the robustness of the particular farming system. In some cases the loss of labour would be as high as 50 per cent, in others rather lower. In some farming systems – for example, those producing tobacco which requires a lot of labour – the loss of cash crop production might be very high; in others there would be an immediate effect on the availability of food. The study concludes that the overall effect would be to reduce cash crop production by about 10 per cent.

Data on labour use and other aspects of agricultural production have been collected for many different farm-management purposes. It might be expected that much of this could be used to undertake simulations such as those outlined. In fact, a study commissioned in 1990 by the FAO indicated that very little of the data which has been collected over the years by agricultural economists, rural sociologists and agronomists does lend itself to such straightforward simulation experiments. There may be, however, sources of usable data for such simulation exercises resting in the archives of various ministries of agriculture in Africa. For example, data collected for the Ugandan Ministry of Agriculture identified 50 farming systems in Uganda.[12] Secondary analysis of this data, which the authors freely admit is not of the highest order of accuracy, allowed us to make the following general analysis of the vulnerability of Ugandan farming systems to labour loss. We addressed the following questions to the data.

1. Does the farming system already have a shortage of energy or protein? (While it may be possible for individual producers to adapt successfully to labour loss in a variety of ways, the existence of systemic food shortage in the first place suggests a lack of access to land, labour, or capital, making adaptations more difficult.)
2. Is labour supply currently less than demand at any time during the

agricultural calendar? (The product-mixes of different farming systems vary in their labour demand profile. In general terms the more seasonally peaked the demand, the more vulnerable the system will be to labour loss. Such peaking is, of course, closely related to the rainfall regime in an area.)
3. Are there substitutable staple crops requiring a lower level of maximum labour input, which will provide sufficient energy and protein?

We identified these three characteristics as being the main determinants of the degree of vulnerability of a farming system to labour loss. Our conclusions were that of the 50 farming systems identified by Johnson and Ssekitoleko, nine were considered very vulnerable, having both existing shortages of protein and energy as well as of labour. Seventeen were identified as vulnerable either on the criterion of existing or potential labour shortages or of experiencing existing protein and energy deficits. The remainder were not vulnerable within the criteria adopted in this method.

One source of data which could be used for similar purposes in connection with a very important sub-Saharan African country, Kenya (in which AIDS is already well-established), is that collected by the government of Kenya in the late 1970s and early 1980s.[13] It may be the case that in the archives of ministries of agriculture and overseas development, similar data sets can be found which will enable this type of simulation to be effected. However, such simulations do, of course, have their limitations. They tell us something about the vulnerability of farming systems (a theoretical and semiotic concept) whereas we know that within even robust farming systems, such as that of Buganda, households will be differentially affected depending upon their resource base.

We undertook limited field studies in Buganda in two communities. One of these is on the Lake Victoria foreshore and is a banana–coffee system. The other, about 40 km inland, is more marginal for bananas and coffee and has a large cattle component. The first system is located in an area of high and dependable rainfall (between 1021 and 1226 mm per year, distributed fairly evenly over between 132 and 140 days per year). In these communities, husbandry is characterised by low seasonal variations in the demand for labour (reflecting the distribution of rainfall), and a wide variety of crops is grown on the rich alluvial soils. The labour demand for perennial tree crops (bananas and coffee) is virtually constant throughout the year, while the annual crops (cassava, sweet potato, Irish potato, groundnuts, beans, yams and several others) usually have a two-peak demand for labour. Given the wide range of crops, there is no great problem in responding to labour shortage by means of a decremental retreat strategy. Such a retreat can be expected to result in a smaller variety of foods rather than in any immediate fall in nutritional status. Thus, because of its robustness, the Lake Victoria foreshore system is an important test case for the impact of AIDS-related labour loss on subsistence communities in sub-Saharan Africa. In the past two decades there has been marked social and economic disruption in this area and, while cash crop production has clearly declined, there have been no major famines or widespread food shortages. For these reasons, this farming system can be said to be very resilient to disturbance and also potentially resilient to labour loss given the range of crops and the abundance and distribution of rainfall. However, even in this area, in some households the impact of AIDS is such as either to reduce farm activity or to require changes in the way that labour is used.

The second system which we studied, the adjoining Ankole cattle-banana system, borders the previous one but receives markedly less rainfall (annual total around 773 mm) extending over fewer days of the year (88 days as opposed to 132–140). In addition, soils are less fertile. There is also a labour constraint, as the present maximum demand for labour already slightly exceeds the maximum supply. Production is predominantly based on cattle and small stock, with minor banana and annual crop cultivation where local soil moisture conditions allow. However, the range of crops grown is restricted by the rainfall constraint. While the remarks about banana cultivation made above apply here too, they are of limited relevance because only a minority of households have access to land suitable for this crop. Here, then, in contrast to the Lake Victoria foreshore system, the farming system is already more constrained by rainfall, potential range of crops and labour supply. Faced with additional labour constraints, there are fewer agricultural production strategies available to the people of this area than to those on the Lake Victoria foreshore.

Of these two production systems, it is the Ankole cattle–banana system which is most likely to be vulnerable to labour loss. This is because it is relatively drier than the other two systems and soils are poorer, resulting in an existing labour constraint as well as fewer opportunities for changing cropping strategies in response to labour loss.

Rainfall and existing labour constraints are to be found in other parts of Uganda, and certainly in other parts of sub-Saharan Africa. Thus, the Lake Victoria foreshore system could be said to represent the more favoured end of a continuum of agricultural systems both in Uganda and in Africa as a whole, while the sorghum systems of the central Sudan (not described here), with limited and concentrated rainfall, might represent the other extreme. It can be assumed that the other more vulnerable systems in Uganda and elsewhere in Africa will show labour-related stress at an earlier stage of the epidemic.

Policy Implications

The ultimate aim of studies such as these, whether they are derived from field data or from the analysis of data collected for other purposes, must be seen as predictive. They provide a rough-and-ready method of classifying the farming systems and communities of a region in terms of their relative vulnerability to the loss of labour as a result of the AIDS pandemic. Such data may be used to develop agricultural planning responses and new input mixes which take account of the loss of agricultural labour.

SOCIO-ECONOMIC DIFFERENTIATION AND IMPACT

The differential impact of the disease on households with different levels of resource endowment provides a potentially important policy tool by enabling identification of those households which, even in robust farming systems such as that on the Lake Victoria foreshore, are likely to be particularly vulnerable. We explored this aspect of AIDS impact by means of three distinctions which allowed us to examine differences in household responses through case studies. The analytical distinctions between households are: unaffected, AIDS-affected and AIDS-afflicted.

1. Unaffected: these are households in which no member is ill or has died from AIDS and which has not been affected by the illness or death of a member of any related household. The notion of being affected can be specified as describing a situation in which no additional burden, either of time or economic or financial resources, has to be devoted to a member of this household or another. This is, of course, a relative term. Most households are in some sense affected in a milieu in which the disease is so widespread.

2. AIDS-afflicted: in this type of household, the impact of the epidemic has been direct. A member of the household is either ill or has died from the disease. Resources have to be reallocated in order to deal with the problem.

3. AIDS-affected: this type of household has been affected by the disease either through the death of a family (not necessarily household) member who was contributing cash, labour or other support, or because the death or illness of a family member has meant that orphans have come to join the household, for example. These are all events which place additional demands on existing resources.

Each of these types of household circumstance will require different strategies for coping with the AIDS pandemic. In some cases households can, of course, be both afflicted and affected.

Social Differentiation

We divided households into three broad categories of rich, middle and poor. These are relative terms. In practice, they are distinguished as follows:

Rich — these households will have some or all of the following attributes: adequate or surplus land, ability to hire labour, involvement in trade or other non-agricultural occupation

Middle — this type of household may have non-agricultural sources of income, may occasionally employ labour, and will certainly have adequate land or sufficient non-agricultural income to be able to rent land or purchase food

Poor — in these households there will be land shortages, labour shortages which cannot be met by hiring, and few if any sources of cash income or, alternatively, the land resources may be so low as to require that household labour is sold

Developmental Cycle

Households go through processes of development and change. The stages of this cycle can be broadly indicated by the ages of the founding partners. Thus we identify young, mature and terminal households. This is roughly indicated by the age of the household head. We may say that in a young household the household head is aged less than 30, a mature household between 30 and 55, and a terminal household over 55 years of age. However, this is only a very rough guide. A very old man who has married a young woman and started a new family has characteristics of both a terminal and a young household. Indeed, one way in which old men can cope with old age is to remarry and thus effectively prolong the mature stage of the household.

There are 18 logical combinations of these characteristics and each of these types of household has different coping responses to the impact of the disease, and each of these, as we will see below, raises different issues for social policy.

Rich household, AIDS-affected, terminal stage: can cope through remarriage (man can marry an additional wife to help with child care, domestic and farm work). Also, earlier investment in children's education means that an adult child is able to make a contribution to the cash requirements of younger siblings and half-siblings, orphaned nephews and nieces from a salaried employment.

Rich household, AIDS-afflicted, mature stage: loss of one income-earner/labour unit does not necessarily have a serious impact (can be replaced by hired labour) and, in any case, given the mature stage of the developmental cycle, productive labour resources are likely to be at their peak in such a household. It is also possible for household members to increase self-exploitation (note that a large family is a safeguard at this stage), to move to intercropping (but probably possible in part because stress is not excessive due to size of family); there may also be additional self-exploitation (in case of women) through cash earning activities, such as weaving mats.

Rich, AIDS-afflicted and aids affected, terminal: the combination of affected and/or afflicted households (pooling resources) is a possibility here. It allows for both labour needs and also care requirements of sufferers. Household combination may also allow pooling of finances in order to hire labour. Even so, withdrawal of children from school has been necessary in some cases in order to cope with labour constraints.

Middle, AIDS-afflicted, mature: frequent decrease of cultivated area, and increase of handicraft production particularly among women in this category. The removal of children (particularly girls) from school, decrease in range of crops cultivated, sale of some of food surplus to raise cash (possible because land is not a constraint) are likely coping responses.

Middle, AIDS-afflicted, terminal: responses include reducing cultivate area, reducing crop range, take children out of school, combine

households, sending some dependent children to other related household.
Poor, AIDS-afflicted, mature: general reduction of level of life, crops, area, domestic environment, sale of labour, petty trade for men.
Poor, AIDS-afflicted, terminal: withdraw children from school, reduce crop range, increase self-exploitation (both domestic and farm work), reduce time spent farming.

This partial summary of some of the patterns found in our case material demonstrates that differences in the two variables – social status and developmental cycle – do affect the range of coping mechanisms available to a household.

It is likely that male-headed and female-headed AIDS-afflicted and AIDS-affected households will in some respects have different coping strategies available to them. This is most clearly the case with wealthier male-headed AIDS-affected housholds, where a man can marry a new wife as part of the coping strategy. This option is unlikely to be available to even a wealthy, female-headed, AIDS-affected household, even if the woman concerned thought it a desirable option.

Detailed analysis of more cases would indicate that the stage of AIDS-affliction or of AIDS-affectedness (how many deaths in a household, how many additional dependants) is another important variable. Thus there is bound to be a point at which even a wealthy, AIDS-afflicted or AIDS-affected household in the mature stage of its development will find it difficult to cope as its resources become depleted and it ceases to be wealthy.

Policy Implications

Four major policy implications can be derived from this analysis. The first is that the coping capacity of households within the same farming system will vary; the second is that, as the epidemic progresses, the customary coping strategies of households will cease to be sufficient to deal with the problem; the third is that in Uganda (and in most other countries of sub-Saharan Africa), the legal and social status of women is of the greatest importance for effective coping to be possible, particularly their rights to land. A fourth policy implication is that, insofar as households and communities are finding ways to cope, they are undertaking experimentation. Government and NGO (nongovernmental organisation) responses should attempt to build on and support these experiments rather than assume that completely new approaches are necessary.

HOUSEHOLD STRUCTURE CHANGES

It appears to be the case that household structure is changing in Buganda. We assume that this is at least in part a response to the epidemic. Table 12.4 shows the distribution of different types of household between households unaffected by AIDS and those affected or afflicted by AIDS in 1989. The cell sizes in this table (derived from a randomly selected sample of households) are small and the data are only suggestive. However, it appears that the two/three generation plus orphan household and the single person living by him/herself are more common in afflicted and affected households.

In terms of overall numbers of households in our survey of the villages worst hit by AIDS, 14 out of a total of 69 (20 per cent) were

Table 12.4 Household structure in two sets of villages in Rakai district

Type of household	Unaffected households Number	%	AIDS-afflicted or AIDS-affected Number	%
Single person	0	0	1	7.1
Couple	3	5.5	1	7.1
2-generation*	40	73.0	8	57.1
Polygenous with male in residence	4	7.3	0	0
3-generation	2	3.6	1	7.1
2/3-generation plus additional members (orphans)	5	9.1	3	21.4
Other	1	1.8	0	0
Total[†]	55	101.3	14	99.8

* Including single-person households, usually female headed but occasionally male headed, and polygynous households where the man may not always be in residence.

[†] Totals do not sum to 100 per cent as cell values have been rounded to take account of the small sample size.

Table 12.5 Household types in a Ganda village in the late 1950s

Type of household	Number	%
Couples living with children	60	36.3
Couples without children	35	21.2
Men living alone	25	15.2
Men living with an older son or daughter	3	1.8
Women living alone	9	5.5
Women living with children	11	6.7
Women living with an adult relative	4	2.4
Couples living with an adult relative	11	6.7
Others	7	4.2
Total	165	100

Source A.I. Richards, *The Changing Structure of a Ganda Village: Kisozi 1892–1952* (Kampala: East African Institute of Social Research, 1966), p. 71.

either AIDS-afflicted or AIDS-affected. Another census carried out by the project of some other communities revealed 49 AIDS-afflicted or AIDS-affected households out of a total of 185 surveyed (26 per cent).

To provide some perspective to these observations, it will be useful to compare these data with an analysis of household structure in a village in Buganda in the late 1950s. In a survey of 165 households it was found that the structure of households was distributed as shown in Table 12.5.[14]

These categories are not directly comparable with our own. However, certain observations can be made. The largest categories of household in the table are couples with children (37 per cent) followed by couples without children (21 per cent). This contrasts sharply with our own data in Table 12.4 where couples without children ('couple') make up only about 5 per cent of households in the unaffected Ganda households in our sample. Richards does not note any polygamous co-resident households, whereas these make up nearly 8 per cent of the total in our material. Perhaps the most significant difference between the two sets of data is the absence of any mention of orphans in Richards's data. She was not interested in the problem, and so does not categorise them separately. There is also no mention of three-generation households where grandparents are looking after children. These may have been included within her category 'couples with children'. If this were so, then we might have expected that category to be larger than it is. We must therefore conclude tentatively that the presence of a significant percentage of households in which grandparents care for orphans is a new development,[15] at least in part a response to the pandemic. Also of significance is the number of households in the category 'couples without children'. We can assume that the majority of these would have been newly-married couples (they make up 21 per cent of the households in Richards's sample). By contrast, in our own sample, they make up only 5 per cent in the unaffected households.

The question must which must be addressed is whether this indicates that in Buganda young people are now hesitating to marry, and hence that there are fewer newly-married couples in the sample. That this may be the case is supported by anecdotal data that there are now very few marriages taking place in Rakai district,[16] as well as by data from our own survey which suggests that young people are delaying marriage. Data in Tables 12.1 and 12.2 suggest that in the villages we surveyed there were fewer children than would be expected from a stable population in a country like Uganda. The reasons for this might include higher mortality due to vertical transmission of the disease to children; raised mortality of very young orphans; and possible underrecording of the existence of children due to the migration of very young children accompanying women who have deserted sick husbands or have migrated. Additionally, it has been suggested by some of the people from Rakai that the lack of children is due to increased celibacy. We met cases where mothers have strongly counselled their children not to marry, and a local midwife (one of our informants) said that she was almost put out of a job by the lack of births. Some women reported growing tensions between spouses over the problem of unwanted sex where it was suspected that a male partner might be already infected.

Policy Implications

Two broad areas of policy are raised by these changes in household structure. The first is the care of orphans, which we have discussed above, and the other is the care of the elderly. In societies such as those we are describing, the present middle generation is losing its teenage and young adult children. This will mean that they themselves may lack care as they grow old.

Results from the research which has been undertaken suggests that communities are being affected in a number of ways, and that those effects can be sensed by means of the robust indicators which we have described. These include: structural changes in households, changes in agricultural production strategies, pressure on farming systems, and the presence of very large numbers of orphans. The indications are that, even on the Lake Victoria foreshore (a comparatively well-endowed area of rural Africa), traditional community coping mechanisms are beginning to show strains at the margins, and that new coping strategies and mechanisms are being developed by the most seriously affected communities.

Projections from the data collected in Uganda – and, to some extent, from Kenya – as well as unpublished information about rates of seropositivity throughout Uganda and Kenya lead us to suspect that similar stresses may be developing in those as well as other African countries (for example, the Kagera region of Tanzania). In particular, it seems very likely that in the next five years a number of farming systems will begin to confront serious labour constraints, possibly leading to declines in food production. These effects are the result of the cohort-specific impact of the disease.

The two simulation exercises which have attempted to examine the impact of AIDS on farming systems in Tanzania and Rwanda have indicated that declines in food production are likely to appear in some systems around 15 years from the initial introduction of AIDS into the community. Such a conclusion should not lead us to believe that there are 15 years in which to examine the possible impacts and to act on the conclusions of such studies. The best informed opinion suggests that many communities in East and Central Africa may already have reached 15 years or more[17] from the start of the epidemic.

We know little of the detail of the socio-economic impact in other parts of the continent.[18] However, the rates of seropositivity which can be inferred from published sources suggest that the kinds of impact observed in Uganda are likely to be found in many other countries.

It is therefore important that a wide-ranging programme of research, education of policy makers and politicians and policy development be undertaken now if the worst downstream effects of this epidemic are to be mitigated. The disease is likely to affect many societies, but the African continent faces very specific problems associated with its heavy dependence on subsistence agriculture, its food situation and the debt burden which makes few African countries able to cope with a disaster of this magnitude. The following areas of research ought to be undertaken as a matter of some urgency.

MAJOR RESEARCH AREAS

Given the unevenness of data sources mapping the sensitivity of African subsistence agricultural systems to labour withdrawal will require an eclectic and pragmatic approach to data collection and use. The aim will be to assemble farming system, land use and seropositivity data into an atlas which will then form the basis of an early warning system. This system will indicate which areas of Africa – and, in particular, which food production systems – are most likely to be affected by AIDS-related labour loss.

The kind of methodology which we have developed for addressing secondary data, plus the simulation exercises we have described, suggest ways in which this data may be used. Additional techniques might include remote sensing combined with selected ground checking, field studies, and the use of government reports produced for other purposes. Additional information to be included in such an atlas would be major population movements such as established labour migration routes and refugee movements.

Macro-Impacts on Labour Markets

There has been some speculation about the impact of AIDS on skill availability in some African countries. However, as far as is known, little if any work is being done on this problem. As well as simple labour market accounting, it may also be important to examine the possible flows of labour in response to local and regional labour shortages arising from AIDS mortality and morbidity.

Such analyses are important for two reasons: first, to identify possible future skill shortages (manual, technical and administrative); and second, to form a view as to possible major local and regional population movements associated with labour market adjustments which might actually affect the rate and direction of spread of the disease. Such information might be important for disease control programmes.

Studies along these lines might use existing demographic projections, sero-data and labour market information, combined with limited field studies of labour market operation, in order to identify and predict possible effects of the epidemic on local and regional labour markets. In addition, attempts will be made to identify and quantify major population movements, whether for economic or political reasons, with a view to feeding this information into epidemiological models.

There are already anecdotal reports (from Zaire) of plantation managements finding it difficult to recruit labour because of the numbers of people dying from AIDS, and (from Zambia) of very high levels of seropositivity among mine workers.[19] If there is any truth in such reports we need to identify the possible effects of the disease on cash-crop production and the mining sector, given the centrality of cash crops and mining to many Central and southern African economies.

Environmental Impact

There is one environmental impact which may be of great importance in some areas. If there is a decline in population, then this might lead to the spread of tsetse fly as farm land is abandoned. This may seem dramatic, but our evidence from Uganda suggests that farm land is already being abandoned in the worst affected parts of Buganda.[20] Spread of the tsetse fly could make additional demands on health sectors which are already stretched by AIDS, as well as adding an additional turn to the ratchet of labour decline and changes in farming practice.

Identification, Recording and Supporting Local Coping Experiments

We have suggested elsewhere that, as communities learn to cope, it is important that such efforts are evaluated and supported where appropriate by government and NGO programmes.[21] It is therefore necessary to ensure that successful coping mechanisms are communicated between different parts of the continent as they evolve. It is important to document the results of such 'experiments' as they develop in the affected parts of Africa. The aim of this research should be to evaluate their effectiveness and communicate the results between affected countries, regions and communities.

Urban 'Plant' Studies

While many and probably most sero-surveys have been of urban populations,[22] little is currently known about the impact of the disease in the urban and industrial sectors as well as in the government sector. Such research is now necessary, particularly if we are to improve our understanding of how the industrial and urban sector is coping with AIDS deaths and illness in the workplace. Such studies would feed into the labour market studies outlined above, the aim being to understand how people with AIDS are treated in the workplace, how their families cope in the urban situation, and how management goes about recruiting replacements for people no longer able to work. An important part of such research would be to encourage administrative audits of skills and death rates within the infrastructure of the state.

A BROADER VIEW: WHERE DOES THIS ALL LEAD TO?

The seventh International AIDS Conference in Florence in June 1991 brought out clearly two features which have been apparent to those working in the field of downstream impact for some time. These two features are concerned with two great divisions, that between medical and social scientists and that between treatment, care and concern for the wealthy and the opposite for the poor. Each of these divisions is to be seen on a local, national and (perhaps most worryingly of all) on an international scale.

In this chapter we have discussed some of the downstream issues raised by the AIDS pandemic. These are issues of social and economic life. To state the obvious, AIDS affects people. However, most of the resources are being put into very sophisticated medical research. This is quite right as the search for a cure or a vaccine must take the highest priority, but not to the total exclusion of funding for projects aimed at confronting the social and economic impact. In the absence of either a vaccine or a cure, and given the long wave nature of the crisis, we must begin to take seriously the problems of long-term responses to the social and economic effects. The kind of medical responses which are likely are very expensive. Some suggested treatments which might keep a person with AIDS alive for 20 years will cost in the region of $85 000 per person. Such sums are an enormous burden even for the few very rich countries; they are an impossibility for all other countries. Africa (as well as most other parts of the world) is going to be terribly affected. The falling price of commodities to pay for even the basic medicines and testing equipment, poor health, and the lack other infrastructure to prevent further spread, all makes Africa particularly vulnerable. In the meantime, there is an undercurrent of opinion which is beginning to suggest that AIDS is under control in Europe and North America, that it can now be seen as 'just' another tropical disease – like malaria – against which the people of Europe and North America can protect themselves by means of simple precautionary measures. Such attitudes are easy to adopt because they fit well with established prejudices along class, gender and ethnic lines. They insidiously penetrate research agendas. For those reasons, those of use who are concerned about confronting the social and economic impact of this pandemic face a considerable struggle to have the problem recognised as a legitimate one for funding. As Jonathan Mann said recently: 'The pandemic not only remains dynamic, volatile and unstable, but it is gaining momentum – and its major impacts, in all countries are yet to come. Public complacency is rising and societal commitment against HIV and AIDS is declining'.[23] The kind of measures and indicators discussed here may make some small contribution to shaking that public complacency about the situation within Africa and towards Africa.

Notes and References

1. Such estimates of seropositivity have usually turned out to be very conservative. Even in countries where the reporting system is fairly well developed (such as the UK), estimates may vary by several orders of magnitude. In most countries in sub-Saharan Africa the estimates are bound to be even less accurate. For Uganda, where there has been a fairly full sero-survey, the estimates are probably better than most. These indicate that over 1 million people out of a total population of around 17 million are HIV positive.
2. We are grateful to Simon Mollison for bringing this point to our attention.
3. T. Barnett and P.M. Blaikie, *AIDS in Africa: The Relevance of the Uganda Case* (London: Belhaven Press, 1991).
4. The main part of this research was funded by the UK Government's Overseas Development Administration (under grant 4491 – Uganda), and also by the Ford Foundation (under grant APP 677G – Kenya). Neither of these organisations nor the governments of Uganda or Kenya necessarily agrees with the views or interpretations expressed here.
5. S. Hunter, 'Social Aspects of AIDS in Uganda in perspective', unpublished page, 1989; S. Hunter, untitled paper given at the NGO AIDS Coordinating Committee Conference, 1 December 1989. Institute of Education, University of London, 1989; S. Hunter and A. Dunn, 'Enumeration and needs assessment of children orphaned by AIDS in Uganda', poster 292 at the sixth International Conference on Aids and Associated Cancers in Africa, 18–20 October 1989, Marseilles.
6. Inclusion of children with only one parent dead does, of course, inflate the number of orphans in a national statistic. This must be borne in mind when considering Ugandan orphan data.

7. S. Hunter, 'An update of the orphan situation in Uganda', paper given to the Conference on AIDS: Community Coping Mechanisms in the Face of Exceptional Demographic Change, International Conference Centre, 20 November 1990, Kampala.
8. On some projections, it seems that in a country where the AIDS epidemic has reached the magnitude which it has in Uganda, in order to have one person aged 50 surviving from the current cohort receiving education and training, 17 will have to be trained now: personal communication from Jane Rowley.
9. S. Gillespie, 'Potential impact of AIDS on farming systems: a case study from Rwanda', Land Use Policy, 6 (1989), pp. 301–12; S. Gillespie, *The Potential Impact of AIDS on Food Production Systems in Central Africa* (Rome: UN FAO, 1989).
10. WHO, 'Epidemiologically based HIV/AIDS projection model', mimeo (Geneva: WHO, 1988).
11. Overseas Development Natural Resources Institute *Potential Impact of AIDS on Food Production and Consumption: Tabora Case Study* (London: for the Overseas Development Administration, Eland House, Stag Place, 1989), contract no. C 0863.
12. D.T. Johnson and Q.W. Ssekitoleko, *Current and Proposed Farming Systems in Uganda* (Entebbe, Uganda: Ministry of Agriculture, Planning Division, Farm Management and Economic Research Station, 1989).
13. R. Jaetzold and H. Schmidt, *Farm Management Handbook of Kenya*, 3 vols (Nairobi, Kenya: Ministry of Agriculture in cooperation with the German Agency for Technical Cooperation, 1982).
14. A.I. Richards, *The Changing Structure of a Ganda Village: Kisozi 1892–1952* (Kampala: East African Institute of Social Research, 1966).
15. This assumption is given additional weight by the report from Susan Hunter in her untitled paper that 30 per cent of children in Rakai district are being cared for by their grandparents.
16. Susan Hunter, personal communication, reports that the country clerk in Rakai told her that there had not been any marriages in the area in the two years previous to 1989.
17. Roy Anderson of Imperial College, University of London, stated at the NGO-AIDS meeting, 1 December 1989, that in 'the central band' in Africa the epidemic may be 20–30 years into its development.
18. There is patchy reporting from a number of countries in sub-Saharan Africa but, apart from our work in Uganda and Kenya, one IBRD study now in progress in Uganda and an FAO study in progress in Malawi, there have been no other systematic studies of the situation. In part this reflects political reluctance to confront the issues as well as resource constraints.
19. There are apparently several unpublished reports on the situation among Zambian mine workers. These have been commissioned by the mining companies but the results are unavailable because of their political sensitivity.
20. H. Kjekshus *Ecology Control and Economic Development in East African History: The Case of Tanganyika 1850–1950* (London: Heinemann, 1977) and other sources indicate the importance of subsistence farming

as a means of control of sleeping sickness. The main reference on this is J. Ford, *The Role of the Trypanosoniases in Africa Ecology: A Study of the Tsetse-Fly Problem* (Oxford University Press, 1971). Reports from Buganda in the early decades of this century show clearly how devastating the impact of sleeping sickness can be.
21. T. Barnett and P.M. Blaikie, 'Community coping mechanisms in circumstances of exceptional demographic change: some methodological and conceptual issue'. Overseas Development Administration Conference on Appropriate Research Methodologies in the Study of AIDS, Brunel University, 11–12 May 1990.
22. Sero-surveys are collated by Peter Way of the US Bureau of the Census, Centre for International Research, AIDS/HIV databases.
23. *Guardian*, 26 June 1991, p. 21.

Part V

Facing up to AIDS in South Africa

13 Lessons from Tropical Africa for Addressing the HIV/AIDS Epidemic in South Africa
Alan Fleming

INTRODUCTION

The main epidemic of HIV and AIDS, in the majority population of South Africa, is the geographical extension southwards of the pandemic in East and Central Africa. Heterosexual contact is the dominant mode of transmission. This one fact determines the pattern of impact of AIDS on society, on demography and on the economy: the clinical expression in adults and children is affected largely by the mode of transmission, so society's response and its attempt to contain the epidemic will be meaningful only insofar as there is an understanding of the heterosexual partner contact networks in South Africa.

There is a wealth of experience and knowledge gathered already in sub-Saharan countries, where the epidemic is much further advanced than it is at present in South Africa. This knowledge is well documented in both international and national medical-scientific journals; it is wholly reprehensible of clinicians and other workers in South Africa to ignore it.

SEXUAL TRANSMISSION

In all parts of the world, the pandemic of HIV has shown up ignorance as to common sexual practices in the population. Africa is no exception but, as a generalisation, *mores* governing sexual behaviour lie between two extremes in traditional African society.[1] At one extreme are patriarchal societies, often polygamous, in which virginity of women is demanded at first marriage. At the other extreme, female chastity before marriage is not expected; unmarried girls are freely available to male guests of the family, and often pregnancy as a demonstration of fertility is the first step towards formalised marriage. Male chastity is not valued especially in either type of society, although nowhere is tolerated what is judged to be excessive sexuality or adultery with married women. To meet the demands of males in strict patriarchal societies, there tends to be a well-defined sub-group of girls and women who are full-time prostitutes, but in 'freer' societies this sub-group does not form.

Traditional attitudes still influence behaviour, despite the profound changes of lifestyle which are the consequences of modern urban and industrial developments. The system of migrant labour and the spontaneous rural – urban drift of population appear to have two opposing effects. Male migrant labourers are often married, but life in hostels without their families inflates greatly the demand for female prostitution[2] which is a feature of patriarchal societies. On the other hand, spontaneous urban drift of young people of both sexes helps create a society in which bar-girls give sexual favours freely or for small presents, while better educated women in salaried jobs are entertained ostentatiously and lavishly by their men friends.

The prevalence of HIV seropositivity in women reflects these two patterns of behaviour. In the first situation, female prostitutes have rates of seropositivity reaching to around 90 per cent – for example, in Nairobi (Kenya) and Kigali (Rwanda) – whereas women attending antenatal clinics have much lower seroprevalance. In the second situation, the rate of seropositivity in women at the antenatal clinic and at the STD clinic may be about the same: for example, around 20–30 per cent in Zambian cities.[3] The latter presents a more immediate threat to society, although in the first pattern, as an increasing number of married women become infected from their husbands, the distinction becomes blurred.

Even in the early stage of the epidemic in South Africa these two differing patterns are seen. In the Baragwanath Antenatal Clinic, HIV seroprevalence amongst pregnant women had reached about 1 per cent by the end of 1990, and about 4 per cent by mid-1992: there is little to distinguish socially the seropositive from the seronegative women since neither admit to multiple sex partners, and both frequently perceive that they are at risk of HIV infection due to their husbands' extramarital sexual contacts with prostitutes, amongst whom there is a high rate of seropositivity (K. Klugman, unpublished observations). In the Durban area, on the other hand, the risk of infection is high amongst young women who are not engaged in full-time or permanent prostitution.[4]

The lower perceived value of women than of men leads to females in Africa being exposed to HIV and other STDs, which act as co-factors in the transmission of HIV more often and at an earlier age (even adolescence or pre-adolescence), through being forced into prostitution, through being allowed to drift into a life of casual sexuality for trivial rewards, or through rape, especially in times of unrest and war.

An estimated 10 million people in the world had been infected by HIV by 1990, of whom 3 million were women. About 80 per cent of infected women are in sub-Saharan Africa, where the overall prevalence is 2.5 per cent in women aged 15–49 years, with up to 40 per cent in some cities in central Africa.[5]

More women than men are infected in Africa:[6] for example, in three population-based studies in Uganda the female to male ratio was 1:4 for the whole country, rising to 1:8 in the capital, Kampala.[7] Infection by HIV is occurring on average much earlier for females than males: for example, in the semi-rural population of Uganda, the peak incidence of seropositivity (nearly 20 per cent) was in 15–19 year old females. In Zambia, HIV-related disease is seen most frequently in women aged 20–24 years, and in men aged 25–35 years (see Figure 13.1).[8] A comparison of fatality rates (deaths per 1000 admissions) in the major hospitals in Abidjan (Côte d'Ivoire) showed an increase of 54 per cent between 1983 and 1988 in the adult medical wards, ascribed to the AIDS epidemic: the largest age-specific increases were in men aged 20–39 years (approximately 100 per cent, or a two-fold rise) and in women aged 20–29 (up 199 per cent, a three-fold rise; see Figure 13.2).[9]

The dynamics of transmission of the heterosexual epidemic of HIV and AIDS and its demographic impact are dependent largely on three factors: a high rate of sexual partner change in the young, men's preference for having sexual contact with women younger than themselves, and a higher efficiency of HIV transmission from male to female than *vice versa*.[10] Transmission of HIV to females in Africa is largely a phenomenon of adolescence, but AIDS is a disease of young adulthood, with a peak of frequency coinciding with the age when women are most often pregnant.

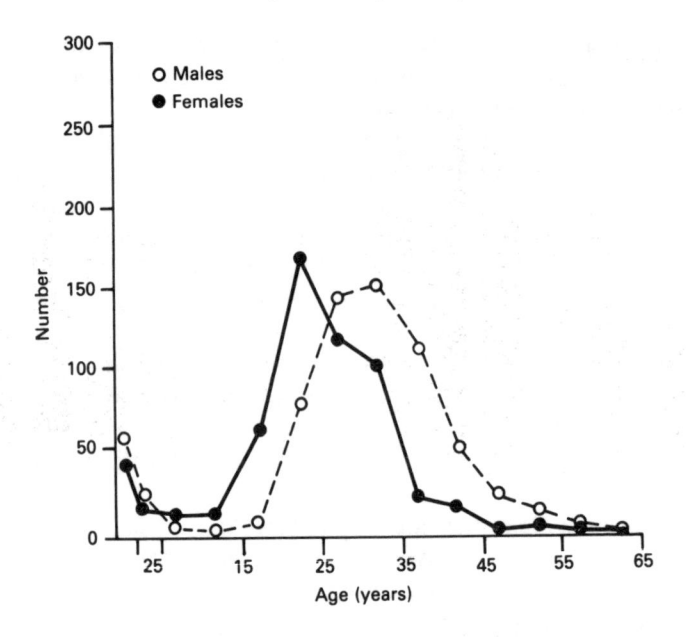

Figure 13.1 Age and sex distribution of 1245 Zambians with HIV-related disease confirmed by anti-HIV-1 seropositivity during 1986

Source A.F. Fleming, 'AIDS in Africa', *Baillière's Clinical Haematology*, 3, 1990, 177–203. Reproduced with permission of Baillière Tindall.

INFANTS OF HIV-INFECTED MOTHERS

Vertical transmission of HIV to infants occurs transplacentally in 24–33 per cent of pregnancies when the mothers are infected: vertical infection during delivery and in infancy (for example, by breast-feeding) may happen, but these do not appear to be major risks. There is a greater chance of transplacental transmission when the mother has advanced disease, as is seen more often in Africa than in developed countries.[11] HIV I DNA sequences were detected by the polymerase chain reaction in 20 (64 per cent) of 31 babies born to infected women in Kinshasa,[12] but this high rate of transmission needs to be confirmed.

Infection of the infant is only one part of the impact of maternal HIV on pregnancy, infancy and childhood. There is increased foetal wastage:[13] for example, 28 per cent of 64 HIV-seropositive and 15 per cent of 311 seronegative women in Malawi gave a history of previous

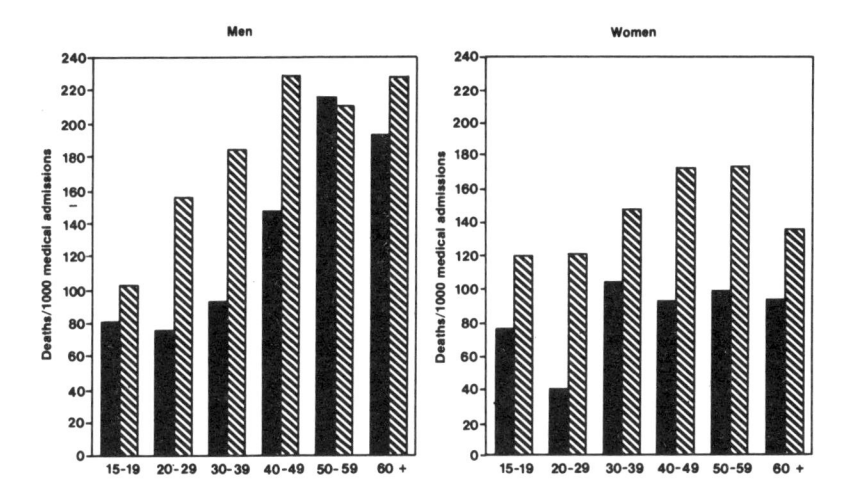

Figure 13.2   Age-specific death rates (deaths/1000 admissions) for medical patients in two hospitals, Abidjan, Côte d'Ivoire, in 1983 and 1988

Source   K.M. de Cock, B. Barrere, M.F. Lafontaine *et al.*, 'Mortality Trends in Abidjan, Côte d'Ivoire, 1983–1988', *AIDS*, 5 (1991), pp. 393–8. Reproduced with permission of Current Science Ltd and authors.

spontanous abortion. There is intra-uterine growth retardation with lower than expected birthweight, reduced period of gestation at delivery,[14] possibly increased frequency of stillbirth, and low Apgar scores (a measure of health of the neonate).[15] Regardless of the HIV status of the infants, there are high rates of neonatal death (6.2 per cent versus 1.3 per cent in controls) and of infant mortality, so that about one-third of all live-born infants have been lost by the age of one year (see Figure 13.3). Of those who survive the first year, up to 10 per cent are infected with HIV.

Already the AIDS epidemic is negating or reversing the gains of childhood survival achieved in Africa in the past few decades.[16] It is predicted that in Central and East Africa, the annual childhood mortality (under 5) will rise to 159–189 per 1000 live births by the year 2000, compared to an expected 132 per 1000 without AIDS and a UN target of 78 per 1000.[17]

Adult (20–49 years) mortality rates are rising, and it is estimated that between 1.5 and 2.9 million women of reproductive age in East and Central Africa will die of AIDS during the 1990s, leaving between 3.1 and 5.5 million AIDS orphans: that is, 6–11 per cent of

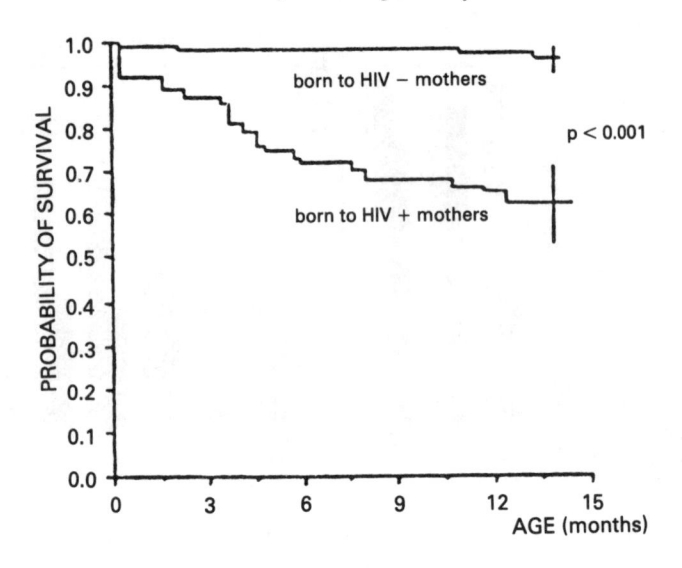

Figure 13.3 Survival curves of children born to HIV+ and HIV− mothers in Brazzaville

Source M. Lallemant, S. Lallemant-Le Coeur, D. Cheynier *et al.*, 'Mother–child transmission of HIV-1 and infant survival in Brazzaville, Congo', *AIDS*, 3 (1989), 643–6. Reproduced with permission of Current Science Ltd and authors.

children under 15 years of age will be orphans. Many of these children could be driven to prostitution, so completing a cycle of transmission of HIV during adolescence within one generation.

CLINICAL MANIFESTATIONS

HIV-related disease is essentially the same in all parts of the world and regardless of the mode of transmission, but the prevalence of different micro-organisms in the environment and carried by the population determines the patterns of disease arising from reactivated infections, invading pathogens and opportunistic infections.[18] Some latent infections are so highly prevalent in Africa (for example, TB and *herpes zoster*) that it is not surprising that they are seen frequently complicating the course of AIDS. Others also have high rates of transmission in Africa, especially during childhood, but are seen only rarely complicating AIDS, either because there is no apparent interaction, as with *Plasmodium falciparum*, or possibly because acquired immunity is so 'solid' that breakthrough is unusual during the clinical course of AIDS, as with *Pneumocystis carinii*, hepatitis B and *Strongyloides stercoralis* (see Table 13.1).

Adults

The commonest presentations of HIV disease in African adults are the loss of weight often associated with chronic water diarrhoea (a syndrome recognised and named 'slim' by the Ugandans), or generalised lymphadenopathy and chronic cough (see Figure 13.4).[19] The fifth commonest presentation is *herpes zoster*, which is seen in about 15 per cent of patients and often precedes all other clinical manifestations by months or even years, and has a specificity of 99 per cent and a positive predictive value of 95 per cent for HIV seropositivity.[20] The WHO clinical case definition of AIDS in adults in Africa is based on the common experiences of many workers (Table 13.2) and has been found to be most useful in diagnosis, to have reasonable sensitivity (59 per cent) and good specificity (90 per cent);[21] it is also a powerful tool in the education of clinicians.

Gastro-intestinal tract
The chronic water diarrhoea of 'slim' is associated with intestinal infection with *Cryptosporidium* and *Isospora belli* in a combined frequency of about 60 per cent,[22] although it is not certain that these organisms actually cause the diarrhoea. Preliminary observations of patients at Baragwanath Hospital imply that 'slim' is relatively uncommon, occurring in only about 11 per cent of adults with AIDS (A. Karstaedt, unpublished observations); if this difference of clinical presentation between tropical and sub-tropical Africa is confirmed, it contains valuable epidemiological clues as to the aetiology of 'slim'.

Oral lesions occur commonly and are often florid in Africans with AIDS; candidiasis and pharyngitis are seen frequently, while aphthous ulcers, Kaposi's sarcoma and tuberculous ulcers are less common.[23] Hairy leukoplakia is reported in 43 per cent of patients in Tanzania,[24] but is strangely absent or rare in Zaire[25] and Zambia (unpublished observations). Once more, observations on the frequency of oral leukoplakia in South Africa could be epidemiologically valuable.

Table 13.1 Infections of clinical or epidemiological interest in AIDS in Africa

	High prevalence	'Missing' infections
Gastro-intestinal tract	*Cryptosporidium* *Isospora belli*	
Lower respiratory tract	*Mycobacterium tuberculosis*	*Pneumocystis carinii* *M. avium intracellulare*
Viruses	*Herpes zoster* Measles Hepatitis C	Hepatitis B
Bacteria	*M. leprae* *Salmonella* *Streptococcus pneumoniae*	
Protozoa	*Leishmania spp* *Toxoplasma qondii*	*Plasmodium falciparum* Trypanosoma brucei Entamoeba histolytica
Helminths		*Stronglyloides stercoralis*
Fungi	*Cryptococcus neoformans*	*Histoplasma duboisii*

Sources O.O. Simooya, R. Mwendapole, S. Siziya and A. F. Fleming, 'Relation between falciparum malaria and HIV seropositivity in Ndola, Zambia', *British Medical Journal*, 297 (1988), pp. 30–1; A.F. Fleming, 'Opportunistic infections in AIDS in developed and developing countries', *Transactions of the Royal Society of Tropical Medicine and Hygiene*, 84 (1990), suppl. 1, pp. 1–6; S.B. Lucas, 'Missing infections in AIDS', *Transactions of the Royal Society of Tropical Medicine and Hygiene*, 84 (1990), suppl. 1, pp. 34–8; C.P. Conlon, A.J. Pinching, C.U. Perera *et al.*, 'HIV-related enteropathy in Zambia: a clinical, microbiological, and histological study', *American Journal of Tropical Medicine and Hygiene*, 42 (1990), pp. 83–8; A.E. Pitchenik, 'Tuberculosis control and the AIDS epidemic in developing countries', *Annals of Internal Medicine*, 113 (1990), pp. 89–90; F. de Lalla, G. Rizzardini, E. Rinaldi *et al.*, 'HIV, HBV, delta-aent and *Treponema pallidum* infections in two rural African areas', *Transactions of the Royal Society of Tropical Medicine and Hygiene*, 84 (1990), pp. 144–7; M. Giovanni, A. Tagger, M.L. Ribero *et al.*, 'Maternal–infant-transmission of hepatitis C virus and HIV infections: a possible interaction', *Lancet*, 335 (1990), p. 1166; B. Carme, A. Ngoler, B. Ebikili and A.I. Ngaporo, 'Is African histoplasmosis an opportunistic fungal infection in AIDS?', *Transactions of the Royal Society of Tropical Medicine and Hygiene*, 84 (1990), p. 293; C.F. Gilks, R.J. Brindle, L.S. Otieno *et al.*, 'Life-threatening bacteraemia in HIV-1 seropositive adults admitted to hospital in Nairobi, Kenya',

Lancet, 337 (1991), p. 604; R.J. Leaver, Z. Haile and D.A.K. Walters, 'HIV and cerebral malaria', *Transactions of the Royal Society of Tropical Medicine and Hygiene*, 84 (1990), p. 201; J.P. Louis, J. Jannin, C. Hengy *et al.*, 'Absence d'interrelations épidémiologiques entre l'infection rétrovirole à VIH et la trypanosomiase humaine africaine (THA)', *Bulletin de la Société de Pathologie Exotique*, 84 (1991), pp. 25–90.

Lower respiratory tract

In striking contrast to the Western world, where PCP occurs in over 60 per cent of patients with AIDS, many studies of series of patients who have been investigated thoroughly have shown that PCP is a rare complication of Africans with AIDS.[26] Instead of *Pneumocystis*, in Africa reactivated *Mycobacterium tuberculosis* is the supreme infection complicating the course of AIDS: up to 60 per cent of all patients newly diagnosed as having pulmonary TB are HIV I seropositive in East and Central Africa, while HIV II has been shown to have a similar interaction in West Africa.[27] HIV positivity rates are even higher in patients with extrapulmonary TB. The numbers of patients diagnosed with TB is rising rapidly: for example, from 239 patients admitted to Ndola Central Hospital (Zambia) in 1984 to 505 in 1988;[28] with the increased pool of infection in young adults, transmission is increasing to children who are predominantly HIV negative.[29] These facts should have a profound influence on the TB control programme of South Africa.

Infants and Children

The most common clinical presentations of AIDS in infancy in Africa are (i) failure to thrive, progressing to severe weight loss and wasting; (ii) chronic fever; (iii) chronic diarrhoea; (iv) pulmonary infections; and (v) hepatosplenomegaly.[30] In children after infancy, generalised lymphadenopathy, oral candidiasis and skin rash are also common.[31] None of these presentations is specific for AIDS, and all can occur as a result of other common diseases of infancy. As a consequence the WHO clinical case definition of AIDS in children (see Table 13.2) has been found to be both insensitive and unspecific.[32] There is a need to redraft the clinical case definition of AIDS in children in tropical Africa; in South Africa, a clinical case definition is required which takes cognisance of the African experience, rather than the criteria of the Center for Disease Control in Atlanta, Georgia, USA.[33]

Table 13.2 WHO clinical case definition of AIDS proposed at WHO Workshop on AIDS in Central Africa, Bangui, 1985

ADULTS
AIDS in an adult is defined by the existence of at least two of the major signs associated with at least one minor sign, in the absence of known causes of immuno-suppression (such as cancer) or severe malnutrition or other recognised aetiologies.

*Major signs**
  Weight loss >10% of body weight
  Chronic diarrhoea > 1 month
  Prolonged fever > 1 month (intermittent or constant)

Minor signs
  Persistent cough for > 1 month
  Generalised pruritic dermatitis
  Recurrent *herpes zoster*[†]
  Oropharyngeal candidiasis
  Chronic progressive, disseminated *herpes simplex*
  infection.

The presence of generalised Kaposi's sarcoma or cryptococcal meningitis are sufficient by themselves for the diagnosis of AIDS.

CHILDREN
Paediatric AIDS is suspected in an infant or child presenting with at least two major signs associated with at least two minor signs in the absence of known causes of immuno-suppression.

Major signs
  Weight loss or abnormally slow growth
  Chronic diarrhoea > 1 month
  Prolonged fever > 1 month

Minor signs
  Generalised lymphadenopathy
  Oropharyngeal candidiasis
  Repeated common infections (otitis, pharyngitis, etc.)
  Persistant cough[‡]
  Generalised dermatitis
  Confirmed maternal HIV infection[§]

Proposed modifications

* Add 'asthenia or body weakness' as major sign.
† Replace by '*herpes zoster* during previous 5 years'.
‡ Promote to major sign.
§ Replace by 'Mother with at least one of the following: weight loss of more than 10% of normal body weight, diarrhoea or fever lasting more than 1 month'.

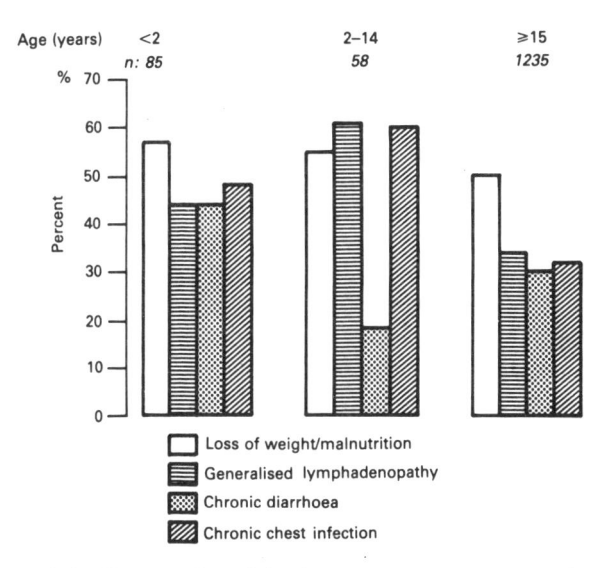

Figure 13.4 Frequencies of the four commonest presentation of HIV-related disease in 1378 Zambians (confirmed anti-HIV-1 positive)

Source A.F. Fleming, 'AIDS in Africa', *Baillière's Clinical Haematology*, 3, 1990, 177–203. Reproduced with permission of Baillière Tindall.

SERODIAGNOSIS

The first generation of anti-HIV I enzyme-linked immunosorbent-assays (Elisas) gave many false positive results with African sera, but the newer commercially available tests are highly sensitive as well as highly specific. Confirmatory tests, such as the Western Blot or radio immuno-assay precipitation, are expensive and technologically complex. When the epidemic is advanced and, for example, about 60 per cent of patients suspected clinically of being infected prove to be HIV seropositive, it is not feasible to confirm every Elisa-positive serum with a Western Blot. Fortunately, it has been shown in Central Africa that testing sera with two simple and inexpensive tests in sequence performs just as well as the more usual procedure of using one screening test followed by confirmatory tests on screen-positive sera.[34] The application of the algorithm (see Figure 13.5) with Serodia-HIV (Fujirebio) as the first and HIVCHEK (Du Pont de Nemours) as the second test had a sensitivity of 100 per cent and specificity of 98.5 per cent, while the cost of reagents was reduced from about US$25 to $7.80 per test. This scheme could be applied

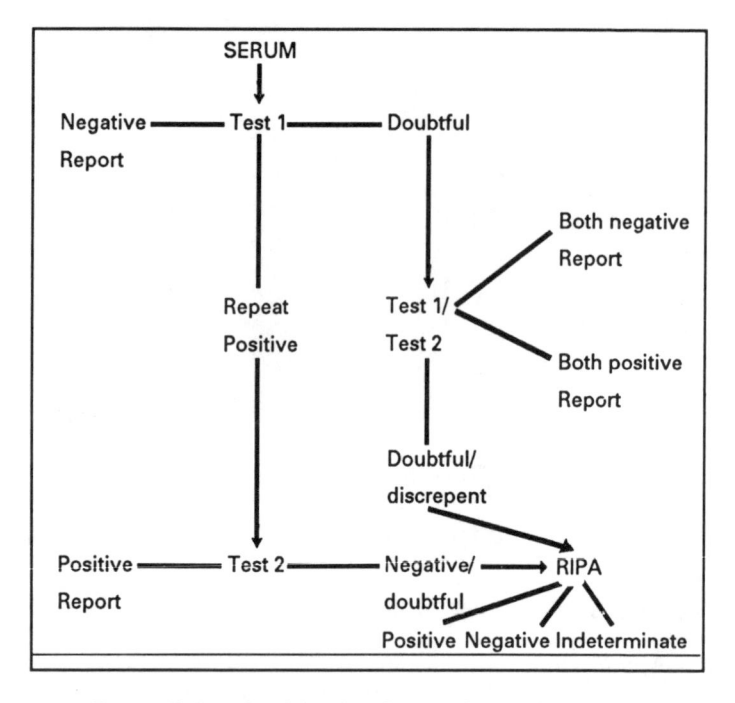

```
                        SERUM
                          ↓
   Negative ——— Test 1 ——— Doubtful
   Report
                                              Both negative
                                              Report
                             ↓
              Repeat      Test 1/
              Positive    Test 2
                                              Both positive
                                              Report

                          Doubtful/
                          discrepent

   Positive ——— Test 2 ——— Negative/ ——→ RIPA
   Report                  doubtful
                                    Positive Negative Indeterminate
```

Figure 13.5 Algorithm for the serodiagnosis of HIV-1
using two simple tests

Note Test 1 could be Serodia-HIV and test 2 HIVCHECK. Radio mimunoassay RIPA or western Blotting could be the confirmating test.

Source Nick *et al.*, 'Simple and inexpensive detection and confirmation of anti-HIV-1 in sera from Africa', *AIDS*, 5 (1991), 232–3. Reproduced with permission of Current Science Ltd and authors.

for all purposes – epidemiological, clinical and blood transfusion – on a national scale in South Africa. The first test should be the simplest, cheapest and most sensitive, and Serodia-HIV is suitable: this could be established in even the smallest peripheral laboratories. The second test should have a higher specificity (for example, HIVCHEK) and should be set up in first referral laboratories for supplementary testing of all sera repeat positive on the first test. The great majority of sera will give unequivocal negative or positive results on the algorithm: only those few sera which give discordant or doubtful results on the two tests need to be referred to a virological or specialist serology laboratory for Western Blot. The selection of tests employed can change with advances in technique, or with the detection of HIV II in sentinel populations, such as female prostitutes or STD clinic attenders.

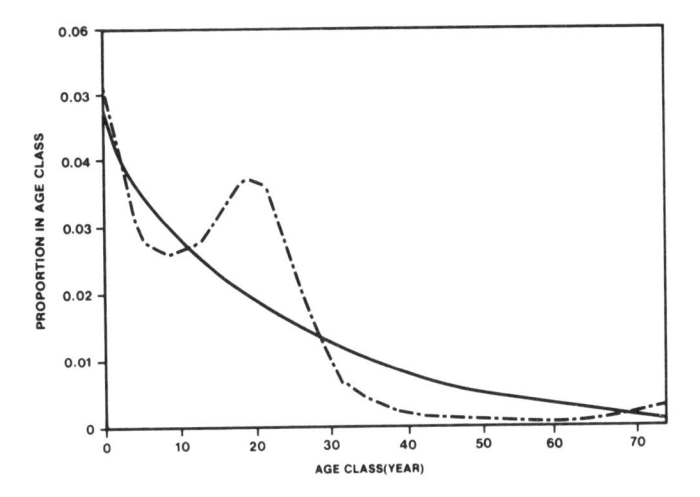

Figure 13.6 Temporal changes in age structure of the total population (males and females combined) at the year 50 of the epidemic of HIV

Source J.T. Rowley, R.M. Anderson and T.W. Ng, 'Reproducing the spread of HIV infection in Sub-Saharan Africa: some demographic and economic implications', *AIDS*, 4 (1990), 47–56. Reproduced with permission of Current Science Ltd and authors.

THE IMPACT OF AIDS ON AFRICA

The pandemic of HIV is having devastating effects on infected individuals, their families, communities and nations. The impact of the knowledge of infection and of disease on the individual does not need to be emphasised any more. The families with infected members are subjected to great emotional distress, disruption of family life and economic strain.[35] The direct costs of health care and death of one AIDS patient can be several hundred US dollars, equivalent to the earnings of many months for the chief wage-earner.[36] The direct costs are overshadowed, however, by the indirect costs from the loss of healthy productive life, amounting to US$5000 or more. The sickness and death of the main provider can lead to destitution in the survivors. Sickness and death of a mother can lead to the neglect of children, or the young family might become a burden on ageing grandparents.[37] The extended family may reject members because of the perceived disgrace, or be unable to cope with the need for food, housing and education of the many orphans.[38]

Industry will be affected adversely through decreased productivity from illness and early retirement or death of employees; at the same time costs will rise due to the need for medical care, sickness benefits and pensions for early retirement and widowhood.[39]

There have been many wild and a few sane predictions as to the demographic impact of the AIDS epidemic. It is probable that the total population of a Central African country will level off or go into slow negative growth after about the thirtieth year of the HIV epidemic,[40] and a similar prediction has been made for South Africa.[41] What is of greater consequence is the temporal changes in the age structure: it is predicted that by the fiftieth year of the epidemic, if there is no control, society will be dominated numerically by 33 per cent of the population being aged between 15 and 25 years, and there will be only 15 per cent aged more than 25 years (see Figure 13.6), as compared to about 30 per cent at present. Relative to the total population, there will be only half the expected manual skill and professional competence: industry and food production must decline catastrophically unless there are successful interventions.[42]

So far, little attention has been paid to the social consequences of one-third of the population being aged between 15 and 24 years (see Figure 13.6), the needs of this relatively large number of adolescents and young adults, and the possible destabilising effects if these needs are not met. Individuals at this age switch from dependency to productivity, a switch which occurs earlier in poorer families and in underdeveloped communities, but somewhat later when the young go on to tertiary education. There is a danger that the lack of older adults, both as producers and as teachers, will force more of the young into being providers – either in subsistence farming or at poorly paid jobs – at an early age, to the detriment of national development. This should be countered by planning and investment to provide job opportunities for the young, and to maintain or develop secondary and tertiary education. Education concerning the epidemic of AIDS is vital, addressed especially to those on the upward slope of the curve of the 15–24 year old bulge (see Figure 13.6), as this will include many who are not yet sexually active. These needs will be greatest amongst the 10 per cent (approximately) who will be orphans. Failure to plan for this age group could expose the young to the influences of the unscrupulous, who for their own gain will encourage socially disruptive behaviour, including substance abuse, prostitution, urban violence or, in the worst scenario, banditry and civil war.

MEANINGFUL RESPONSE

The epidemic of HIV and AIDS will permeate the whole community of South Africa unless there is a response involving the whole of society. All the necessary control strategies are well known so that only those which are particularly relevant and based on the experiences of tropical Africa will be discussed.

Development of Health Care

The burden of the care of infected people will be huge and beyond the capabilities of the existing health delivery systems. These must be developed, but the community itself is also an invaluable resource which must be called upon. A model from which we should learn is the integrated community approach at Mazabuka, Zambia, which involves home-based care and prevention, inpatient care at Chikankata Hospital when required, and collaboration with PHC, leprosy, TB, nutrition and other departments.[43] It is visualised and planned that care of patients in and around Soweto can be coordinated to involve home-based care, the Soweto Clinics, a referral outpatients clinic and inpatient care at Baragwanath Hospital. Cooperation with the TB control programme is essential, as is the development of STD clinics (there is none at present in Baragwanath Hospital).

Antenatal clinics are in a key position as they are centres for (i) the education of the community through the contact with all pregnant women and their families; (ii) sero-epidemiological surveys to monitor the epidemic in the sexually active age group of the general population; (iii) the identification, counselling and management of HIV-infected women and their families; (iv) the management of other STDs; (v) the prevention of vertical and horizontal transmission; and (vi) the reduction of the need to transfuse blood through the prevention and treatment of anaemia, and the identification and management of women at risk of obstetric complications.

Educational programmes for all cadres of health care workers is required, with the objective of (i) improving compassionate and effective medical care, (ii) allaying fears as to the risk of transmission and introducing appropriate preventive measures, and (iii) instructing all, including the lowest-paid workers, as educators of the public. The debate in South Africa has been dominated recently by surgeons to the exclusion of other matters which are at least as important as the safety of the health-care workers: a deep skin puncture with a hollow needle contaminated by a patient's blood is by far the most likely cause of nosocomial infection at the place of work, and instruction on the safe use and disposal of sharp instruments should be given high priority. A new cadre of counsellors also needs to be recruited and trained. At Baragwanath Hospital there is an active programme of staff education and counsellor training.

Recommended protocols for the treatment of the common complications of AIDS need to be prepared, together with lists of relatively inexpensive drugs. Ugandan experience has shown that a high degree of palliation can be achieved with the use of nine drugs – cotrimoxazole, metronidazole, ketoconazole, chlorpromazine, chloroquine, aspirin or acetaminophen, codeine, calamine lotion and petroleum jelly – plus anti-tuberculous chemotherapy.[44]

Prevention of Sexual Transmission

Women and children bear the brunt of the AIDS epidemic in Africa. Women are also a major resource, as carers, providers and educators. In the absence of any sex education in the schools, women's groups are the best hope there is for educating the young. AIDS education for schoolchildren has been successful in informing and altering sexual behaviour in Zambia;[45] as 85 per cent of Zambians attend primary school and only a minority continue to secondary school, the programme has been directed mostly towards children before they become sexually active, and it is immediately obvious from the curves of age-specific incidence (see Figure 13.1) that this is the age when intervention is essential. African experience has shown that programmes of education can be effective with schoolchildren,[46] married couples[47] and high-frequency STD transmitters.[48]

Prevention of Transmission by Blood Transfusion

In tropical Africa, blood transfusion continues to contribute to probably about 10 per cent of all transmissions, with anaemic children and women being amongst the highest risk groups.[49] HIV was transmitted by blood and blood products in South Africa before the recognition of the virus and the introduction of antibody screening in 1985, but there is now a high degree of safety due to the careful choice of donors and to antibody screening.[50]

However, the risk of a donor being in the 'window' between the time of infection and the time of seroconversion remains real. There are two strategies which should reduce this risk. First, new criteria for recruitment of blood donors are necessary: these must include intensive AIDS education preceding recruitment amongst young adults as they are most likely to be in the window, and exclusion of such groups as long-distance lorry drivers and all uniformed service men, as these are known to have higher prevalence of infection than the general population. Second, the transfusion of blood should be restricted to situations when patients are at risk of death or major morbidity.[51]

CONCLUSIONS

As the epidemic of HIV and AIDS in South Africa is at the beginning of the exponential expansion, many lessons can be learnt and many questions can be asked as a result of the experiences of tropical African countries which are further advanced into the epidemic.
1. We are all ignorant of the heterosexual partner contact networks of Africa. In some societies, there are recognisable sub-groups of the female population who are full-time prostitutes, and who now have extremely high seroprevalence of HIV. In other societies, there is a genteel form of female prostitution, which is part-time, temporary and for trivial reward, and HIV seroprevalence is more evenly distributed in all sectors of the sexually active.
2. Approximately three women are being infected with HIV for every two men in Africa, as a consequence both of social factors and the biologically greater efficiency of the male – female transmission more than *vice versa*. Transmission of HIV is a phenomenon of adolescence, especially in girls, so that the peak incidence of AIDS coincides with that of pregnancy.
3. The impact of the epidemic on female fertility has been underestimated because, besides transplacental transmission of HIV, there are adverse effects on the foetus regardless of its HIV status: pregnancies in HIV-infected women show increased frequency of foetal wastage, intra-uterine growth retardation, premature delivery and (possibly) stillbirth: the infants have a high frequency of low Apgar scores, neonatal deaths and infant mortality, so that about one third of live-born infants die before one year.
4. The immuno-deficiency following HIV infection leads to the reactivation of latent TB, so that about one-third of AIDS patients have pulmonary TB and, where the HIV epidemic is advanced, up to 60 per cent of all new patients with TB are HIV positive. The rate of

new infections with *M. tuberculosis* is rising as the children, predominantly HIV negative, are exposed to the increased pool in young adults. The secondary epidemic of TB is one of the most serious consequences of the HIV epidemic, and will have a major impact on society and the health services, especially the TB control programmes.

5. The clinical case definition of AIDS in Africa has proved to be a useful tool in diagnosis, epidemiology and education. On the other hand, the clinical case definition of AIDS in children is almost valueless. South Africa needs to define its own clinical case definitions, taking cognisance of both African and Western experiences.

6. The orthodox practice of serodiagnosis – that is, one screening test followed by confirmatory testing of positive sera – has been found impractical in African countries at the height of the epidemic because of the high cost of Western Blot or other confirmatory tests. A practical alternative is the application on a national scale of an algorithm involving two inexpensive tests in sequence, with confirmatory testing only of the few sera which give discrepant or doubtful results.

7. Demographic predictions show that there could be a slowing of population growth, possibly a levelling-off of total population, but probably not negative population growth. However, the age structure of the population will show considerable distortion, with deficiencies in early childhood and after the age of 25 years due to early death from AIDS, and an excess of 15–24 year olds, perhaps amounting to 33 per cent of the total population. Attention is being given to the economic and social consequences of the shortage of adults in the productive age range, but so far little thought has been spared for the education and employment needs of relatively large numbers of adolescents (of whom about 10 per cent will be orphans) and young adults; unless these needs are met, this bulge in the population could prove to be socially disruptive.

8. Direct costs of the care of illness and death of patients with AIDS will be huge, and cannot be met by existing health delivery systems. Planning should be directed towards developing integrated care in the home and community, PHC units, hospital outpatient clinics and hospital wards. Investment and development is required also in antenatal clinics, STD clinics and TB control programmes.

9. The best hope there is of diminishing transmission of HIV and decreasing the impact of the AIDS epidemic is education in primary and secondary schools. To this end there must be a mobilisation of government, schools, womens' groups and community leaders.

10. The transmission by blood transfusion is being controlled largely by the exclusion of donors with high-risk behaviour, the screening of donors and the inactivation of virus in blood products. However, transmission of HIV from donors who are in the window between infection and seroconversion remains a very real risk, especially during the exponential phase of the epidemic. At present, this risk can be reduced only by intensive AIDS education of potential donors, especially young adults, by restricting donor recruitment amongst long-distance lorry drivers and the uniformed services, and by avoiding the inappropriate transfusion of blood and blood products.

Acknowledgement

I thank Miss Gayle Spring for her dedicated work in the preparation of the typescript.

Addendum

Observations from the experience at Baragwanath Hospital, Soweto, quoted on pp. 296 and 309, have been published since the preparation of this text.[52–55]

References

1. P. Piot and M. Caraël, 'Epidemiological and sociological aspects of HIV-infection in developing countries', *British Medical Bulletin*, 44 (1988), pp. 66–8; A.F. Fleming, 'AIDS in Africa', *Baillière's Clinical Haematology*, 3 (1990a), pp. 177–205.
2. C.W. Hunt, 'Migrant labour and sexually transmitted disease: AIDS in Africa', *Journal of Health and Social Behaviour*, 30 (1989), pp. 353–73.
3. Fleming, 'AIDS in Africa'.
4. C.R.B. Prior and G.C. Buckle, 'Blood donors with antibody to human immunodeficiency virus – the Natal experience', *South African Medical Journal*, 77 (1990), pp. 623–5.
5. J. Chin, 'Current and future dimensions of the HIV/AIDS pandemic in women and children', *Lancet*, 336 (1990), pp. 221–4.
6. S. Berkley, W. Naamara, S. Okware *et al.*, 'AIDS and HIV infection in Uganda – are more women infected than men?', *AIDS*, 4 (1990), pp. 1237–42; Chin, 'Current and future dimensions'; Rwandan HIV Seroprevalence Study Group, 'Nationwide community-based serological

survey of HIV-1 and other human retrovirus infections in a central African country'. *Lancet*, i (1989), pp. 941–3.
7. Berkley et al., 'AIDS and HIV infection'.
8. Fleming, 'AIDS in Africa'.
9. K.M. de Cock, B. Barrere, M.F. Lafontaine et al., 'Mortality trends in Abidjan, Côte d'Ivoire, 1983–1988', *AIDS*, 5 (1991), pp. 393–8.
10. R.M. Anderson, S. Gupta and W. Ng, 'The significance of sexual partner contact networks for the transmission dynamics of HIV', *Journal of Acquired Immune Deficiency Syndromes*, 3 (1990), pp. 417–29.
11. R.W. Ryder, W. Nsa, S.E. Hassig et al., 'Perinatal transmission of the human immunodeficiency virus type 1 to infants of seropositive women in Zaire', *New England Journal of Medicine*, 320 (1989), pp. 1637–42.
12. P. Paterlini, S. Lallemant-Le Coeur, M. Lallemant et al., 'Polymerase chain reaction for studies of mother to child transmission of HIV-1 in Africa', *Journal of Medical Virology*, 30 (1990), pp. 53–7.
13. M. Lallemant, S. Lallemant-Le Coeur, D. Cheynier et al., 'Mother-child transmission of HIV-1 and infant survival in Brazzaville, Congo', *AIDS*, 3 (1989), pp. 643–6; P. Lepage, F. Dabis, D.-G. Hitimani et al., 'Perinatal transmission of HIV-1: lack of impact of maternal HIV infection on characteristics of livebirths and on neonatal mortality in Kigali, Rwanda'. *AIDS*, 5 (1991), pp. 295–300; P.G. Miotti, G. Dallabetta, E. Ndovi et al., 'HIV-1 and pregnant women: associated factors, prevalence, estimate of incidence and role of foetal wastage in central Africa', *AIDS*, 4 (1990), pp. 733–6; M. Temmerman, F.A. Plummer, N.B. Mirza et al., 'Infection with HIV as a risk factor for adverse obstetrical outcome', *AIDS*, 4 (1990), pp. 1087–93.
14. M.R. Braddick, J.K. Kreiss, J.E. Embree et al., 'Impact of maternal HIV infection on obstetrical and early neonatal outcome', AIDS, 4 (1990), pp. 1001–5.
15. Ryder et al., 'Perinatal transmission'.
16. Chin, 'Current and future dimensions'.
17. E.A. Preble, 'Impact of HIV/AIDS on African children', *Social Science and Medicine*, 31, 6 (1990), pp. 671–80.
18. A.F. Fleming, 'Opportunistic infections in AIDS in developed and developing countries', *Transactions of the Royal Society of Tropical Medicine and Hygiene*, 84 (1990), suppl. 1, pp. 1–6; S.B. Lucas, 'Missing infections in AIDS', *Transactions of the Royal Society of Tropical Medicine and Hygiene*, 84 (1990), suppl. 1, pp. 34–8.
19. Fleming, 'AIDS in Africa'.
20. Fleming, 'Opportunistic infections'.
21. R. Widi-Wirski, S. Berkley, R. Downing et al., 'Evaluation of the WHO clinical case definition of AIDS in Uganda', *Journal of the American Medical Association*, 260 (1988), pp. 3286–9.
22. C.P. Conlon, A.J. Pinching, C.U. Perera et al., 'HIV-related enteropathy in Zambia: a clinical, microbiological, and histological study', *American Journal of Tropical Medicine and Hygiene*, 42 (1990), pp. 83–8; Fleming, 'Opportunistic infections'.
23. Fleming, 'Opportunistic infections'; Z. Mugaruka, J.H. Perriëns,

B. Kapita and P. Piot, 'Oral manifestations of HIV-1 infection in Zairian patients', *AIDS*, 5 (1991), pp. 237–8.
24. M. Schiodt, I. Bygbjerg, P. Bakilana *et al.*, 'Oral manifestations of HIV-infection in Tanzania'. Second International Symposium on AIDS and Associated Cancers in Africa, Naples, 7–9 October 1987, Abstracts, p. 106.
25. Mugaruka *et al.*, 'Oral manifestations'.
26. Fleming, 'AIDS in Africa'; Fleming, 'Opportunistic infections'.
27. Fleming, 'AIDS in Africa'; Fleming, 'Opportunistic infections'; K.M. de Cock, E. Gnaore, G. Adjorlolo *et al.*, 'Risk of tuberculosis in patients with HIV-I and HIV-II infections in Abidjan, Ivory Coast', *British Medical Journal*, 302 (1991), pp. 496–9; A.E. Pitchenik, 'Tuberculosis control and the AIDS epidemic in developing countries', *Annals of Internal Medicine*, 113 (1990), pp. 89–90.
28. O.O. Simooya, M.N. Maboshe, R.B. Kaoma *et al.*, 'HIV infection in newly diagnosed tuberculosis patients in Ndola, Zambia', *Central African Journal of Medicine*, 37 (1991), pp. 4–7.
29. B. Standaert, F. Niragira, P. Kadende and P. Piot, 'The association of tuberculosis and HIV infection in Burindi', *AIDS Research and Human Retroviruses*, 5 (1989), pp. 247–51.
30. F. Davachi and N. Mayemba, 'AIDS in infancy', *Postgraduate Doctor Caribbean*, 7 (1991), pp. 56–63.
31. F.K. Nkrumah, R.G. Choto, J. Emmanuel and R. Kumar, 'Clinical presentation of symptomatic human immunodeficiency virus in children', *Central African Journal of Medicine*, 36 (1990), pp. 116–20.
32. H.J. Lambert and H. Friesen, 'Clinical features of paediatric AIDS in Uganda', *Annals of Tropical Paediatrics*, 9 (1989), pp. 1–5; P. Lepage, P. van de Perre, F. Dabis *et al.*, 'Evaluation and simplification of the World Health Organization clinical case definition for paediatric AIDS', *AIDS*, 3 (1989), pp. 221–5; O. Müller, P. Musoke, G. Sen and R. Moser, 'Paediatric HIV-1 disease in a Kampala hospital', *Journal of Tropical Paediatrics*, 36 (1990), pp. 283–6.
33. R.A. Bobat, H.M. Coovadia and I.M. Windsor, 'Some early observations on HIV infection in children at King Edward VIII Hospital, Durban', *South African Medical Journal*, 78 (1990), pp. 524–7.
34. F. Spielberg, C.M. Kabeya, T.C. Quinn *et al.*, 'Performance and cost-effectiveness of a dual rapid essay system for screening and confirmation of human immunodeficiency virus type 1 seropositivity', *Journal of Clinical Microbiology*, 28 (1990), pp. 303–6; S. Nick, E. Chimfuembe, G. Hunsmann and A.F. Fleming, 'Simple and inexpensive detection and confirmation of anti-HIV-1 in sera from Africa', *AIDS*, 5 (1991), pp. 232–3.
35. G.A. Lloyd, 'HIV-infection, AIDS, and family disruption', in A.F. Fleming, M. Carballo, D.W. FitzSimons, M.R. Bailey and J. Mann (eds), *The Global Impact of AIDS* (New York: Alan R. Liss, 1988), pp. 183–90; M. Carballo and M. Caraël, 'Impact of AIDS on social organizations', in Fleming *et al.*, *The Global Impact*, pp. 81–93.
36. M. Over, S. Bertozzi, J. Chin, B. N'Galy and K. Nyamuryekung'e. 'The

direct and indirect cost of HIV infection in developing countries: the cases of Zaire and Tanzania', in Fleming *et al.*, *The Global Impact*, pp. 123–35; F. Davachi, P. Baudoux, K. Ndoko, B. N'Galy and J. Mann, 'The economic impact on families of children with AIDS in Kinshasa, Zaire', in Fleming *et al.*, *The Global Impact*, pp. 167–9.
37. C. Beer, A. Rose and K. Tout, 'AIDS – the grandmother's burden', in Fleming *et al.*, *The Global Impact*, pp. 171–4.
38. P. Onyanga and P. Walji, 'The family as a resource', in Fleming *et al.*, *The Global Impact*, pp. 301–6.
39. B.M. Nkowane, 'The impact of human immunodeficiency virus infection and AIDS on a primary industry: mining (a case study in Zambia)', in Fleming *et al.*, *The Global Impact*, pp. 150–60.
40. J.T. Rowley, R.M. Anderson and T.W. Ng, 'Reducing the spread of HIV infection in sub-Saharan Africa: some demographic and economic implications', *AIDS*, 4 (1990), pp. 47–56.
41. R. Schall, 'On the maximum size of the AIDS epidemic among the heterosexual black population of South Africa', *South Africa Medical Journal*, 78 (1990), pp. 507–10.
42. N. Abel, T. Barnett, S. Bell, P. Blaikie and S. Cross, 'The impact of AIDS on food production systems in east and central Africa over the next ten years: a programmatic paper', in Fleming *et al.*, *The Global Impact*, pp. 145–54.
43. C.M. Chela, I.D. Campbell and Z. Siankanga, 'Clinical care as part of integrated AIDS management in a Zambian rural community', *AIDSCare*, 1 (1989), pp. 319–25; I.D. Campbell, 'AIDS care and prevention – a community approach. Part I: structuring a response', *Postgraduate Doctor Middle East*. 13 (1990), pp. 641–6; I.D. Campbell, 'AIDS care and prevention – a community approach. Part II: structuring a response', *Postgraduate Doctor Middle East*, 13 (1990), pp. 722–4.
44. R.W. Goodgame, 'AIDS in Uganda – clinical and social features', *New England Journal of Medicine*, 323 (1990), pp. 383–9.
45. Panos Institute and Save the Children, *AIDS and Children: A Family Disease – Mini-Dossier 2* (London, 1989), p. viii.
46. Ibid.; S.H. Kapiga, G. Nachtigal and D.J. Hunter, 'Knowledge of AIDS among secondary school pupils in Bangamayo and Dar-es-Salaam, Tanzania', *AIDS*, 5 (1991), pp. 61–7.
47. R.W. Ryder, M. Ndilu, S.E. Hassig *et al.*, 'Heterosexual transmission of HIV-1 among employees and their spouses at two large businesses in Zaire', *AIDS*, 4, 8 (1990), pp. 725–32; M. Kamnega, R.W. Ryder, M. Jingu *et al.*, 'Evidence of marked sexual behaviour change associated with low HIV-1 seroconversion in 149 married couples with discordant HIV-1 serostatus: experience at an HIV counselling center in Zaire', *AIDS*, 5 (1991), pp. 61–7.
48. S. Moses, F.A. Plummer, E.N. Ngugi *et al.*, 'Controlling HIV in Africa: effectiveness and cost of an intervention in a high-frequency STD transmitter core group', *AIDS*, 5 (1991), pp. 407–11.
49. A.F. Fleming, 'Prevention of transmission of HIV by blood transfusion in developing countries', in Fleming *et al.*, *The Global Impact*, pp. 357–67.
50. A. du P. Heynes, E. Kuun and R.L. Crookes, 'The risk of transmitting

HIV by blood and blood products from the South African Blood Transfusion Service', 31st Annual Congress of the Federation of South African Societies of Pathology, Warmbaths, 30 June–3 July, Abstract H18 (1991), p. 125.
51. Global Blood Safety Initiative of the WHO and League of the Red Cross and Red Crescent Societies, *Guidelines for the Appropriate Use of Blood*, WHO/GPA/INF/89, 18, WHO/LAB/89.10 (Geneva: WHO, 1989).
52. I.R. Friedland, K.P. Klugman and A.S. Karstaedt *et al.*, 'AIDS – the Baragwanath experience. Part I. Epidemiology of HIV infection at Baragwanath Hospital, 1988–1990', *South African Medical Journal*, 82 (1992), pp. 86–90.
53. I.R. Friedland and J.A. McIntyre, 'AIDS – the Baragwanath experience. Part II. HIV infection in pregnancy and childhood', *South African Medical Journal*, 82 (1992), pp. 90–4.
54. A.S. Karstaedt, 'AIDS – the Baragwanath experience. Part III. HIV infection in adults at Baragwanath Hospital', *South African Medical Journal*, 82 (1992), pp. 95–7.
55. C.W. Allwood, I.R. Friedman, A.S. Karstaedt and J.A. McIntyre, 'AIDS – the Baragwanath experience. Part IV. Counselling and ethical issues', *South African Medical Journal*, 82 (1992), pp. 98–101.

14 Facing up to AIDS
Sholto Cross

This volume has presented a number of approaches to the study of AIDS which as yet form a distinctly minor part of the global research effort directed at the containment and treatment of the disease. The utilisation of the methods of the social and behavioural sciences in addressing this epidemic is still in its infancy, despite universal recognition that – as yet – behaviour modification is the only effective defence against AIDS which we possess. This book is a modest contribution towards such global studies, and the first of its kind in southern Africa. What is needed now is a large programme of action-oriented research to carry this forward.

While relying on the established techniques of epidemiology to outline the scale of the impact, the authors who have investigated statistical methods for assessing the demographic implications have created new tools for the use of health planners. These, it is hoped, may replace the crude rules-of-thumb which have given AIDS-impact estimation such a deservedly bad name. As the data builds up and becomes more extensive and reliable, it should be possible to refine the techniques presented here further, enabling robust analytical procedures to be developed which can assist in the detailed tracking of the disease according to a wide range of factors, of which social cohort and locality are only a beginning.

Further research in demography and epidemiology is needed to fine tune the methodology and to build up the flow of useful information. It would clearly be of great interest to establish a national database of the HIV incidence in South Africa utilising a modified geographical information system (GIS). This country has the research skills, the academic institutions and existing data sources to enable a task of this magnitude to be attempted with the confidence that the results could prove of great significance not only here but also in other countries with potentially massive AIDS invasion, such as India. If all HIV data-reporting centres around the country were integrated into a GIS, supported by specific sampling of socio-economic profiles, transmission modes, and a host of co-factors of both a medical and social type, questions on the nature and spread of the disease could be asked and answered which would have the effect of bringing public health policy to a new level of refinement and usefulness.

Associated with this is the need to push ahead with studies of sexual behaviour in the various sub-cultures of the land, to enable the most effective interventions to be made in terms of modifying behaviour. This research would be of interest and relevance not only to those formally concerned such as psychologists, anthropologists and sociologists, those responsible for national education and health policies, and sectoral groups such as employers and unions who have statutory or other requirements to attend to the welfare of their constituencies; it is also of vital importance that the communities and households amongst whose ranks this deadly virus is moving should see themselves as concerned and committed activists, equally involved in the business of research. A systematic programme of such research is required whereby each institution of higher learning in South Africa should take a regional area, a group of organised communities, and a thematic aspect of AIDS-related behaviour as their focus of study, with regular sharing of insights and findings between the research teams and their supporting communities. The mounting of such a programme should be seen as a priority by university-based public-sector health programmes.

It is probable that studies of the economic and financial aspects of AIDS will increasingly take the road of examining specific sub-sectors, as has already been the case with the life insurance industry. This is not to say that the macro-level analyses of the type presented in this volume do not have a role. They have a general importance for shaping overall development thinking about endemic disease and economic growth, but perhaps the most relevant studies will be those which are sharply focused on specific target communities. As a country which has recently been undergoing labour-shedding in some of its key sectors, South Africa may not be the most appropriate model to develop analytical techniques of precise comparative relevance to, say, Brazil and Indonesia, but clearly the development of methods of analysis of direct and indirect costs, and the establishment of linkage effects resulting from AIDS which run throughout the economy, are important exercises.

These studies should help to address some of the most difficult of the forthcoming questions in health policy. What share of the national budget should be allocated to health, and should there be a ceiling on this despite the burgeoning problems resulting from AIDS? How far should public-sector provision be allowed to treat AIDS as a priority, overriding other areas – both related and unrelated – such as malaria, malnutrition and TB, which may have better prospects for prevention and cure? How far can community care of the dying actually cope with the situation of AIDS sufferers, and what should the balance be between public and private provision of hospices?

The lessons of other African countries which are further along the AIDS road suggest that, over the medium term, one of the major social problems which will result from the epidemic will be the increase in orphans. South Africa already has a major social crisis with 'street children', despite having on the Witwatersrand one of the largest programmes in the world attempting to cope with this. Research and planning involving professionals in the social services, community organisations and NGOs should be mounted to address the questions of the most effective means of coping with a dramatic rise in orphans in both urban and rural contexts. Effective strategies for coping will involve not only national policies, but will also require a much greater understanding of the impact of morbidity and death on the household in general.

It is a tragic historical irony that South Africa, on the brink of a new political dispensation, should also be facing the onslaught of the most devastating plague of modern times. The expectation that this disease will have a differential impact along existing lines of cleavage will intensify the difficulties. If only for this reason, the allocation of sufficient resources to the mounting of research into understanding and modifying the behavioural dimensions of the disease is fully justified. There are also major potential benefits for many other areas globally which may result from the development of new models and planning techniques for confronting AIDS. South Africa has the reality of Third World poverty, urban ghettos and rural slums, together with an urban industrial infrastructure and sophisticated centres of learning and administration, which uniquely may enable new approaches to the management of an epidemic to be developed. These may be of great value to other such countries, notably in Asia and Latin America, which have not yet gone as far down the AIDS road.

Finally, South African society is nothing if not politicised to a fault. It is inconceivable that the course of the epidemic will not add fuel to an already fiery political debate. This underlines the need for an integrated and systematic national research effort which can help to puncture the myths and misinformation surrounding AIDS, and which can lead to effective strategies of caring and coping. In the absence of a miracle vaccine costing less than a bottle of beer, this is the most practical way we have of facing up to AIDS.

Index

Abidjan 297, 299
Africa 295–316
  AIDS and HIV infection in southern 7–9
  blamed as source of AIDS epidemic 15
  clinical manifestations 300–4; adults 301–4, 305; children 303, 304
  demographic effects of AIDS 30–1, 307–8
  estimated HIV infection 261
  impact of AIDS 307–8
  infants of HIV-infected mothers 298–300
  meaningful response 308–10; development of health care 309–10; prevention 310
  monitoring in sub-Saharan *see* monitoring
  projections 22, 23
  reported AIDS cases 16, 17–18
  serodiagnosis 305–7
  sexual *mores* 295–6
  sexual transmission 295–8, 299
  vulnerability and complacency 289–90
African National Congress 73
age
  AIDS deaths in Zimbabwe 229, 230, 231
  death rates 297, 299
  distribution of new HIV infections in South Africa 97
  HIV-related disease 297, 298
  medical aid societies' beneficiaries 245–6
age structure of population
  distortion and 'bulge' of young people 308, 312
  non-'greying' of African 258
  population pyramids in Buganda 265–7
  South Africa and AIDS 108, 110, 138, 140–5
  Zimbabwe and AIDS 242–3
agricultural impact simulation studies 264, 274–9, 286
  Buganda 277–9

  policy implications 279
  Rwanda 274–5
  Tabora in Tanzania 275–6
agriculture 146, 148
  see also rural–urban dependency
AIDS
  cases in southern Africa 7, 8; South Africa 7, 8, 62–4, 103–4, 105, 133; Zimbabwe 8, 218–21, 243
  costs *see* costs
  global epidemic 15–22
  modes of transmission 6–7
  nature of 4
  patterns of spread 5, 63–4, 88
'AIDS-related complexes' (ARC) 4, 7
American Red Cross 26
Americas 16, 18–19
Anderson, R. 116
Angola 8, 9
Ankole cattle-banana farming system 278
antenatal clinic data
  South Africa; differing patterns 296–7, Doyle model compared with 99–101; first national HIV survey 67–8
  Zimbabwe 223, 224
antenatal clinics 309
Asia
  projections 22, 23, 31
  reported AIDS cases 16, 19–20
attendance registers 234
Auguste-Viktoria, K. 40
awareness-raising 236
  see also health education
AZT 36, 47, 162
  costs research 46
  Zimbabwe's medical aid societies 249, 253

Bailey, N.T.J. 61
banana-coffee farming system 277–8, 279
banking industry 225
Baragwanath Antenatal Clinic 296
Baragwanath Hospital 309
behaviour change 318
  health education and 69, 72–3
  prevention and 47

321

behavioural research 27
Belgium 24
Bell, G. 54
Bernard, Roger 16
black population in South Africa
  demographic impact of AIDS
    113–34; input data 117–20;
    modelling 114–17; projection
    results 120–8
  dependency ratio 143, 144–5
  dual society 70–1
  environment for 69–70
  migration 145
  occupational advancement 150, 151
  TFR (total fertility rate) 142–3, 144
Blaug, M. 194, 213
blood donors
  HIV data 66, 68; Zimbabwe 222,
    223, 243–4
  medical aid societies and testing 247
  restricting recruitment 310, 312
blood transfusions
  global pandemic 24, 26
  transmission by 6–7, 25; minor in
    South Africa 116, 118;
    prevention 310, 312
  window period 6, 26
Bloom, D.E. 37
body fluids 7
  see also blood donors; blood
    transfusions; sexual transmission
Botswana 8, 9, 12
Brand, S.S. 146
Brazil 40, 178
breast milk 26
Brett, Vincent 76
Buganda
  agricultural impact simulation
    studies 277–9
  farm land abandoned 288
  household structure changes 283–6
  parenting 273
  population pyramids 265–7
building industry 54

Cabral, A.J.R. 69, 70
cancer 28–9, 259
candidiadis 301, 303, 304
Carliner, G. 37
cash crop production 276, 288
  see also agricultural impact simulation
    studies
cattle-banana farming system 278

celibacy 285
children
  clinical manifestations 303, 304
  fewer than expected in Rakai 285
  see also infant mortality; infants;
    orphans
Chin, James 24–5
China 31
cholera 71
CIMAS 254
  AIDS research unit 246
  claims expenditure 247–52
  drugs expenditure limited 236
  reserve fund 235
  STD claims 252–3, 254–8
cities see urban employment; urban
  'plant' studies; urban–rural
  dependency
clinical case definitions 301, 303,
  311–12
clinical manifestations 300–4
  adults 301–4, 305
  children 303, 304
clinics, community 259
clothing 273
Coale, A.J. 141, 156
Commercial Farmers Union
  (CFU) 224, 236–7
community care 259, 309
  economics of 45–6
  orphans 273
community clinics 259
community political structures 73
complacency 289–90
condom use 120, 130–1, 133
Confederation of Zimbabwe Industries
  (CZI) 233–4, 236, 237
confidentiality, HIV testing and 246–7
coping strategies 262, 264, 286
  farming systems 274–9
  households 280–3, 285
  need for research into
    experimental 288
  orphans 273
cost bearers 48–9
cost–benefit analysis 193–5, 213
cost-effectiveness 193–4
cost shifting 48
costs of AIDS/HIV 10–11
  data variability 35–6
  developed countries 37–8, 39, 40,
    41–2
  developing countries 38, 39–41, 42
  direct see direct costs

indirect *see* indirect costs
medical *see* medical costs
personal *see* personal costs
South Africa 160–75; and overall economic impact 184–7; per person treated 178–9; total 169–75, 184–7, 187
Zimbabwe *see* Zimbabwe
Côte D'Ivoire 297, 299
coughs, persistent 301, 304
cover-up, Zimbabwe 218–19
Crookes, R.L. 78–9
crop range 281–2
 see also agricultural impact simulation studies; agriculture; cash crops
crowding out 41, 232
cryptosporidium 301, 302
Cunningham, D. 40
current cost calculations 170–1, 172–4, 184

data reliability 35–6
Davies, R. 230–1
De Beer, C. 70, 71
death benefits, lump sum 236
demographic cohort models 79–80
demographic impact
  Africa 307–8
  global pandemic 30–2
  South Africa 307–8, 312; *see also* black population; Doyle model
  Zimbabwe 227–31
 see also age structure of population
dependency ratios 143, 144–5
  at household level 145–9
dermatitis 303, 304
developed countries 179
  AIDS and society 29–30
  current research 37–8, 39, 40, 41–2
developing countries
  AIDS and society 30–1
  current research 38, 39–41, 42
  economic impact 179–80, 185
  reductions in TFR 143, 144
development, economic
  population growth and 140–5
  South Africa and AIDS/HIV 52–5
Devlin, A.C. 234
diagnosis, economics of 47–8
 see also serodiagnosis
diarrhoea, chronic 301, 304, 305
didanosine 28
direct costs 307
  current research 39–43; non-

personal medical care 42–3;
personal medical care 39–42
South Africa 50–2, 161–2, 178–81; components of 167; contribution to total costs 172–3, 174–5; cost per person treated 178–9; total direct costs 163–7, 179–81
Zimbabwe 232–3
 see also costs; indirect costs; medical costs
discount rate 203–6
Doomsday predictions 75–6, 185–6
doubling times 22, 65, 78, 131
Doyle, P. 77, 78
Doyle model 79–80, 81, 87–112, 159
  background to development of 87–8
  calibration 99–102; geographic spread of infection 99–101; spread by risk group 101–2
  details of structure and inputs 94–9; age distribution of new infections 97; AIDS mortality 98–9; demographic data 94; distribution of population into risk groups 95; incubation period 98; mother-to-child transmission 98; probability of infection per contact 95–6; sexual contact patterns 96–7
  scenarios for South Africa 102–9
  structure and basic principles 88–94; HIV infection 92–3; imports 93–4; risk groups 90–2
drugs 28, 46–7, 310
 see also AZT
dual society 70–1
Durban 75, 296–7

early warning systems 262, 287
earnings
  human capital approach 201; rate of increase 203–6, 214
  lost 31, 161, 163, 172, 182–3
  and medical aid societies' contributions 241
economic development *see* development
economic impact model 158–90
  direct cost model 161–2; components of 167; implications 178–81; results for total direct costs 163–7
  indirect cost model *see* indirect costs
  methodological approach 160–3; problems 162–3

economic impact model *cont.*
  simulating effects of policy measures 175–7
  total costs of HIV/AIDS 169–75; contribution of direct and indirect costs 174–5; and overall economic impact 184–7
economic sectors 49, 53–5
  see also industry
economies, collapse of 52, 53
Edelston, K. 71, 75–6, 77, 81–2
education
  'bulge' in population needing 308, 312
  expenditure: compared with health expenditure 192–4; Zimbabwe 233
  for health care workers 309
  household coping strategies and withdrawal from 281–2
  human capital theory 191–2; lost investment 195–200
  orphan population 272–3, 291
  see also health education
elderly, care of 285
Elisa 223, 305
employment 146
  urban 149–53
  see also labour; unemployment
employment agency fees 208, 214
employee benefits 235–6
environment
  impact on and abandoned land 288
  South African and black population 69–70
epidemic(s)
  defining 64–6
  global 14–22; *see also* global pandemic
  maximum size in South Africa 80
  monitoring 262
  predicting 9
epidemiological data 36
Epstein, P. 69
Europe 22, 24, 40, 48
  AIDS cases 16, 20–1
  complacency 289–90
  hospitalisation 45–6
exploitation 70
  self- 281–2
exponential growth 64–5, 226
extended families 273, 307

factory workers 228

families 229
  costs to 48–9, 188, 307
  disruption 108–9, 110, 307
  extended 273, 307
  medical aid society cover 253
  see also orphans
farmers 236–7
  see also agricultural impact simulation studies; agriculture; rural–urban dependency
fertility rate
  reduction in developing countries 144
  South Africa 141–3, 144; black population 117–18, 132–3; Doyle model 106–8
financial costs 171–2
foetal wastage 298–9, 311
food production 262, 286
  see also agricultural impact simulation studies
Fraser-Mackenzie, Peter 224, 236, 237
future cost calculations 171, 174, 175, 184–5

Gallo, Robert 14
gastro-intestinal tract 301, 302
gender differences 297, 298, 299
genital ulcers 117, 120
geographical information system (GIS) 317–18
geographical spread of infection (South Africa) 99–101
Gillespie, S. 274–5
gleaners 147–8
global pandemic 13–33
  AIDS and society 28–32
  epidemic 14–22
  transmission patterns 22–7
GNP 170–4
government policy *see* policy
Graaff, J. 147
grandparents 273, 284–5
Griffith, S.F. 40
Groeneveld, H. 93

haemophiliacs 22–4
Harare AIDSTECH workshop 226–7
Harding, Peter 234
Hardy, A.M. 40, 44
Hay, J.W. 40
health care
  availability in South Africa 74
  development of 309–10, 312
  managed and cost reduction 236

Index

politics of 153–5
primary (PHC) 26, 70–1, 72–3, 83
health-care workers
  education for 309
  transmission by 25, 27
health education 27, 312
  South Africa 72–3
  workplace 236
  Zambia 310
  Zimbabwe 236, 258
health expenditure 179–80
  education expenditure compared with 192–4
  politics 154–5
  South Africa 185; proportion spent on AIDS/HIV 164–7, 179–80
  US 37–8
  Zimbabwe 232, 233
  see also costs of AIDS/HIV
health services
  South Africa and economic impact 180, 187
  Zimbabwe 232–3
'healthy life years' lost 201–3
  see also life expectancy
Hellinger, F.J. 37, 40
herpes zoster 300, 301, 302, 304
heterosexual transmission 6, 113
  see also sexual transmission
HIV infection 4, 66, 113–14, 114–15
  costs *see* costs; direct costs; indirect costs; medical costs; personal costs
  data 218, 221–4
  Doyle model 92–3, 109–10; age distribution of new 97; geographic spread 99–101; infection probability 95–6; scenarios 102–3, 104–5; spread by risk group 101–2
  global pandemic 7, 16–22, 23, 64
  insurance and 55
  labour quality and 192–3
  South Africa 66–8; black population 120–3, 128–9, 133; economic impact modelling 160; first national survey 67–8; projections 75–82 *passim* and TB 74
  transmission routes: and efficiency 24–5; infants of HIV-infected mothers 298–300; sexual 296–7
  Zambia 297, 298
  Zimbabwe: data 221–4; medical aid societies' monitoring 246–7, 253–4, 255; risk groups and incidence 243–5
HIV I 4, 25
  serodiagnosis 305–7
HIV II 4, 25
HIVCHEK 305, 307
Hoima district 268
home nursing 258–9
homosexual men 22–4, 29, 113
hospital accommodation, low-cost 176, 177
hospitals, Zimbabwe 258
hospitalisation 162, 180–1
  effects of reduction 176–7
households
  dependency ratios 138, 145–9
  labour use and agricultural impact simulation studies 264, 274–9
  socio-economic differentiation and impact 279–83; developmental cycle 280–2; policy implications 282–3; social differentiation 280
  structure changes 264–5; Buganda 283–6
human capital approach 43, 161, 163, 191–214
  lost educational investment 195–200
  mortality cost estimates 200–6
  recruitment adjustment and retraining costs 206–11
  theory 191–5
Hunter, S. 268

'imports', Doyle model and 93–4, 97
incubation period 4, 116, 132
  Doyle model 98, 99
  Zimbabwe 252
India 31, 72
indirect costs 14, 231–2, 307
  current research 43–5
  economic impact model 161, 167–9, 181–3; adjustment for replacement of workers 168; contribution to total costs 174–5; formal and informal sector 169; lost production 168, 168–9; lost work years 167–8
  see also costs; direct costs; medical costs
industry 11, 307
  and AIDS in Zimbabwe 233–8, 239
  labour market planning 212
  South Africa: economic

industry: South Africa *cont.*
    development 53–5;
    restructuring 153, 155
infant mortality 299, 300, 311
    South African black population 124–5
infants 7
    incubation period 98, 99
    life expectancy of infected in Zimbabwe 252
    vertical transmission of HIV to 25, 25–6, 98, 298–300
infection, probability of 95–6
infectivity 116–17
informal sector 169, 201
inheritance 274
insurance industry
    current research 49, 54–5
    Zimbabwe: AIDS data 219, 220, 221; AIDS deaths 228–9, 230, 231; HIV data 222–3
    see also medical aid societies
International Monetary Fund 14
intravenous drug abuse 6, 24, 25, 26–7
investment
    lost educational 195–200
    skills as 191–2
    see also human capital approach
Isospora belli 301, 302
Izoniazid (INH) 47

Jackson, H. 234
Jamaica 40
Johnson, M. 40
Joubert, P. 147

Kagamba sub-county 269, 270
Kaiser Permanente 40
Kakuuto sub-county 268–71
Kalisizo sub-county 268–71
Kampala 297
Kaposi's sarcoma 14, 301, 304
Kenya 277, 286
Kizer, K.W. 40
Kyakabanda sub-county 269, 270
Kyebe sub-county 268–71

labour 30, 53
    loss; agricultural impact simulation studies 274–9; household coping strategies and 281–2
    quality and health expenditure 192–3
    supply shortages 52, 186; planning and 211–12

urban employment 149–53
    Zimbabwe industry and AIDS 234–8
    see also employment; unemployment
labour market research 287–8
Lafferty, W.F. 40
Lake Victoria foreshore farming system 277–8, 279, 286
land, abandoned 288
land rights 274, 282
landlords 274
latent phase 4
    see also incubation period
Latin America 22, 23
Lesotho 7, 8, 9, 12
Lesthaege, R. 142
leukoplakia 301
life expectancy
    South Africa's black population 118, 124, 126, 127
    Zimbabwe's AIDS cases 252
life years lost 201–3
lifetime costs 35, 36
    see also costs
limits, severe on claims 235–6
lost earnings 31, 161, 163, 172, 182–3
lost educational investment 195–200
lost production *see* production
lost work years 167–8
lump-sum death benefits 236
Luwero area 272
Lwamagwa sub-county 269, 270
Lyantonde sub-county 269, 271

Mabiyasu sub-county 269, 271
MacBarry, Brian 224–5
Malawi 6, 7
    AIDS incidence 8, 15
    HIV infection 100, 101
manifestations, clinical *see* clinical manifestations
Mann, Jonathan 29, 290
marital status 229, 230, 231
market shrinkage 52
marriage
    frequency decreasing 285, 291
    remarriage as coping strategy 281, 282
Mazabuka community aproach 309
McCormick, J. 72
medical aid societies 241–2, 245–59
    AIDS data 219, 220
    case histories 248–52
    claims expenditure 247–8; impact of AIDS 254–8; reducing costs 258–9

identification of AIDS cases 247
options and policies 235-6
medical costs 289
current research: non-personal 42-3; personal 39-42; in pre-AIDS phase 41-2; South Africa 50
Zimbabwe *see* Zimbabwe
see also costs; direct costs
Medley, G.F. 116
Merson, Michael 16, 22, 31
migration, rural-urban 296
research needed 287
South Africa 69-70, 73-4, 130, 145-7
Zimbabwe 229-31
mine worker 130, 133-4, 134, 288, 291
mobilization, political 73
monitoring 261-92
agricultural impact simulation studies 264, 274-9
broader view 289-90
data sources and techniques 263-5
household structure changes 264-5, 283-6
major research areas 287-9; environmental impact 288; labour markets 287-8; local coping experiments 288; urban 'plant' studies 288-9
orphan studies 263-4, 268-72
policies for large orphan populations 272-4
population pyramids 263, 265-7
results from studies 265-72
socio-economic differentiation and impact 264, 279-83
Montagnier, Luc 14
mortality costs 182, 200-6, 210-11
mortality rates 141
African 297, 299
black population in South Africa 117-18, 124, 125
Doyle model and 98-9, 106, 107
educational level 196, 197, 198-200
global pandemic 13, 30
infant *see* infant mortality
Zimbabwe 221, 242, 243, 245; insurance industry 228-9, 230, 231
mother-to-child transmission 98, 298-300
global pandemic 25, 25-6
Mozambique 8, 9
Mpumudde sub-county 269, 271

Mycobacterium tuberculosis 302, 303
see also TB

Namibia 8, 9, 10, 12
Natal 100, 101, 102
natural increase of population (RNI) 127-8
NBTS 243-4
neonatal death 299, 300
non-personal costs 42-3, 162, 164, 167
see also costs; direct costs; personal costs
North America 289-90
see also Americas; United States
nursing, home 258-9
nutrition, orphans' 273

occupational advancement 150, 151
occupational exposure 25, 27
see also health-care workers
occupation groups, AIDS deaths by 229, 230, 231
Oceania 16, 21
Old Mutual insurance group 76, 77, 220
opportunity costs 193
oral lesions 301, 304
orphan studies 263-4
Uganda 268-72, 290
orphans 109, 110, 231, 262
estimated numbers 49, 299-300
household structure changes 284-5
need for planning care of 308, 319
policies for large populations 272-4; education 272-3; legal protection of property 274; nutrition, shelter and clothing 273; parenting 273
Ortmann, G.F. 146
Osborne, E. 51, 52
O'Sullivan, E. 78-9
outpatient care settings 45-6
outpatients, general 223, 224
Over, M. 40, 44

Packard, R.M. 69
Padayachee, G.N. 75-6, 79, 114
projections 77, 78, 81, 120
parenting 273
parents' deaths 268-71, 272
see also orphans
Pascal, A. 40
patriarchal societies 295-6
patterns of spread 5
Pattern I 5, 63, 88

patterns of spread *cont.*
  Pattern II 5, 63–4
  Pattern III 64
pension benefits 236
pantamidine 46
perinatal transmission 25, 25–6
  see also mother-to-child transmission
personal costs
  current research 39–42; in the pre-AIDS phase 41–2
  economic impact model 161–2, 164, 167
  see also costs; direct costs; non-personal costs
pharyngitis 301
Pneumocystis carinii pneumonia (PCP) 14, 46, 303
policy
  applicability of research 35
  issues and orphans 272–4
  simulating effects of 175–7
  Zimbabwe 237–8
political mobilisation 73
politics of health care 153–5
population pyramids 263
  Buganda 265–7
population screening 47–8
population size 126–8
  see also demographic impact
population structure *see* age structure of population; demographic impact
PRAY model 115
pregnant women 67–8
  see also antenatal clinic data
Prentice, G. 76, 77
pressure groups 28–9
prevention
  economics of 47
  of sexual transmission 310
  of transmission by blood transfusion 310
primary health care (PHC) 26, 70–1, 72–3, 83
private sector
  South Africa 164–7, 181; changing role 175–7
  Zimbabwe 241; *see also* medical aid societies
probability of infection 95–6
production, lost 43
  economic impact model 181–3
  human capital approach 201–6, 210–11
Project SIDA 15

projections
  South Africa 75–82; black population 120–31; demographic cohort models 79–80; Doomsday 75–6; Doyle model 102–9; economic sectors 53–5; maximum epidemic size 80; other high projections 76–8; short-term medical forecasts 78–9
  Zimbabwe 224–7, 244–5
promotion, replacement by 208–10
property, orphans' 274
prostitution 72, 296–7, 300, 311
protocols, treatment 309–10
psychological impact 11–12, 29, 71
Public Health Act, Zimbabwe 238
public sector
  South Africa 164–7, 181; changing role 175–7
  Zimbabwe 241
Puerto Rico 259

racial groups, South Africa
  dual society and AIDS 70–1
  lost educational investment 195–200
  mortality cost estimates 201–3
  population structure 95, 142–5
  STDs 91
rainfall 277–9
Rakai district 267
  household structure changes 283, 285, 291
  orphans 268–72, 274
recruitment
  costs 206–11
  screening and 234–5, 238
Rees, M. 40
remarriage 281, 282
remitted incomes 146–7
replacement of workers 44–5, 53
  economic impact model 163, 168, 182–3
  human capital approach: mortality cost estimates 203–63; recruitment and retraining costs 206–11, 214
research 34–57
  direct costs of HIV/AIDS 39–43
  indirect costs 43–5
  major areas needing 287–9
  recent trends 34–8; developed countries 37–8; developing countries 38; limited policy

applicability 35; limited
  scope 36–7; variability of
  results 35–6
South Africa 49–55; direct
  costs 50–2; economic implications
  of HIV/AIDS 49–50; impact on
  economic development 52–5
specific issues in the economics of
  HIV/AIDS 45–52; cost-bearers
  48–9; diagnosis 47–8; impact on
  specific economic sectors 49;
  prevention 47; treatment 45–7
resource allocation 10–11, 139, 159–60
  economic impact model 179–80
  see also health expenditure
respiratory tract, lower 302, 303
retraining costs 206–11
Rice, D.P. 37, 40, 44
Richards, A.I. 284–5
risk groups
  Doyle model 90–2; distribution of
  population into 95; pattern of
  sexual contacts with other 96–7;
  spread of infection between 101–2
  Zimbabwe 243–5
rural prevalence rates 73–4
rural–urban dependency 139, 145–9
  see also dependency ratios
rural–urban migration see migration
Rwanda 274–5

'S' curve 225–6
salaries see earnings
scenarios see projections
Schall, R. 75, 78, 79, 114
  projections 77, 80, 81, 120
Schoub, B.D. 66, 68, 70
Scitovsky, A.A. 37, 40, 44
screening
  population 47–8
  pre-employment 234–5; 238
Seage, G.R. 40
Seekings, J. 147
self-exploitation 281–2
sentinel surveys
  South Africa 66–8
  Zimbabwe 223–4
seroconversion phase 4
serodiagnosis 305–7, 312
Serodia–HIV 305
seroprevalence studies 66–7
sexual behaviour
  changed see behaviour change

mores in Africa 295–6
  need for research 318
  networking and black
  population 129–31, 133–4
  risk groups in Doyle model 90–1
  South Africa 69–70
sexual transmission 6, 24–5, 295–8
  black population in South
  Africa 113, 116; sexual
  activity 118–20
  efficiency 25
  prevention of 310
  see also STDs
Shapiro, M. 77, 78–9
sharp instruments 25, 309
shelter 273
short-term medical forecasts 78–9
skills 191–2, 272
  distribution and mortality cost
  estimates 200–5
  replacement costs 207–11
  see also training
Skrabanek, P. 72
sleeping sickness 291–2
'slim' 14, 301
Smith, Adam 191–2
social change 72
social epidemic 11–12, 29–71
society, AIDS and 28–32
socio-economic analysis 137–57
  dependency ratios at household
  level 145–9
  politics of health care 153–5
  population structure 140–5
  projecting urban employment
  levels 149–53
socio-economic differentiation 264,
  279–83
socio-economic impact 9–11
  monitoring see monitoring
socio-economic status 152, 227–8
South Africa 10, 295
  black population see black
  population
  contaminated blood 6–7
  current research see research
  Doyle model see Doyle model
  economic impact of AIDS epidemic
  see economic impact model
  facing up to AIDS 317–19
  human capital approach see human
  capital approach
  meaningful response 308–12;

South Africa: meaningful response *cont.*
    development of health care
        309–10; prevention 310
    population distribution 94, 95
    reported cases 7, 8, 62–4, 103–4,
        105, 133
    sexual transmission patterns 296–7
    'slim' 301
    social implications of AIDS 11–12,
        307–8
    socio-economic analysis of long-run
        effects *see* socio-economic analysis
    special nature of 69–75; dual
        society 70–1; environment
        69–70; health care availability 74;
        health education and behaviour
        change 72–3; rural prevalence
        rates 73–4
    trends and projections of HIV
        infection 61–86; AIDS cases and
        deaths data 62–4; epidemics
        64–6; first national HIV
        survey 67–8; projections 75–82;
        using HIV data 66–7
Southern African Development
    Coordination Conference 154
Soweto 309
Spiegel, A. 147
Spier, A. 50, 51
Stamps, Timothy 219
STDs (sexually-transmitted
    diseases) 117, 296, 297, 309
    South Africa 74, 109; doubling
        times 131; risk groups 90–1, 91;
        socio-economic status 152
    Zimbabwe 223–4, 243;
        monitoring 247, 252–3
stockmarket 54
sub-Saharan Africa 22, 23, 297
    monitoring *see* monitoring
sugar-growing industry 54
Swaziland 8, 9, 12
syphilis 74
    see also STDs

Tabora region 275–6
Tanzania 8, 180
    agricultural impact simulation
        studies 275–6, 286
    costs of AIDS/HIV 38, 40, 42, 44
    Doyle model calibration 100, 101, 102
    reported AIDS cases 8, 15
    targeting assistance 274

Taylor, G. 50, 51
TB (tuberculosis) 42, 45, 302, 303
    secondary epidemic 13, 311
    South Africa 74; development of
        health care 309
    Zimbabwe 243, 247
Thailand 31
therapeutic interventions *see* drugs
Thormeyer, T. 146
T-lymphocytes 4
Toms, I. 70
tourism 54
trade unions 237–8
training 234–5
    retraining costs 206–11
    see also education; skills
transmission, modes of 6–7
    see also under individual names
transmission patterns 22–7
    South Africa 63–4
transplacental transmission 298
treatment
    economics of 45–7; settings 45–6;
        therapeutic intervention *see* drugs
    protocols 309–10
tsetse fly 288

Uganda 7, 286, 290
    agricultural impact simulation
        studies 276–7, 277–9
    Doyle model 100, 101
    gender and HIV infection 297
    orphan studies 268–72, 290
    policies for large orphan
        populations 272–4
    population pyramids in
        Buganda 265–7
unemployment 44–5, 53, 163, 214
    human capital approach 201;
        mortality cost estimates 203–6;
        recruitment and retraining
        costs 206–11
    projections 149, 150–1
United States (US) 22, 43, 45
    cost-bearers 48
    costs 35, 37–8; direct 39, 40, 42,
        43; indirect 44
    insurance 49
    transmission patterns 22–4, 29–30
urban employment 149–53
urban 'plant' studies 288–9
urban–rural dependency 139, 145–9
    see also dependency ratios

vaccines 28, 289
see also drugs
Van den Berg, S. 146
Van der Merwe, J.A. 50, 51
Van Niekerk, W.A. 50, 51
variability of research results 35–6
  South Africa 50–1
Viravaidya, Mechai 31
vocational schools 272
Volkskas Bank 76

weight loss 301, 303, 304, 305
Western Blot tests 223, 305
'window period' 6, 26
women
  lower perceived value 296–7
  prevention by education of 310
  status 282
work years lost 167–8
workers, replacement of *see* replacement of workers
workplace discrimination 188, 238
World AIDS Day 28
World Bank 14, 115, 141
World Health Organisation (WHO) 261
  clinical case definitions 301, 303
  Global Programme on AIDS 15, 16
'worst-case' scenario 80

Zaire 101, 288

costs 38, 40, 42, 44, 48; proportion of health expenditure 179–80
Project SIDA 15
Zambia 7, 8
  Doyle model 100, 101, 102
  Mazabuka community care 309
  mine workers 288, 291
  sexual transmission 296, 297, 298
zidovudine 28, 74
Zimbabwe 9, 10, 214, 217–60
  age structure of population 242
  AIDS cases 8, 243; data 218–21
  HIV data 221–4
  implications 227–33; costs 231–3; demographic 227–31
  industry and AIDS 233–8
  medical costs 241–60; case histories 248–52; medical aid societies 245–7; overall implications 253–9; research findings 247–8; risk groups and HIV incidence 243–5
  projections 224–7; comments on modelling 225–7
  Public Health Act 238
Zimbabwe Congress of Trade Unions (ZCTU) 237–8
Zimbabwe Owner Drivers' Organization 223
Zwi, A.B. 69, 70